AI, Machine Learning, and IoT for Communication and Medical Applications

Altaf O. Mulani
https://orcid.org/0000-0002-2692-336X
SKN Sinhgad College of Engineering, Pandharpur, India

Korhan Cengiz
Istinye University, Turkey

Suman Lata Tripathi
https://orcid.org/0000-0002-1684-8204
Department of E and TC, Symbiosis Institute of Technology, Symbiosis International University, Pune, India

IGI Global
Scientific Publishing
Publishing Tomorrow's Research Today

Vice President of Editorial Melissa Wagner
Director of Acquisitions Mikaela Felty
Director of Book Development Jocelynn Hessler
Production Manager Mike Brehm
Cover Design Jose Rosado

Published in the United States of America by
IGI Global Scientific Publishing
701 East Chocolate Avenue
Hershey, PA, 17033, USA
Tel: 717-533-8845 | Fax: 717-533-7115
Website: https://www.igi-global.com E-mail: cust@igi-global.com

Library of Congress Cataloging-in-Publication Data

Names: Mulani, Altaf, editor. | Cengiz, Korhan, editor. | Tripathi, Suman Lata, editor.
Title: AI, machine learning, and IoT for communication and medical applications / edited by Altaf Mulani, Korhan Cengiz, Suman Tripathi.
Description: Hershey, PA : Engineering Science Reference, [2026] | Includes bibliographical references and index. | Summary: "The book provides a comprehensive and insightful exploration of the intersection of these advanced technologies, with a focus on their applications, challenges, and contributions to the fields of communication and healthcare"-- Provided by publisher.
Identifiers: LCCN 2024010192 (print) | LCCN 2024010193 (ebook) | ISBN 9798369338643 (hardcover) | ISBN 9798369348802 (paperback) | ISBN 9798369338650 (ebook)
Subjects: LCSH: Medicine--Data processing. | Artificial intelligence--Medical applications. | Internet in medicine.
Classification: LCC R858 .A393 2024 (print) | LCC R858 (ebook) | DDC 610.285--dc23/eng/20240313
LC record available at https://lccn.loc.gov/2024010192
LC ebook record available at https://lccn.loc.gov/2024010193

British Cataloguing in Publication Data
A Cataloguing in Publication record for this book is available from the British Library.

Table of Contents

Detailed Table of Contents

The accurate differentiation between PD and other forms of Parkinsonism is crucial for appropriate treatment, management, and patient care. However, clinical overlap among these conditions often leads to diagnostic challenges and potential misclassification. This chapter proposes an in-depth exploration of the utilization of Support Vector Machine (SVM) for enhancing the differentiation process. It will discuss the ethical considerations, potential benefits, challenges, and the impact of SVM-based diagnosis on patient care, diagnosis accuracy, and cost-effectiveness. By delving into these aspects, this chapter aims to contribute significantly to the advancement of Parkinson's disease diagnosis and management through the application of machine learning techniques.

Retracted Chapter 3

A. Aruna, Sri Ramachandra Faculty of Engineering and Technology, SRIHER, India

A. Sathya, Sri Ramachandra Faculty of Engineering and Technology, SRIHER, India

The emergence in the development of sensory equipment endorses the expansion of the Internet of Things (IoT) across the globe. The usage of diversified applications and IoT devices generates massive sensor data which in turn need analytics or intelligent processing system. IoT, Machine Learning, and Fog Computing are utilized to achieve healthcare assistance and diagnosis progression in diverse aspects, Machine Learning is a kind of data analysis technique that retrieves the needed information without performing any explicit program. This chapter focuses on two diverse paradigms such as machine learning and fog computing which concern the processing and analysis of sensor data. The taxonomy of Machine Learning algorithms, significant aspects of Machine Learning in IoT data analytics and applications of Machine Learning based IoT techniques are elaborated. This chapter also elucidates fog computing and its tiered computing architecture for healthcare. The major issues and the future research directions of IoT Data analysis are also explained in this chapter.

Brain tumours pose significant health challenges, necessitating accurate detection for effective treatment planning. This research explores deep learning architectures, including CNN, MobileNetV2, and EfficientNetBO, in brain tumour detection. Evaluated across glioma, meningioma, nontumor, and pituitary classes, EfficientNetBO outshines with a 99.16% test dataset accuracy, superior precision, and minimized errors. Its efficacy highlights transfer learning's dominance in medical imaging, leveraging pre-trained datasets for enhanced feature extraction. EfficientNetBO's reliability in brain tumor identification underscores transfer learning's significance, offering potential for improved medical diagnoses and treatments. Future research might delve into advanced techniques or practical integrations, promising enhanced brain tomour detection and treatment efficacy.

The unification of Internet of Things (IoT) technologies in healing requests has revolutionized healthcare by permissive authentic-time listening, disease, and treatment. This chapter investigate the deep impact of IoT in medical sciences, stressing its act in embellishing patient care, optimizing resource exercise, and reconstructing healthcare outcomes. Leveraging pertain instruments and sensors, IoT facilitates detached patient listening, personalized situation plans and predicting analytics. Moreover, IoT authorizes healthcare artists to make dossier-compelled decisions expeditiously, superior to timely mediations and full of enthusiasm healthcare management. As IoT resumes to advance, allure transformative potential in healing uses remains superlative, hopeful a future of efficient, patient-in the middle healthcare transmittal.

Ocular diseases are a global public health concern, demanding precise diagnostic methods. This study tackles the challenge of accurate recognition from low-resolution ocular images using a combined approach of Super-Resolution Generative Adversarial Networks (SRGAN) and Convolutional Neural Networks (CNN). Our method involves enhancing image quality through SRGAN to create high-resolution versions of low-quality ocular images. Subsequently, a CNN-based recognition model is trained on these enhanced images, learning discriminative features for precise classification of various ocular diseases. Performance evaluations on the Ocular disease dataset demonstrate the practicality and effectiveness of our approach. Beyond diagnostics, this SRGAN-CNN combination holds potential for telemedicine, enabling swift and reliable eye disease diagnosis, especially in remote areas. This synergy not only improves diagnostic accuracy but also streamlines analysis, enhancing treatment efficiency and patient outcomes.

The integration of cutting-edge technologies like 5G and IoT has led to innovative applications, particularly in healthcare, revolutionizing patient care through real-time monitoring. Healthcare IoT applications have the potential to improve patient outcomes and the caliber of care given by physicians, nurses, clinicians, and pharma companies, to name a few. However, this convergence raises concerns regarding ethics, regulation, and privacy. Consumer-facing medical devices enable automatic data collection for early intervention but often overlook security hazards. Despite the potential for improved patient outcomes, robust security and privacy safeguards are necessary. Healthcare IoT has revolutionized the medical industry but requires careful consideration of security measures. Wearable IoT gadgets simplify

Preface

INTRODUCTION

The rapid convergence of Artificial Intelligence (AI), Machine Learning (ML), and the Internet of Things (IoT) is redefining the landscape of communication systems and healthcare technologies. Advances in sensing, computation, connectivity, and intelligent analytics have enabled a paradigm shift from reactive healthcare models to predictive, personalized, and preventive medical solutions. Simultaneously, intelligent communication frameworks powered by AI and IoT are enhancing accessibility, efficiency, and reliability across diverse application domains.

The book *AI, Machine Learning, and IoT for Communication and Medical Applications* brings together contemporary research contributions from academicians, researchers, and practitioners that collectively highlight the transformative potential of intelligent systems in healthcare and communication. This edited volume aims to bridge the gap between theoretical foundations and real-world applications by presenting data-driven methodologies, intelligent architectures, and emerging paradigms such as fog computing, federated learning, and ethical AI.

A key strength of this book lies in its multidisciplinary perspective, encompassing assistive technologies, medical image analysis, disease prediction, remote patient monitoring, stress and cognitive assessment, data privacy, and ethical considerations. The chapters emphasize not only algorithmic innovation and performance evaluation but also practical deployment challenges, societal impact, and regulatory concerns.

This volume is intended for graduate students, researchers, healthcare technologists, data scientists, and industry professionals seeking insights into the design and application of intelligent systems for modern healthcare and communication infrastructures. By consolidating state-of-the-art techniques and future research directions, the book aspires to serve as a valuable reference for advancing intelligent, ethical, and secure digital health ecosystems.

CHAPTER OVERVIEW

Chapter 1: AI Powered Assistive Solution for Navigation of Visually Impaired Persons

This chapter presents an AI-enabled assistive navigation system designed to enhance the mobility and safety of visually impaired individuals. Using Raspberry Pi, computer vision, ultrasonic sensing, and deep learning–based object detection (SSD MobileNet), the system provides real-time audio feedback. The chapter demonstrates how multimodal sensing and edge intelligence can significantly improve independence and situational awareness.

Chapter 2: Differentiation Between Parkinson's Disease and Other Forms of Parkinsonism Using Support Vector Machine

Focusing on clinical decision support, this chapter explores the application of Support Vector Machines (SVMs) for distinguishing Parkinson's Disease from other Parkinsonian disorders. It addresses diagnostic challenges, ethical implications, and the potential of ML-based classification systems to enhance accuracy, cost-effectiveness, and patient outcomes.

Chapter 3: Enabling Computational Intelligence in Healthcare using IoT, Machine Learning and Fog Computing

This chapter provides a comprehensive overview of IoT-driven healthcare systems supported by machine learning and fog computing. It discusses ML taxonomies, IoT data analytics, and fog-based architectures that enable low-latency, scalable, and efficient healthcare data processing, along with key challenges and future research directions.

Chapter 4: Exploring Parkinson's Disease Pathophysiology Through Random Forest Analysis

By employing Random Forest classifiers on multimodal medical datasets, this chapter demonstrates highly accurate Parkinson's Disease detection. The work highlights acoustic feature analysis and innovative data partitioning strategies, showcasing the effectiveness of ensemble learning in early diagnosis and disease management.

Chapter 5: Forecasting Gestational Hypertension: Insights for Maternal Health Planning

This chapter addresses maternal healthcare through the prediction of gestational hypertension using stacking-based machine learning classifiers. The proposed approach supports early detection, personalized prenatal care, and risk mitigation, emphasizing the role of predictive analytics in improving maternal and fetal health outcomes.

Chapter 6: Improved Brain Tumor Detection using CNN and Transfer Learning Techniques for MRI Images

Focusing on medical image analysis, this chapter evaluates deep learning architectures such as CNN, MobileNetV2, and EfficientNetB0 for brain tumor classification. The superior performance of transfer learning models underscores their importance in accurate diagnosis and clinical decision-making.

Chapter 7: IoT in Medical Applications

This chapter examines the transformative role of IoT in healthcare, including real-time monitoring, remote diagnostics, and personalized treatment. It highlights how interconnected medical devices and sensors enable data-driven clinical decisions while improving operational efficiency and patient care delivery.

Chapter 8: Ocular Disease Recognition Using Deep Learning

This chapter introduces a hybrid SRGAN–CNN framework for ocular disease recognition from low-resolution images. By enhancing image quality prior to classification, the approach improves diagnostic accuracy and supports telemedicine applications, particularly in resource-constrained and remote regions.

Chapter 9: Safeguarding Data Privacy and Security in Healthcare IoT

Focusing on security and ethics, this chapter analyzes privacy risks associated with healthcare IoT systems. It emphasizes the need for robust security frameworks to protect sensitive patient data while enabling the benefits of wearable devices, real-time monitoring, and connected healthcare infrastructures.

Chapter 10: Ethical and Legal Implications of Artificial Intelligence in Health Care

This chapter explores the ethical, legal, and regulatory dimensions of AI adoption in healthcare. It discusses transparency, bias, accountability, and trust, emphasizing responsible AI development to ensure safe, fair, and human-centered medical applications.

Chapter 11: Revolutionizing Health Management Through Federated Learning and AI

Addressing privacy-preserving intelligence, this chapter investigates federated learning as a solution for collaborative healthcare analytics without centralized data sharing. It explores applications in remote monitoring and personalized care, alongside enabling technologies such as edge computing and next-generation connectivity.

Chapter 12: The Impact of Artificial Intelligence on Human Cognition and Thinking Processes

The final chapter examines the cognitive and psychological implications of AI integration. It discusses both augmentation and potential dependency concerns, highlighting the importance of transparency, ethical design, and continuous human–AI collaboration to maintain cognitive balance and trust.

Acknowledgement

We would like to express their sincere gratitude to all the authors who contributed their valuable research, time, and expertise to this edited volume. Their scholarly efforts and commitment to academic excellence have been instrumental in shaping this book and ensuring its technical depth, interdisciplinary relevance, and overall quality.

We are deeply thankful to the reviewers for their constructive feedback, insightful suggestions, and rigorous evaluation, which significantly enhanced the clarity, accuracy, and scholarly rigor of the chapters. Their dedication to maintaining high academic standards is sincerely appreciated.

We also extend our appreciation to the editorial and production team at IGI Global for their professional guidance, timely support, and meticulous coordination throughout the submission, review, and publication processes. Their assistance has been invaluable in bringing this project to completion.

Special thanks are due to our respective institutions and research organizations for providing a supportive academic environment and necessary resources that facilitated the successful completion of this book. We are also grateful to colleagues, collaborators, and students whose discussions and encouragement contributed, directly or indirectly, to the development of this work.

Finally, we acknowledge the continued support and encouragement of our families and well-wishers, whose patience and motivation were essential throughout this endeavor.

Introduction

The rapid convergence of Artificial Intelligence (AI), Machine Learning (ML), and the Internet of Things (IoT) has ushered in a transformative era across communication systems and medical technologies. These intelligent paradigms are redefining how data is acquired, processed, and utilized, enabling smarter decision-making, enhanced connectivity, and improved healthcare outcomes. This edited volume, *AI, Machine Learning, and IoT for Communication and Medical Applications*, arrives at a crucial time when interdisciplinary innovation is essential to address complex technological and societal challenges.

The chapters presented in this book collectively explore cutting-edge methodologies, architectures, and applications that integrate AI and ML techniques with IoT-enabled systems. The contributions provide a balanced blend of theoretical foundations, algorithmic advancements, and real-world implementations, highlighting how intelligent systems are revolutionizing areas such as wireless communication, smart healthcare, medical imaging, remote monitoring, predictive diagnostics, and personalized treatment solutions. By bridging communication engineering and medical informatics, the book emphasizes the growing importance of cross-domain collaboration in modern research.

One of the key strengths of this volume lies in its comprehensive scope and diversity of perspectives. The contributing authors—drawn from academia, research institutions, and industry—offer insights into emerging trends, challenges, and future directions. Topics such as intelligent sensing, data-driven decision systems, secure communication frameworks, IoT-based healthcare platforms, and ethical considerations of AI deployment are addressed with scholarly rigor and practical relevance. This makes the book valuable not only for researchers and postgraduate students, but also for professionals seeking to apply intelligent technologies in real-world environments.

Furthermore, the book underscores the role of AI and IoT in enabling scalable, efficient, and patient-centric medical solutions, while also advancing next-generation communication infrastructures. As healthcare systems and communication networks become increasingly data-intensive and interconnected, the approaches discussed in this volume contribute meaningfully to building resilient, adaptive, and intelligent systems.

I commend the reviewers and contributors for their dedication in curating a high-quality scholarly work that reflects both depth and breadth. I am confident that this book will serve as a valuable reference for researchers, educators, and practitioners, and will inspire further innovation at the intersection of AI, Machine Learning, IoT, communication technologies, and medical applications.

Chapter 1
AI Powered Assistive Solution for Navigation of Visually Impaired Persons

Yamini Singh
VIT Bhopal University, India

Ghananjani Saini
https://orcid.org/0009-0008-3749-571X
VIT Bhopal University, India

Sahaj Jain
VIT Bhopal University, India

Akshat Singh
https://orcid.org/0009-0000-7124-5812
VIT Bhopal University, India

Swagat Kumar Samantaray
VIT Bhopal University, India

ABSTRACT

This paper explores the development of smart navigation stick for the visually impaired. The innovation provides crucial audio feedback and precise object location information, significantly improving the overall security of blind users. The specific functionalities of each component and the speculation for the choices are specified. The arrangement that has been recommended takes processing power of the Raspberry Pi 3 Model B to check the Raspberry Pi camera V2. The camera captures real-time images for object detection and recognition. Furthermore, an ultrasonic sensor (HC-SR04) is incorporated To determine how far away obstacles are, providing a

DOI: 10.4018/979-8-3693-3864-3.ch001

complementary layer of spatial awareness. To enhance object recognition accuracy, the author utilizes the SSD MobileNet algorithm alongside OpenCV libraries. After detecting objects, they are converted to audio feedback for the user via the Python eSpeak module. This multi-modal approach caters to diverse user preferences and environmental conditions.

INTRODUCTION

Think of a society, in which orientation in space, from roads of large cities to narrow corridors of schools, is possible without help and fear. The Intelligent Navigation Stick is about to bring this into reality for the visually impaired persons. This revolutionary assistive technology means that the future would be a much freer and mobile one. This articulate communication equips users with perfect situation awareness so that they are able to make decisions at their comforts. Think about walking in a crowded sidewalk, the INS not only warns that there is an object in your way but tells you 'You have a fire hydrant on your right. ' Such information proved to be extremely helpful in avoiding change collisions and having a sense of direction with ease.

Loss of vision refers to visual impairment and it can be as a result of heredity, disease, or an accident. Based on (Flaxman et al., 2017), the major causes for sightlessness are uncorrected refractive error, cataract, age related macular decline, glaucoma, and diabetic retinopathy. Blindness also can be caused by accident among the various causes of instance blindness.

According to the World Health Organization (2018) global estimates reveal that 253 million plus people have some form of vision impairment. Vision as a disability hinders the performance of the routine activities of the day and impacts the attribute of life, the user's capability to engage with the existing environment, hence discourages the use of unfamiliar spaces (Akhila et al., 2016). The walking impaired have it really bad when it comes to getting around in the community. The conventional white canes are essential aids, yet they do not relay much information regarding the surroundings. Hence, the need to tackle this problem is immensely significant because a significant proportion of the world population is suffering from visual impairments (National Academies of Sciences, Engineering, and Medicine [NASEM], 2016). Thus, the purpose of this proposition is to offer a contingency system that aids blind individuals to construct a mental map of the environment and be ready to take appropriate actions if encountering some obstacles. The implications of visual impairment extend beyond mere inconvenience, discouraging individuals from navigating unfamiliar environments. Recognizing the pressing need for innovative solutions, we set out to develop a navigation device designed to assist blind individuals in detecting obstacles and enhancing their overall visual experience (Dhaygude & Waghmare, 2023).

At the heart of our motivation is a deep belief in the transformative power of technology to bridge the gap and create freedom opportunities. Visually impaired individuals often face barriers that go beyond physical barriers; They face the challenge of navigating a world that seems out of control and unpredictable. With new independence and confidence, our proposed policy represents a considerable improvement to safety of the blind and sighted. Furthermore reducing the inherent risks associated with cataracts, our device holds some hope for individuals facing these challenges. This chapter details the development, use, and potential impact of the device, demonstrating its potential to change the lives of the visually impaired and contribute to an inclusive and accessible society. Combining these factors, this discussion aims to develop a comprehensive and user-centered navigation system.

LITERATURE REVIEW

The SmartCane is a low cost electronic travel assistance for the visually impaired created by the Assistive Technology (Assistech) lab at IIT Delhi. It is a component or appliance that is relatively light, portable, and easily affixed to a conventional folding white cane. It adopted ultrasonic ranging to determine the obstacles in front of or above the knee level within a 3-meter distance. Its compulsion enables it to consider objects that are coming close at a high speed such as vehicles within 3 meters of distance which can allow for a reflex move. Distance information is communicated through a variation of frequency which changes proportionally with the distance to obstacles; thus, the SmartCane can equally be used by persons with impaired hearing and vision (Singh et al., 2010).

A device that serves as a walking stick for the visually impaired with features of obstacle detection, navigational aid, and fall detection is also presented in (Singh et al., 2010). This stick incorporated ultrasonic sensors, infrared sensors, and gyroscope to identify obstacles in front of /over/under the person holding the stick. The stick equally contains a GPS module, which serves the purpose of a navigator to the user. Also, the smart stick has the feature of a fall identification algorithm that can attract the attention of emergency services also (Akhil et al., 2022).

This paper comprehensively shows the efficiency of technology in helping the visually impaired. The intelligent stick moves and leans forward when there are obstacles on its path and has sensors on its handle. The smart walking stick not only helps the user with navigation but also is aware about the obstacles through electronic sensors and modern technology; therefore the customer feels confident while using the walking stick and reduces the chances of instantiating an accident (Thakur et al., 2018).

In enabling the visually impaired, the paper provides a unique solution for that category of people. Thus, with the help of attached ultrasonic detectors, GPS module, and voice output, this system helps them to move around safely and without assistance.

The product that was developed by them was a small-sized, cost efficient and comfortable to wear navigation system.

This special walking stick does two main things: it will assist you to choose where one would like to be, similar to identifying a destination, and it assists you in navigation at the point of destination, for instance, on the sidewalks and corridors. It is really brilliant in averting any object that it doesn't want to hit, which includes chairs and tables; and others that do move, such as people. Rather than inventing a new type of walking stick that could be used exclusively to toy with the minds of the Blue Man's observers, Malm and his team came up with a different concept. They came up with a camera that is worn like an appliance at the chest area, sort of like a small selfie camera. They also developed a tiny computer that one had to carry in a bag hanging on the shoulder or pocket. In order to hear what the device wants to communicate to you, you only have to plug one earpiece or a small speaker. It is nearly invisible and thus people will not consciously pay much attention to it, and your movement won't be hindered by it if you use a standard walking stick. It also will not drown out the external noises so you will be able to hear the events happening in the surrounding (Sahoo et al., 2019).

They developed a cane that is capable of notifying the users through voice and vibrating the cane as well. They employ ultrasonic sensors which are fairly accurate in the identification of objects in front of it most preferably within a few meters. Once these sensors detect an obstacle, what lies in its path, a message in the form of an audible voice warning is produced. This message is then played audibly through a speaker for the user to listen to. In this way, people with the loss of vision can move more freely, having information on what is present in their way and receiving signals when the obstacles are detected, which is considerably more effective than the use of ultrasonic sensors (Dada et al., 2017).

They developed what is known as the electronic long cane, particularly for the blind and those with poor vision to help with their navigation.

This has an easy to use interface and also contains an electronic device that is easily insertable into the handle of a normal long cane. With regards to the lower part of the body, the system employs haptic sensors to discern obstacles situated above the waste line. If an obstacle is detected the vibration or an audio cue is felt through the handle of the cane. Nonetheless, it is vital for one to understand that this system is capable of perceiving obstacles that are above the waist level (Yohannan & Shyam, 2020).

The publication (Xu et al., 2023) known as VibroCap, which can assist visually-challenged people to move safely and freely. The device is a hat mounted device that works on ultrasonic sensors to sense barriers in the path of the user. It also employs a 'tactile interface' that communicates information to the user by specific vibrations. It is lightweight, simple to use and is best worn with other accessories (Xu et al., 2023).

Presenting a tool to assist blind or visually challenged people to move around, this paper proposes a smartstick. This helps the challenged blind people face perceiving hindrances in their environment or the physical space around them. Ultrasonic sensors are the first components of the smart stick for obstruction detection, a vibration motor for providing haptic feedback; a water sensor for hazard perception; a light sensor for using it as a touch sensor; and an Arduino Uno R3 board for processing signals from the sensors and making alarm signals. The stick is supposed to act as a vision and alarm substitute. The technology has been found to help direct the users in unfamiliar locations since the gadget could incorporate a mobile's device global positioning system (Mohite et al., 2018).

This paper proposes a concept of a new smart cane intended to enhance the standard of living of the people with blurred visions or complete blindness.The cane has GSM (Global System for Mobile) that can be utilized in case of an emergency and Built-in GPS to locate its user. Notably, the system can locate traffic lights and learn objects with the help of connection with a Raspberry Pi. It can also give out speech alerts through a headset. An alert system is incorporated thus assisting in the retrieval of the cane and dealing with misplaced canes. It is created to interface with the user's mobile phone. This smart cane intends to make the lives of visually impaired people easier and safer while performing routine tasks, as these characteristics (Subbiah et al., 2019).

METHODOLOGY

The core of the architecture revolves around custom software modules designed to fulfill specific functionalities. A Raspberry Pi Control Module acts as the central control unit, managing and orchestrating the functionalities of the Raspberry Pi 3 Model B. It encompasses the programming logic for the Pi Camera, ultrasonic sensors, and the SSD MobileNet algorithm. Dedicated to real-time image processing, an Image Processing Module interacts with the Pi Camera to capture and manipulate images. It leverages OpenCV libraries for efficient image manipulation, ensuring accurate object detection within the captured frames.The ultrasonic sensor interface facilitates communication with the ultrasonic sensor (HC-SR04). This module uses sound waves to capture the distance, providing essential data for real-time obstacle detection, especially in situations where the camera may have limited visibility. This proposed strategy of operation entails the combining of the best Machine Learning and Computer Vision approaches, in consolidation with other technologies like Ultrasonic Sensing. An effective audio feedback system is incorporated to give detailed information on such obstacles helping users make the right decisions on how to handle them/us. The Raspberry Pi 3 Model B is the control center, responsible for image interpretation, mathematical equations used in navigation, or audio. Real-time video feed is recorded using a Raspberry Pi Camera V2. An ultrasonic sensor, such as the HC-SR04 Module, reflects sound waves from an object in order to calculate the distance between an object. Current control in a circuit is done by simple electrical parts such as resistors and capacitors while switches allow users to control the circuit's navigating system. All the magic is in consolidation of using machine learning and computer vision algorithms such as SSD MobileNet that execute on Raspberry Pi. This helps in the detection, recognition and identification of objects in real time. Finally, the Python Pyttsx3 module provides the missing link of making the text outputs audible to the users concerning their environments.

AI powered Blind cane devices not only aids in the recognition of obstacles and landmarks but also enhances their visual capabilities. Imagine a world where visually impaired individuals can confidently navigate unfamiliar roads, easily recognizing and responding to objects and landmarks in their path, all thanks to auditory information that is due to the navigation equipment.

- Ultrasonic sensor-based distance calculation: Our system uses ultrasonic sensors to continuously calculate the distance to objects in the user's path. If the distance to an object falls below a predefined threshold, the system will activate the Pi Camera for further analysis.
- Image Capture and Processing: The activated Pi Camera captures an image of the immediate surroundings. This image will then be processed using the SSD MobileNet algorithm for real-time object detection.
- Object Detection and Recognition: The SSD MobileNet algorithm and Tensorflow lite identifies and classifies objects within the captured image, providing vital information about the user's environment.
- Audio Feedback Generation: Detected objects get converted into audio feedback using the Python Pyttsx3 Module. This audio feedback will serve as a real-time assistant for the blind user.

Figure 1. Flowchart of the object detection

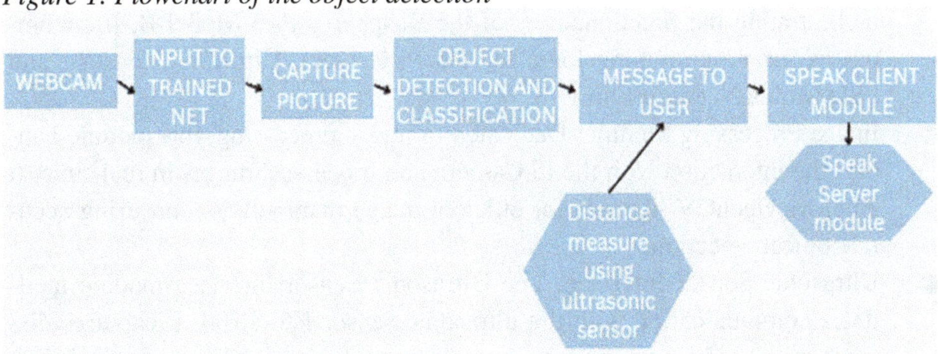

The heart of the software architecture, the Object Detection Module integrates the SSD MobileNet algorithm for object detection. It leverages machine learning and computer vision to identify obstacles above the user's waistline in their surroundings. Finally, a Feedback Generation Module translates the information gleaned from the object detection module into real-time audio feedback. This module essentially translates the nature and location of identified obstacles into audible alerts, empowering users with comprehensive situational awareness. OpenCV libraries and the SSD MobileNet algorithm act as essential tools within this architecture. OpenCV libraries act as a positional role in the image processing and object detection workflows. The architecture incorporates OpenCV to leverage its powerful tools for image deception along with feature extraction, and seamless integration with the SSD MobileNet algorithm. The SSD MobileNet algorithm, a deep learning algorithm, is seamlessly integrated into the software architecture to enhance the precision and rate of object detection. SSD MobileNet excels in real-time processing due to its efficient architecture, making it well-suited for the dynamic conditions of navigation stick.

By combining these software modules with use of powerful libraries for example OpenCV and SSD MobileNet, the system facilitates real-time object recognition and translates this information into audio responses responsive to the visually impaired thereby enabling them to navigate their surroundings more confidently, safely.

IMPLEMENTATION

The software architecture for the Intelligent Navigation Stick is designed to seamlessly integrate and orchestrate various components, ensuring optimal performance and reliability. The architecture revolves around developing custom software to fulfill the specified functionalities. The key components of the software architecture include:

- Raspberry Pi Control Module: This module is responsible for controlling and orchestrating the functionalities of the Raspberry Pi 3 Model B. It encompasses the programming logic for the Pi Camera, Ultrasonic sensors, and SSD MobileNet algorithm.
- Image Processing Module: Dedicated to image processing, this module handles the interaction with the Pi Camera and processes images in real-time. It employs OpenCV libraries for efficient image manipulation, ensuring accurate object detection.
- Ultrasonic Sensor Interface: The Ultrasonic Sensor Interface module facilitates communication with the ultrasonic sensor HC-SR04. It captures distance measurements using sound waves, providing crucial input for real-time obstacle detection.
- Object Detection Module: The heart of the software architecture, this module integrates the SSD MobileNet algorithm for advanced object detection. It leverages machine learning and computer vision capabilities to identify obstacles above the waistline in the user's surroundings.
- Feedback Generation Module: Responsible for generating real-time audio feedback based on the information gathered from the object detection module. This module articulates the nature and location of identified obstacles, empowering users with comprehensive information.
- Utilization of OpenCV Libraries: OpenCV libraries play a pivotal role in the image processing and object detection workflows. The architecture incorporates OpenCV to harness its powerful tools for image processing, feature extraction, and seamless integration with the SSD MobileNet algorithm.
- Integration of SSD MobileNet Algorithm: The SSD MobileNet algorithm is seamlessly integrated into the software architecture to enhance the precision of object detection. This deep learning algorithm excels in real-time processing, making it well-suited for the dynamic requirements of the navigation stick.

SSD (Single Shot Multibox Detector) MobileNet is a DL -based object detection algorithm that incorporates the efficiency of MobileNet, a convolutional neural network (CNN) architecture designed for mobile and embedded vision applications, with the accuracy of the SSD framework for object detection.

SSD MOBILENET

- Object Detection: SSD MobileNet is used for real-time object detection in images and videos. It's proficient in detecting multiple objects within an image in various categories simultaneously.
- Architecture: The SSD MobileNet architecture consists of the MobileNet backbone (acting as a feature extractor) and other convolutional layers responsible for predicting bounding box and class probabilities at different scales
- Efficiency: The mobile net model is known for its efficiency in size and computing requirements, making it suitable for devices with critical features such as smartphones and embedded systems.
- Multi-scale Feature Maps: SSD employs multiple convolutional layers at different scales in the network to detect objects of different sizes, allowing it to handle various object scales and aspect ratios effectively.

Inter-Module Communication: The modules are also integrated through interfaces where the components have well and clearly organized interfaces which govern how data is passed. The Raspberry Pi Control Module acts as the control center of the flow of data and commands between and among image processing, Ultrasonic Sensing, Object detection and feedback generation modules.

Scalability and Adaptability: From the software perspective, that has an architecture that can be easily scaled and then updated in the near future. This means that even the intelligent Navigation Stick will be able to design the additional technologies or enhanced algorithms.

Testing and Iterative Refinement: In addition to this, testing strategies will be incorporated to ensure full functionality as well as efficacy of each module. To improve the functionality and solidity of the navigation stick, the performance feedback from all the users will be incorporated in the successive modifications.

Figure 2. Circuit Diagram

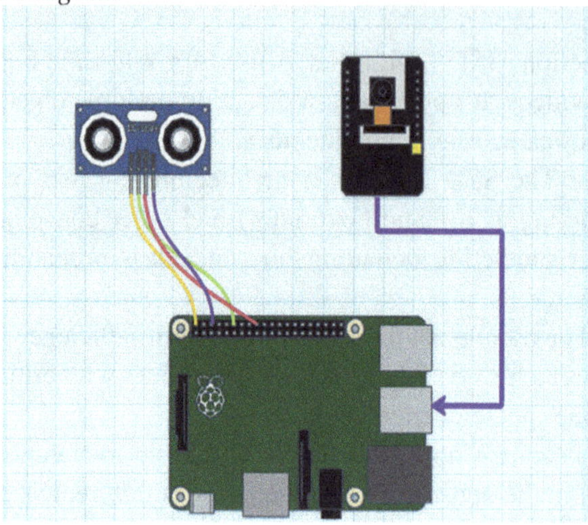

Figure 3. distance monitored between user and object using Ultrasound sensor

The circuit diagram for the object detection system with ultrasonic sensor and camera integration shown in the figure 1.2 explains the ways of essential components required for obstacle detection and navigation help in real time. A Raspberry Pi is also used here as a central processing unit and a system controller of the whole system. As for the circuit connections for this system, the ultrasonic sensor is connected to the Raspberry Pi while the camera module is also connected. The ultrasonic sensor connected with Raspberry Pi's GPIO pins calculates distance to an object by emitting ultrasonic sounds and then analyzing the bounce back from it, essential information for obstacle detection integrated in its design making it an IoT object.

Figure 4. (a) and (b)

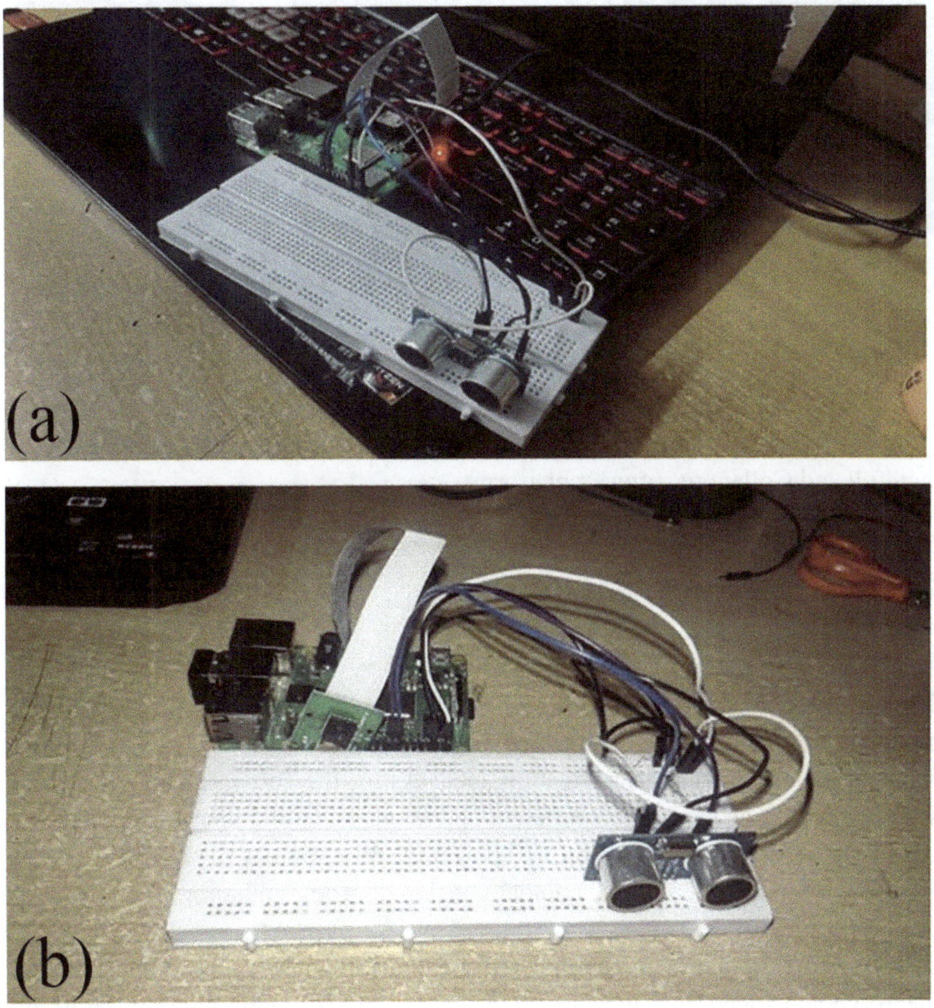

A drawing of the ultrasonic sensor and pi camera. Namely, the ultrasonic sensor will determine the distance between it and the said obstacle in front of it. Thus, when the obstacle is getting closer and when it gets close to the user-set threshold value, a buzzer is activated so as to inform the blind about the existence of the obstacle blocking their path. The stick in the subfigure (a) is expanded with IoT devices and sensors that add more features to it. These IoT based devices may include parts that give information and feedback to the user to enable him/her make a good decision on; say a right turn or the existence of an obstacle such as a wall or any physical barrier.

Figure 5. Stick Design figure, made using notefull and collanote

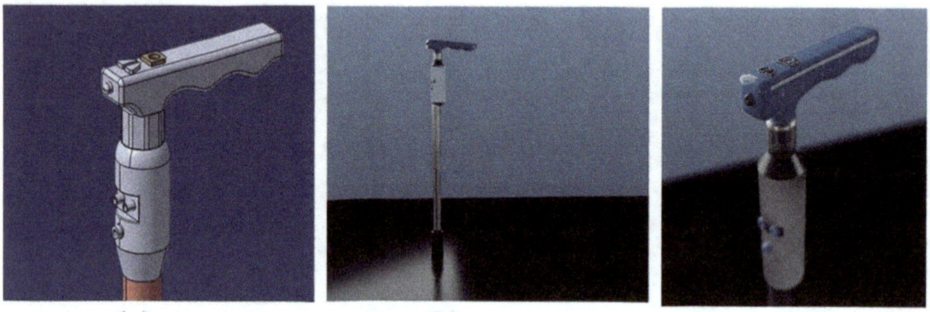

(a) (b) (c)

Specifically, subfigure (a), (b) and (c) show other designs of the stick, made in Notefull and Collanote software platforms.

REQUIREMENT ARTIFACTS

The necessary items of hardware are Raspberry Pi 3 Model B, Raspberry Pi Camera V2, Ultrasonic Sensor HC-SR04, two push buttons, resistor, power bank, breadboard, and jumper wires. All of these components are fabricated affording a functional and integrated navigation stick. As for the software part, functional software is designed to support different operations including image manipulation, Ultrasonic sensor communication, and object identification by the SSD MobileNet algorithm. Various open source computer vision libraries, including OpenCV, have been utilized.

In the constriction of the module requirements, the necessary components are identified and stated with their functions along with the technologies used in the given project. Raspberry Pi 3 Model B acts as a master processing unit for image processing, algorithms, and to give out audio instructions. Raspberry Pi Camera V2 module is used to capture an image to process it in real-time while on the other hand Ultrasonic Sensor HC-SR04 measures distance from the barrier. Real time object recognition is done by resistors and the SSD MobileNet algorithm. The Python Pyttsx3 Module is used to give commands in the following audio feedback converting the text results into speech.

Regarding the project's specifications, the data requisites for YOLO v5, Pyttsx3 module, and video-based applications are established. The function requirements underlines the significance of every single hardware component and software module in the system and provide the screwed vision of a properly and effectively navigated world for the people with low vision. Lastly, the look and feel requirements chiefly address the design specifications, this includes the general layout and size, portability and space efficiency, usability and ease of control and operations, minimalistic and streamline prototype that does not interfere with the display, modifiable features and systems, and well defined response systems.

Hardware Requirements

More so, the requisites required for this project include Raspberry Pi Camera V2, Raspberry Pi 3 Model B, Ultrasonic sensor HC-SR04, Raspberry Pi Camera Module, push buttons, Resistors, Power bank, breadboard and Jumper wires. These will be incorporated into a working navigation stick.

Software Requirements

This involves getting Raspberry Pi to supervise the Pi Camera, Image Processing, and Ultrasonic sensors, SSD MobileNet algorithm for Object Detection. We will also be employing utilization of OpenCV libraries and also the SSD MobileNet Algorithm.

Module Requirements

This section is aimed at describing what constitutes the foundational technologies of an AI-based navigation system. The Raspberry Pi 3 Model B performs the roles of the CPU, or central processing unit, and directs the image processing, algorithm calculations, and audio functionalities. The Raspberry Pi Camera V2 recovers streaming video that is ready to be analyzed at the moment. An ultrasonic sensor uses high-frequency sound waves to measure distances; namely, the HC-SR04 Module does this. capacitors and resistors limit current flow and supplemental push buttons/ switches permit user engagement with the directional system. Lastly, machine learning and computer vision algorithms such as SSD MobileNet executes in the Raspberry Pi for real-time identifying of objects. Finally, the recorded Python Pyttsx3 converts textual outcomes into words for the end user of the proposed speculation to hear about their environment.

- Raspberry Pi 3 Model B: Raspberry Pi is a small computer used to interface with the system in its entirety. This component performs the function of image processing, algorithm processing, and audio output.
- Raspberry Pi Camera V2: This is a camera that captures images and also records video. It is applied to acquire real-time images for further real-time processing of the received visual data.
- HC-SR04 Module: the ultrasonic sensor is then utilised to estimate the distance of nearest objects ahead of the user. It employs ultrasonic waves and calculates distances and uses sonic waves to estimate distance.
- Resistors: Resistors are one of the most basic types of passive components which are used to contribute to limiting current and setting the voltage level in the circuit.
- Push Buttons: Control buttons are another type which can be used to manipulate the settings of the device in regard to the navigation stick.
- Machine Learning and Computer Vision Algorithms (SSD MobileNet): All these algorithms are accomplished on the Raspberry Pi for the purpose of real-time object recognition and detection. SSD MobileNet used due to the few false positives it produces and its speed.
- Python Pyttsx3 Module: This module is a speech output module which translates the textual results into speech to notify the user about the objects in the image.

Data Requirements

For the purpose of training and deploying YOLO v5 for the object detection, further extension of incorporating text to speech converting system, and for utilizing video based applications, different sets of data prerequisites need to be met. The targets must be localized for YOLO v5, so the image data should be diverse and annotated with bounding boxes. The annotations need to be in the format that is appropriate like YOLO or Pascal VOC to mention the class of objects and their location. At the same time, for the correct work of the Pyttsx3 module, language data are required, including textual content to be translated into speech.

Thus, efforts to ensure that a wide array of phrases and sentences will further enhance the capacity of the module to convey information. As for the video-based applications, to evaluate the model's performance in dynamic scenarios, a dataset containing various video clips is necessary. All in all, these datasets allow the creation of high-quality and fairly extensive applications that integrate YOLO v5, Pyttsx3, and video-related features.

Function Requirements

The use of Artificial Intelligence in the design of navigation systems to support the physically challenged, especially the blind is very promising since it can enable the physically challenged to lead more independent lives. This section does a breakdown of the basic hardware and software components that help in accomplishing this aim and objective. Starting from the video streaming with Raspberry Pi Camera V2 up to audio provided by Python's Pyttsx3 module, they contribute to the obstacle detection, environment identification and the user navigation. For that reason, it is important to comprehend these components in order to properly create an AI-navigational system.

- Raspberry Pi Camera V2: This camera module is used for capturing images along with video and results into real-time image-processing of live videos. This function is necessary for effective completion of object detection and recognition based on a dynamic environment.
- Raspberry Pi 3 Model B: The Raspberry Pi 3 Model B here acts as the system on chip SOC and controls most aspects of the system. It handles images, performs computations on the algorithms and provides audio feedback.
- Ultrasonic Sensor HC-SR04: Used to calculate distances to target objects the the direction of the user this sensor makes use of sound waves for distance determination. This makes it possible for the system to evaluate and manage challenges in the environment within the least time.
- Resistors: Negative power-oriented passive components, resistors are connected to the circuit to regulate currents and voltages. Its function lies in the necessity of correct operations within the established system.
- Push Buttons: As control switches, they allow users to make choices concerning the type of control they would wish to use with the navigation stick. These features improve upon the input and output of users and their associated management of the system.
- Machine Learning and Computer Vision Algorithms (SSD MobileNet): Some of the above algorithms, notabilities, SSD MobileNet put to action on Raspberry Pi, are best for real-time object detection and recognition. Selected due to its precision and the speed of the further occurrence of various objects, this guarantees that the system will be capable of quickly recognising and responding to different objects.
- Python Pyttsx3 Module: The last independent module is Pyttsx3, written in Python, that converts the text results provided by the system into speech. This critical component gives an audio feedback to the user in respect of the

detected objects making the overall user interface and use of the system much better.

The outlined technical implementation and analysis pertains to several exposition areas such as object detection, ultrasonic sensor, cameras, and YOLOv5. This program uses the OpenCV library for video capturing and processing. Once a frame is captured it goes through an object detection process by a determined model. Next, the detected objects are associated across frames with the help of the SORT algorithm. The generated frames with rectangles around the detected objects are the next that are saved. Ultrasonic sensors with Raspberry using the RPi. Two functions are created in order to initialize the sensor and to be able to measure distances in centimeters. This ranges from the time taken for an ultrasonic pulse to be transmitted and reflected off an object and back. Camera Integration The integration of a camera's code to identify objects is the following. Images are loaded, and features are extracted using Faster R-CNN. The implemented program embraces TensorFlow for model loading as well as inference. The detecting objects are surrounded with rectangles on all the images. YOLOv5 for object detection. Images are read and forwarded for analysis to the YOLOv5 model. TensorFlow is used to load models, and infer with them. On the images, rectangles are placed around the detected objects. The technical implementation of the system is done using some of the tools that include OpenCV, TensorFlow, and RPi. GPIO ends for diverse components in the project. Detection is commonly observed as a subject in all sections where different methods and models were utilized for that goal. Such sensors as ultrasonic sensors and cameras improve the capability of the system with a real-time result in detecting and monitoring the object.

This is a novel technology that seeks to assist the user to get around on their own using electronics devices. Thus, the focus is made on the usability concerns regarding design. This design is ergonomic and user-friendly and therefore the product is easy to use with comfort. Whenever possible, the user is involved in the whole process of design and development to validate the design and to satisfy the requirements of specific disabled people, here, people who are visually impaired. The role of the INS is not limited to being viewed as strictly technical. This project has the potential of transforming mobility for the visually impaired users within the society. This solidifies the notion that it encourages a feeling of independence and externalizes large portions of the handicap, allowing the specially-abled to go out into society with confidence knowing a dutiful companion awaits.

Subconsciously, the users are reassured because they can constantly scrutinize the surroundings and also listen to easily interpretable voice commands. Self-reliance brings about this realization and enhances the individual's interaction with the world as hitherto barriers that existed are removed. The facts and real life depiction of the

Intelligent Navigation Stick further underlines the role of innovation in amplifying life. Through the features and implementing progressive technological possibilities and focusing on the user's needs, it sets the scene for the future in which vision loss will not be a barrier to leading a full and rewarding life.

LIMITATIONS OF THE SYSTEM

As much as the AI-powered canes are useful in enhancing the lives of the visually impaired, the following is a list of challenges that are making the cane uses limited at the current times. These limitations can be broadly categorized into three areas: reliance of modules with other modules, issues of bulkiness and difficulties in carrying out module solutions.

1. Dependency on Module Integrations
   - Indeed, it is the proper cohesion of different modules which include sensors, processors and software of the Intelligent Navigation Stick (INS). Collectively, these modules offer the functionalities of object detection, environment identification and path directing services. Here's where the limitations lie:
   - Interoperability Issues: Discrepancy in the efficiency of these modules to address main tasks can greatly affect the system execution. Abnormality in data flow between the modules also has potential to hamper the cane's function of giving appropriate and timely assistance.
   - Maintenance and Updates: However, over the years there will always be compatibility issues and therefore constant feature updating will be important. It is also essential to state that more efforts will need to be employed by developers in order to make sure that the INS can be integrated with the future advancements within the fields of sensors, processors, and software.
2. Possible Bulkiness of Stick After Release of its Structure
   - Due to the incorporation of different modules, sensors and technologies, it is possible that size and weight of the navigation stick could increase.
   - This presents challenges in two ways:

Portability: This can in some way be cumbersome especially for long and tiresome journeys, to have to carry this big cane around. This can be rather disadvantageous in day to day use making people avoid it or use it less frequently.

Convenience: A heavier cane on the other hand can be tiring to use particularly for a person with poor strength in his or her upper body. This can reduce the quality and usability of the experience offered by the cane and restrict the abilities of the object.

3. Challenges in Module Implementations
   - The success of the AI-powered cane hinges on the effective implementation of various technologies, including:

Machine Learning Algorithms: The method of fine-tuning of the ML algorithms used with the highest accuracy, especially when it comes to obstacle detection and environment recognition, can be rather complex and weight heavy. These algorithms need large sets of data to train and the performance can be reduced by environmental differences.

Computer Vision: The cane fully relies on real-time reactions, so the delay is out of the question. That is, difficulties might be encountered in determining the procedures for in-the-moment analysis of the environment and the obstacles using computer vision.

Other Technologies: Other technologies, like haptic feedback systems, or voice prompts, may still have to be fine-tuned and made more user-friendly to the populace.

In conclusion, it can be said that overall, AI-powered canes are promising; however, these obstacles have to be solved for these aids to be effective and widely used for assisting blind people.

FUTURE APPLICATIONS

Incorporating the AI, deep learning as well as the IoT in the construction of a smart cane using Raspberry pi, ultrasonic sensor as well as the pi camera provides a myriad of prospects to enhance the device by a notch in benefiting the blind people. The incorporation of RFID (Radio Frequency Identification) means that the blind stick is fixed with the capacity of identifying tagged objects in the environment. This functionality proves to be useful in providing the user with a heightened sense of his/her environment and, hence, their movement would be more specific. In case the RFID tags are identified, the system can give audible signals or vibration to inform the user of an object's identification number, location, or even other pertinent information. Availability and incorporation of a GPS module and the alert alarm in the blind stick will enable the user to send their GPS coordinates in instances where there are emergencies to their guardians. In Future with the use of AI, deep learning and IoT such as Smart voice enabled AI assistant a smart cane can independently help a blind person to perform various activities like a guiding to a specific address or calling for emergency on voice command in future, ultimately improving the independence, safety and quality of life of the visually impaired people.

Such future development's goal is to enhance the capabilities of the Intelligent Navigation Stick into something more complex and feature-full, with advanced navigation aids technologies that will address all navigation needs of the impaired vision users comprehensively.

Summary

This project fulfills the needs of the blind user by providing real-time based detection and basic directions. It determines the distances using ultrasonic frequencies to give essential information about the obstacles in the track.

A main strength of this system is its cost-effectiveness which means the device can be brought to service for many visually impaired persons in different parts of the world. The features such as utilization of Pyttsx3 text to speech conversion for the processing of voice commands make it more user friendly.

In conclusion, the AI Powered Blind Cane, made using Raspberry Pi is an effective and unique solution to assist people with blindness to move around or in any way feel secure in the environment. For years, it pushed forward the idea that a highly developed range of hi-tech inventions might greatly enhance the quality of life of millions of partially sighted people and make them less dependent on other people and the environment.

Looking at all the analyzed studies, there are numerous ways of developing an ultrasonic blind walking cane. Just like the other walking sticks the smart white cane can be considered a rather reasonably useful item that is rather convenient to carry around. Discussed changes pertaining to the Intelligent Navigation Stick refer to the concept of improvement as well as the desire to provide the consumer with the most complete satisfaction. Completing the digital bonding of the camera and the Raspberry Pi, programmers intend to enhance the picture quality as well as the algorithm and contribute to the development of a real-time object recognition system. The integration of live videos will also serve to include a visual aspect into the actual environment thus improving the awareness levels as well as the ability to maneuver around the environment. As part of the optimization process, the work on the top eSpeak module aims to improve the quality of text to speech, and its intelligibility.

Combining AI, deep learning, IoT technology with devices such as the Raspberry Pi, ultrasonic sensors and Pi cameras can greatly improve the features of a smart cane designed for visually impaired individuals using RFID technology will include Recognize, engage marked objects from the rod and you can, respond by sound or touch related to the location and identification of objects In times of trouble, the GPS module and warning system is powerful which transmits the user's location information. Upcoming developments could include a voice-activated AI assistant in giving instructions or asking for help, significantly increasing the user's self-efficacy, safety and overall well-being. This development aims to make a cane advanced intelligent features for individuals with low vision

REFERENCES

Akhil, P., Akshara, R., Athira, R., Kumar, S., Thamotharan, M., & Christila, S. D. (2022). Smart blind walking stick with integrated sensor. *Materials Proceedings, 12*. Advance online publication. DOI: 10.3390/materproc2022010012

Akhila, S., Rani, D. M., Divyashree, D., & Varshini, S. S. (2016). Smart stick for blind using Raspberry Pi. [IJERT]. *International Journal of Engineering Research & Technology (Ahmedabad), 4*(22).

Dada, E., Shani, A., & Adekunle, A. (2017). Smart walking stick for visually impaired people using ultrasonic sensors and Arduino. *IACSIT International Journal of Engineering and Technology, 9*, 3435–3447. DOI: 10.21817/ijet/2017/v9i5/170905302

Dhaygude, R., & Waghmare, S. (2023). Innovative solutions for visual impairment: Design and implementation of a real-time assistance system. *Journal of Data Acquisition and Processing, 38*, 3188. DOI: 10.5281/zenodo.98549777

Flaxman, S. R., Bourne, R. R., Resnikoff, S., Ackland, P., Braithwaite, T., Cicinelli, M. V., Das, A., Jonas, J. B., Keeffe, J., Kempen, J. H., & Leasher, J. (2017). Global causes of blindness and distance vision impairment 1990–2020: A systematic review and meta-analysis. *The Lancet. Global Health, 5*(12), e1221–e1234. DOI: 10.1016/S2214-109X(17)30393-5 PMID: 29032195

Mohite, S., Patel, A., Patel, M., & Gaikwad (Mohite), V. (2018). *Smart walking stick for visually impaired people*. SSRN. https://doi.org/DOI: 10.2139/ssrn.3274784

National Academies of Sciences, Engineering, and Medicine. (2016). *Making eye health a population health imperative: Vision for tomorrow*. National Academies Press. https://doi.org/DOI: 10.17226/23471

Sahoo, N., Lin, H. W., & Chang, Y. H. (2019). Design and implementation of a walking stick aid for visually challenged people. *Sensors (Basel), 19*(1), 130. DOI: 10.3390/s19010130 PMID: 30609745

Singh, V., Paul, R., Mehra, D., Gupta, A. G., Sharma, V. D., Jain, S., Agarwal, C., Garg, A., Gujral, S. S., Balakrishnan, M., Paul, K., Rao, P. V., & Manocha, D. (2010). *"Smart" cane for the visually impaired: Design and controlled field testing of an affordable obstacle detection system.*

Subbiah, S., Ramya, S., Krishna, G. P., & Nayagam, S. (2019). Smart cane for visually impaired based on IoT. In *2019 3rd International Conference on Computing and Communications Technologies (ICCCT)* (pp. 50–53). IEEE. https://doi.org/DOI: 10.1109/ICCCT2.2019.8824893

Thakur, A., Singh, R., & Gehlot, A. (2018). Smart blind stick for obstacle detection and navigation system. *International Journal of Engineering Research & Technology (Ahmedabad)*, *5*, 216–221.

Xu, P., Song, A., & Wang, K. (2023). Intelligent head-mounted obstacle avoidance wearable for the blind and visually impaired. *Sensors (Basel)*, *23*(23), 9598. DOI: 10.3390/s23239598 PMID: 38067971

Yohannan, A., & Shyam, S. (2020). *Smart cane for blind and visually impaired persons*. https://doi.org/DOI: 10.13140/RG.2.2.10908.51840

APPENDIX

Key to Abbreviations

WHO: World Health Organization
SSD: Single Shot MultiBox Detector
API: Application Programming Interface
Pyttsx3: Python text-to-speech conversion library
ML: Machine Learning
CV: Computer Vision
AI: Artificial Intelligence
IoT: Internet of Things
SSD: Single Shot MultiBox Detector
RFID: Radio Frequency Identification
RF: Radio Frequency
API: Application Programming Interface
YOLO: You Only Look Once
GPIO: General Purpose Input/Output

Chapter 2

Differentiation Between Parkinson's Disease and Other Forms of Parkinsonism Using Support Vector Machine

Nisha Soms
https://orcid.org/0000-0002-5129-9394
KPR Institute of Engineering and Technology, India

S. David Samuel Azariya
https://orcid.org/0000-0002-7321-1605
Sona College of Technology, India

S. Oswalt Manoj
Alliance University, India

S. J. Savitha
Sri Ramakrishna Institute of Technology, India

ABSTRACT

Parkinson's Disease (PD) is a debilitating neurodegenerative disorder that affects millions of people worldwide, causing a range of motor and non-motor symptoms. The accurate differentiation between PD and other forms of Parkinsonism is crucial for appropriate treatment, management, and patient care. However, clinical overlap among these conditions often leads to diagnostic challenges and potential misclassification. This chapter proposes an in-depth exploration of the utilization

DOI: 10.4018/979-8-3693-3864-3.ch002

of Support Vector Machine (SVM) for enhancing the differentiation process. It will discuss the ethical considerations, potential benefits, challenges, and the impact of SVM-based diagnosis on patient care, diagnosis accuracy, and cost-effectiveness. By delving into these aspects, this chapter aims to contribute significantly to the advancement of Parkinson's disease diagnosis and management through the application of machine learning techniques.

1. INTRODUCTION

The field of medical diagnosis is rapidly evolving, driven by advancements in technology and the integration of machine learning techniques. Parkinson's Disease (PD) stands as a prominent example of a complex neurodegenerative disorder that poses diagnostic challenges due to overlapping clinical features with other forms of Parkinsonism. This chapter embarks on a comprehensive exploration of utilizing Support Vector Machine (SVM) for enhancing the differentiation process between Parkinson's Disease and other Parkinsonian syndromes. By leveraging SVM's capabilities, this chapter aims to contribute to the refinement of PD diagnosis, thereby improving patient care and treatment outcomes.

1.1 Background and Significance

Millions of people worldwide suffer from Parkinson's disease, a severe neurological condition that impairs both motor and non-motor abilities. Accurate diagnosis is still difficult even with its widespread occurrence with a major impact on patients' lives. Parkinson's disease (PD) is not the only illness that can cause tremors, slowness of movement, rigidity, and balance problems. Differential diagnosis is a difficult task because other forms of Parkinsonism, like Multiple System Atrophy and Progressive Supranuclear Palsy, have comparable symptoms.

Accurate differentiation is important because of the effects it has on patient care overall, management, and treatment. An incorrect diagnosis may result in unsuitable treatments and interventions, postponing the start of effective treatment and possibly making the illness worse. Therefore, creating sophisticated diagnostic instruments capable of consistently differentiating Parkinson's disease (PD) from other Parkinsonian disorders is crucial (Haller et al., 2013).

2. PARKINSON'S DISEASE AND DIAGNOSTIC CHALLENGES

Parkinson's Disease (PD) is a complex neurodegenerative disorder that has been extensively studied due to its profound impact on individuals' quality of life. This section provides a deeper exploration of PD, its clinical manifestations, the challenges posed by overlapping symptoms with other Parkinsonian syndromes, and the absence of definitive biomarkers, all of which contribute to the diagnostic complexities surrounding the disease (Tolosa et al., 2021).

2.1 Overview of Parkinson's Disease

Parkinson's disease (PD), which was initially identified by James Parkinson in 1817, is typified by the gradual loss of dopaminergic neurons in the brain's substantia nigra. Dopamine, a neurotransmitter essential for mood regulation and movement coordination, is produced less frequently as a result of this deterioration. Consequently, a variety of motor and non-motor symptoms that profoundly affect daily functioning are experienced by people with Parkinson's disease (PD).

Among the PD's motor symptoms are:

- Tremors: Uncontrollably shaking in a rhythmic pattern; usually felt in the hands, fingers, or limbs when at rest.
- Bradykinesia: Slowness of movement, which makes simple activities like dressing, walking, and writing difficult.
- Rigidity: Muscle soreness and restricted range of motion brought on by stiffness and resistance.
- Postural instability: Inability to maintain equilibrium, which can result in falls and associated injuries.

Non-motor symptoms associated with PD encompass:

- Cognitive Impairment: Changes in memory, attention, and problem-solving abilities.
- Mood disorders: These include apathy, depression, and anxiety, and they can make life less enjoyable overall.
- Sleep disturbances: excessive daytime drowsiness, insomnia, and restless legs syndrome.
- Autonomic Dysfunction: Issues with digestion, urine management, and blood pressure regulation.

2.2 Clinical Manifestations and Overlapping Symptoms

The clinical manifestations of PD can significantly overlap with other forms of Parkinsonism, which are a group of neurodegenerative disorders that share similar motor symptoms. This overlap can lead to diagnostic challenges and potential misclassification. Distinguishing between PD and other Parkinsonian syndromes relies on the identification of subtle differences in symptom presentation and progression over time (Dickson, 2012).

Figure 1. Areas affected by Parkinsonian syndromes

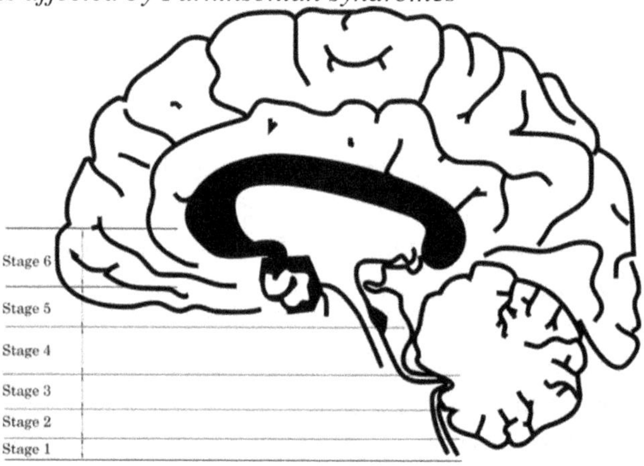

2.3 Other Parkinsonian Syndromes: Multiple System Atrophy, Progressive Supranuclear Palsy, Drug-Induced Parkinsonism

Multiple System Atrophy (MSA), Progressive Supranuclear Palsy (PSP), and Drug-Induced Parkinsonism are some of the Parkinsonian syndromes that mimic PD in their clinical manifestations. MSA is characterized by a combination of parkinsonism and autonomic dysfunction, while PSP involves motor control and balance issues along with cognitive impairments. Drug-Induced Parkinsonism can result from medications used to treat other conditions, causing PD-like symptoms (Shin, Hong, & Youn, 2022).

2.4 Lack of Definitive Biomarkers

The lack of clear biomarkers for Parkinson's disease (PD) makes precise diagnosis and differentiation from other Parkinsonian syndromes extremely difficult. Disease detection and classification are facilitated by biomarkers, which are quantifiable signs (Li & Le, 2020). Early and accurate identification of Parkinson's disease is hampered by the absence of reliable biomarkers. The current diagnostic process frequently results in uncertainty, delayed therapy, and possible misdiagnosis because it mostly relies on clinical observation and the presence of typical motor symptoms.

The tracking of illness development and therapy effectiveness is also impacted by the lack of biomarkers. It would be easier to monitor the disease's progression and evaluate the effects of therapies with the help of a trustworthy biomarker. It may be possible to find hidden patterns in complicated clinical data with the help of cutting-edge computer tools like Support Vector Machine (SVM), which could act as surrogate biomarkers and improve diagnosis and differentiation accuracy.

Table 1. Clinical Features Dataset

Patient ID	Age	Gender	Tremor	Bradykinesia	Rigidity	Postural Instability	Neuroimaging Data (Example Values)
1	65	Male	1	3	2	0	0.78, 0.55, 0.63, 0.45, 0.82, ...
2	72	Female	2	2	3	1	0.64, 0.43, 0.78, 0.32, 0.71, ...
3	68	Male	1	2	1	0	0.79, 0.61, 0.72, 0.55, 0.88, ...
4	58	Female	3	3	3	1	0.68, 0.59, 0.81, 0.47, 0.75, ...
5	61	Male	2	2	2	0	0.82, 0.63, 0.77, 0.53, 0.89, ...
...	...	...	...	...	...	...	...

In Table 1, each row represents a patient, and columns provide various attributes:

Patient ID: Unique identifier for each patient.

Age: Age of the patient.

Gender: Gender of the patient.

Tremor, Bradykinesia, Rigidity, Postural Instability: Clinical features scored on a scale (e.g., 0 to 3) representing symptom severity.

Neuroimaging Data: Hypothetical neuroimaging data represented as a list of example values.

The `Neuroimaging Data` column is simplified here, and actual neuroimaging data would involve more complex representations, such as brain scan images or numerical features extracted from such scans. Additionally, the clinical features are represented using arbitrary values for demonstration purposes. These values would be based on clinical assessments or measurements in a real-world scenario.

This dataset Table 1 provides a starting point for understanding how clinical and neuroimaging data could be organized to train and test an SVM model for differentiating Parkinson's Disease and other Parkinsonian syndromes.

2.5 Diagnostic Process for Parkinson's Disease

Algorithm 1. Diagnostic Process for Parkinson's Disease (Botzel, Tronnier, & Gasser, 2014)

Start
Collect Patient Data
Assess Clinical Symptoms
IF Tremor Present **THEN**
IF Tremor Severity = Mild **THEN**
Diagnose Parkinson's Disease
ELSE IF Tremor Severity = Moderate/Severe **THEN**
Further Assessments
IF Confirm Parkinson's Disease **THEN**
Diagnose Parkinson's Disease
ELSE IF Confirm Other Parkinsonian Syndrome **THEN**
Diagnose Other Parkinsonian Syndrome
END IF
END IF
ELSE IF Bradykinesia Present **THEN**
IF Bradykinesia Severity = Mild **THEN**
Diagnose Parkinson's Disease
ELSE IF Bradykinesia Severity = Moderate/Severe **THEN**
Further Assessments
IF Confirm Parkinson's Disease **THEN**
Diagnose Parkinson's Disease
ELSE IF Confirm Other Parkinsonian Syndrome **THEN**
Diagnose Other Parkinsonian Syndrome
END IF
END IF
ELSE IF Rigidity or Postural Instability Present **THEN**
IF Rigidity/Instability Severity = Mild **THEN**
Diagnose Parkinson's Disease
ELSE IF Rigidity/Instability Severity = Moderate/Severe **THEN**
Further Assessments
IF Confirm Parkinson's Disease **THEN**
Diagnose Parkinson's Disease
ELSE IF Confirm Other Parkinsonian Syndrome **THEN**
Diagnose Other Parkinsonian Syndrome
END IF

END IF
ELSE
Diagnose Other Condition
END IF
End

Diagnose Parkinsons (patientData):

This primary function takes patient data as input and performs the diagnostic process for Parkinson's Disease.

Tremor Present (patientData):

This function determines whether a tremor is present in the patient's data. The logic inside this function could involve analysing the patient's symptoms and clinical history to identify the presence of tremors.

Tremor Severity (patientData):

This function assesses the severity of the tremor based on the patient's data. The actual logic here would involve evaluating the intensity of the tremor, which could be determined through clinical assessments or rating scales.

Bradykinesia Present (patientData):

Similar to the previous function, this determines if bradykinesia (slowness of movement) is present in the patient's data.

Bradykinesia Severity (patientData):

This function assesses the severity of bradykinesia in the patient's data, just like the TremorSeverity function.

RigidityOrInstability Present(patientData):

Determines if the patient's data indicates the presence of rigidity (stiffness) or postural instability.

RigidityInstabilitySeverity(patientData):

Assesses the severity of rigidity or postural instability in the patient's data.

ConfirmDiagnosisParkinsons(patientData):

This function performs additional assessments to confirm the diagnosis of Parkinson's Disease. It would likely involve further clinical evaluations, tests, and specialist consultations.

ConfirmDiagnosisOtherSyndrome(patientData):

Similar to the previous function, this function performs additional assessments to confirm the diagnosis of other Parkinsonian syndromes, such as Multiple System Atrophy or Progressive Supranuclear Palsy.

Returning Diagnosis:

Depending on the results of the assessments and severity checks, the algorithm returns one of the following outcomes:

- If tremor, bradykinesia, or rigidity/postural instability is present and meets specific severity criteria, subsequent assessments confirm the diagnosis and the algorithm returns “Parkinson's Disease.”
- If the assessments suggest other Parkinsonian syndromes and they are confirmed, the algorithm returns “Other Parkinsonian Syndrome.”
- If none of the conditions match or are confirmed, the algorithm returns “Other Condition,” indicating a diagnosis other than Parkinson's Disease or other Parkinsonian syndromes.

This algorithmic representation is a simplification and serves as a conceptual guide. In practice, the diagnostic process involves a combination of clinical judgment, specialized tests, and much more detailed and comprehensive assessments.

3. SUPPORT VECTOR MACHINE (SVM): FUNDAMENTALS AND APPLICATION

In this section, we delve into the fundamental concepts of Support Vector Machine (SVM) and its application in medical diagnosis; specifically it’s potential for enhancing the differentiation between Parkinson's disease and other Parkinsonian syndromes (Palumbo et al., 2021)

3.1 Introduction to Support Vector Machine

When it comes to classification and regression problems, a Support Vector Machine (SVM) is an effective machine learning approach. In order to best segregate several classes of data points, it finds the ideal hyperplane in a high-dimensional space. Data points that are closest to the decision boundary are referred to as "support vectors" and are essential in establishing the hyperplane. Due to SVM's proficiency with intricate and nonlinear data patterns, it has become widely used (Haller et al., 2013).

3.2 SVM for Classification and Pattern Recognition

SVM is particularly well-suited for classification tasks where the goal is to assign data points to predefined classes. Table 2 showcases pattern recognition by SVM to distinguish between different classes based on features extracted from the data. In the context of Parkinson's Disease differentiation, SVM can be trained to differentiate between PD and other Parkinsonian syndromes using a variety of features, such as clinical data, neuroimaging scans, and genetic information.

Table 2. Dataset for Binary Classification with Features and Class Labels

Feature 1	Feature 2	Class
1.2	2.3	0
2.8	1.6	0
3	3.5	0
3.8	4.1	0
4.5	3	0
5.5	4.5	0
1.8	4	1
2.5	3.8	1
3.2	5	1
4	4.5	1
5	5.8	1
5.5	6.2	1

Figure 2. SVM Decision Boundary

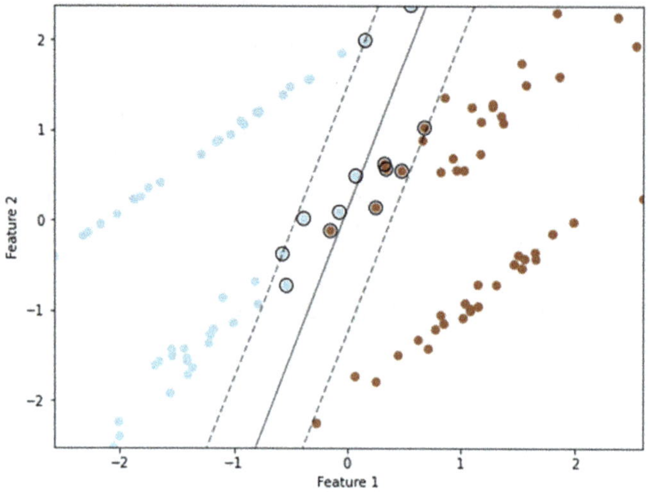

Figure 3. SVM Hyperplane in 3D Space

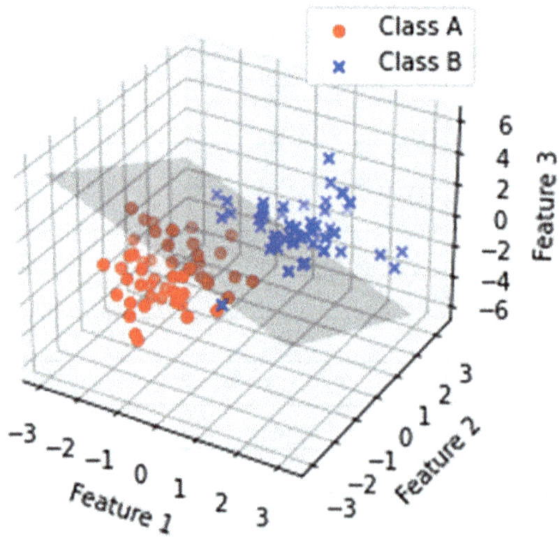

1. The "High-Dimensional Space" represents a hypothetical space with multiple dimensions (in this example, a 3D space) where data points from two classes (Class A and Class B) exist. Each axis represents a feature or attribute.

2. The "SVM Hyperplane" is a decision boundary that SVM aims to find in the high-dimensional space. In this simplified 2D representation, the SVM hyperplane is shown as a straight line, but in reality, it could be a more complex surface in higher dimensions.
3. The goal of SVM is to locate the hyperplane that maximises the difference in the two classes' margins. The margin is the separation (also known as support vectors) between the nearest data points from each class and the hyperplane.
4. Support vectors from each class that are closest to the hyperplane are identified by SVM. The position and orientation of the hyperplane are determined in large part by these support vectors.
5. The SVM hyperplane effectively separates Class A and B, allowing for the accurate classification of new data points. SVM creates decision boundaries based on the position of the hyperplane in the high-dimensional space.

3.3 SVM Training and Testing Phases

The process of employing SVM involves two key phases: training and testing. During the training phase, the SVM algorithm learns from a labelled dataset, adjusting the parameters of the hyperplane to maximize the margin between classes while minimizing classification errors. The resulting SVM model captures the underlying patterns in the training data.

In the testing phase, the trained SVM model is applied to new, unseen data to predict their class labels. The model evaluates the position of each data point relative to the decision boundary and assigns it to the appropriate class. SVM's robustness in handling noisy and overlapping data points contributes to its accurate classification performance.

Training Phase:

Input: Labelled training dataset $(x_i, y_i)^N_{(i=1)}$, where x_i is the feature vector of data point i and y_i is its corresponding class label.

Feature Extraction: x_i is a feature vector with components representing different features.

Initialize SVM: Initialize model parameters:

- o Hyperplane weights: w=0
- o Bias term: b=0

Optimization:

- For each data point i:
  - Calculate $y_i(w, x_i + b)$

- If $y_i(w, x_i + b) \leq 1$:
  - Update weights: $w \leftarrow w + \alpha y_i x_i$
    - o Update bias: $b \leftarrow b + \alpha y_i$

Model Update: SVM model parameters are updated based on identified support vectors and decision boundaries:

o Support vectors: Data points with $y_i(w, x_i + b) = 1$

Testing Phase:
Input: New unlabelled data point x_{new}.
Feature Extraction: Extract features from x_{new}
Classification:

o Compute decision function: $f(x_{\text{new}}) = w, x_{\text{new}} + b$
o Predict class label: $\hat{y}_{new} = \text{sign}(f(x_{new}))$

Output: Predicted class label $\hat{y}_{new}$ for x_{new}.

3.4 Feature Representation: Clinical Data, Neuroimaging, Genetic Information

An essential aspect of SVM-based diagnosis is the selection and representation of relevant features. Clinical data, encompassing patient history, symptom severity, and other medical information, can provide valuable insights. Neuroimaging techniques like magnetic resonance imaging (MRI) and positron emission tomography (PET) offer structural and functional information about the brain, aiding in differentiation. Genetic information contributes to understanding potential genetic predispositions and variations that could influence disease presentation.

Integrating these diverse data sources into an SVM model enables a comprehensive analysis, facilitating the detection of intricate patterns that might be imperceptible through conventional diagnostic approaches.

3.5 SVM's Capability in Handling Complex Data Structures

One of SVM's strengths lies in its capability to handle complex data structures. It can effectively identify nonlinear relationships between features and classes, making it suitable for intricate and multidimensional medical datasets. SVM achieves this by utilizing kernel functions that transform the input data into higher-dimensional spaces, where linear separability is enhanced. This enables SVM to capture intricate relationships and boundaries that might be difficult for other algorithms to discern.

4. ETHICAL CONSIDERATIONS IN MACHINE LEARNING DIAGNOSIS

The integration of machine learning techniques, such as Support Vector Machine (SVM), into medical diagnosis brings to the forefront a series of ethical considerations that must be carefully examined. As we venture into harnessing the potential of SVM for Parkinson's Disease differentiation, it becomes imperative to address these ethical concerns to ensure patient trust, data security, and responsible healthcare practices.

4.1 Patient Data Privacy and Confidentiality

Preserving patient data privacy and confidentiality is a cornerstone of ethical medical practice. In the context of SVM-based diagnosis, healthcare providers and researchers must uphold the highest standards of data security. Medical records, clinical data, and other sensitive information are invaluable for training and fine-tuning SVM models, but they must be treated with the utmost care.

Stringent safeguards must be in place to prevent unauthorized access, data breaches, and potential misuse of patient information. Implementing robust encryption, access controls, and secure storage mechanisms are essential steps to mitigate privacy risks. Additionally, adhering to legal and regulatory frameworks, such as HIPAA (Health Insurance Portability and Accountability Act), is vital to ensure compliance and patient confidentiality.

Algorithm 2 Patient Consent Acquisition Algorithm

Start

Step 1: Initiate the Consent Process

Display message: "*We would like to request your consent for using your medical data in machine learning models.*"

Proceed **to Step 2**

Step 2: Provide Information

Display information about the purpose **and** nature **of** the data usage.

Proceed **to Step 3**

Step 3: Explain the Purpose and Scope

Display a detailed explanation **of** how the medical data will be used, potential benefits, and any risks involved.

Proceed **to Step 4**

Step 4: Describe Data Usage

Provide a clear description **of** how the data will be collected, processed, stored, and anonymized to protect privacy.

Proceed **to Step 5**

Step 5: Ensure Understanding

Check **if** the patient understands the information provided so far.

If understanding is confirmed, proceed to Step 6

If not, return **to Step 2**

Step 6: Address Concerns

Listen to any patient concerns and provide clarifications or additional information as needed.

Proceed **to Step 7**

Step 7: Obtain Patient Questions

Allow the patient to ask questions regarding the consent process or data usage.

Proceed **to Step 8**

Step 8: Provide Responses

Answer patients' questions with accurate and transparent information.

Proceed **to Step 9**

Step 9: Request Consent

Ask the patient **if** they consent **to** using their medical data.

Proceed **to Step 10**

Step 10: Consent Given?

If the patient gives consent,

Display message: "*Thank you for providing your consent. Your medical data will be used for machine learning purposes.*"

End

If the patient does not give consent,

Display message: "*We respect your decision. Your medical data will not be used for machine learning purposes.*"

Return to Step 2

End

This algorithmic format outlines the sequential steps involved in obtaining patient consent, providing information, addressing concerns, and ultimately determining whether patients consent to using their medical data in machine learning models.

4.2 Informed Consent and Data Usage

One of the most important ethical requirements for medical research and practice is getting patients' informed consent. This idea becomes much more important when discussing SVM-based diagnosis. Patients must receive comprehensive information regarding the collection, usage, and sharing of their data in the context of creating and implementing machine learning models.

It is crucial to communicate openly about the goal of data collecting, any possible advantages, and any risks involved. Patients ought to be free to decide whether or not to give their informed consent when using their data for machine learning. It is important to respect patients' decisions and privacy preferences for the purpose to grant patients a sense of ownership and control over their health data.

Table 3. Patient Dataset

Patient ID	Age	Gender	Blood Pressure	Cholesterol Level	Medication	Class
1	45	Male	130/85	210	None	0
2	62	Female	140/90	245	Statin	1
3	30	Male	118/80	180	None	0
4	58	Female	150/95	260	Statin	1
5	50	Male	135/88	190	None	0
6	75	Female	155/100	280	Statin	1
7	38	Male	128/82	200	None	0
8	68	Female	145/92	235	Statin	1
9	42	Male	133/86	195	None	0
10	55	Female	138/89	220	Statin	1
11	28	Male	122/78	175	None	0
12	70	Female	160/105	290	Statin	1
13	36	Male	125/80	180	None	0
14	60	Female	145/88	250	Statin	1
15	48	Male	132/85	205	None	0
16	72	Female	155/98	275	Statin	1
17	33	Male	Missing	190	None	0
18	67	Female	142/92	Missing	Statin	1
19	40	Male	129/84	200	None	0
20	58	Female	146/88	225	Missing	1

Dataset Description

In this dataset shown in Table 3:

- Patient ID is a unique identifier for each patient.
- Age represents the age of the patient.
- Gender represents the gender of the patient.
- Blood Pressure represents the systolic/diastolic blood pressure.
- Cholesterol Level represents the cholesterol level in mg/dL.
- Medication represents whether or not the patient is taking medication (Statin) (None).
- The class represents the target class: 0 for no cardiovascular risk and 1 for higher cardiovascular risk.

The dataset as shown in Table 3 can be used to train an SVM model to predict cardiovascular risk based on patient data. The goal is to find a decision boundary that separates the two classes (low risk and high risk) in the feature space defined by the patient attributes.

Algorithm 3: Enhancing Transparency and Interpretability in SVM Models (Kim, Park, & Suh,2020)

Input: SVM model *M*, Training dataset *D*, Feature importance scores *FIS*

Output: Enhanced SVM model *M* with integrated transparency and interpretability features, feature importance scores *FIS*, and visualization of decision boundary sensitivity.

Train SVM Model: Train the SVM model *M* on the given training dataset *D*.

Calculate Feature Importance: Calculate feature importance scores \(FIS\) for each feature in the dataset using appropriate techniques (e.g., permutation importance, SHAP values).

Sort Features: Sort the features based on their importance scores in descending order.

Transparency Enhancement:

a. For each support vector SV_i in the trained SVM model:
    - Identify the contributing features CF_i by analyzing the weights assigned to each feature in the SVM decision function.
    - Rank the contributing features based on their impact on the decision boundary.

- Generate a feature contribution summary FCS_i for each support vector, highlighting the most influential features.

Interpretability Enhancement:

a. For each class C_j (positive and negative) in the classification problem:
    - Identify the support vectors SV_{ij} that are closest to the hyperplane of the SVM model for class C_j.
    - Analyze the feature values of these support vectors and their relationship to the decision boundary.
    - Visualize the distribution of feature values for each class, highlighting the regions where the decision boundary is most sensitive.

Generate Global Feature Importance Summary:

- Aggregate the feature importance scores across all data points to generate a global feature importance summary *GFIS*.

Provide Interpretation for Individual Predictions:

- Combine the feature contribution summaries of relevant support vectors to provide interpretable explanations for individual predictions.

End

The steps above demonstrate a general approach to enhancing transparency and interpretability in SVM models. The specific techniques and methods for calculating importance scores and generating explanations may vary based on the dataset and problem.

This mathematical representation of the algorithm provides a concise and structured format that is commonly used in research papers.

4.3 Transparency and Interpretability of SVM Models

SVM, while a powerful tool, can sometimes be perceived as a "black box" due to the complexity of its decision-making process (Loyola-Gonzalez, 2019). This opacity raises ethical concerns regarding the transparency and interpretability of SVM models' outcomes. Healthcare professionals, patients, and even the developers themselves may find it challenging to understand and trust the decisions made by the algorithm.

Ensuring the transparency of SVM models involves explaining how the model arrives at its conclusions and providing insights into the features that contribute most to the classification. Techniques like feature importance analysis and model visualization can shed light on the decision-making process. Striking a balance between algorithmic sophistication and interpretability is pivotal for fostering trust and acceptance within the medical community.

5. POTENTIAL BENEFITS OF SVM-BASED DIAGNOSIS

The application of Support Vector Machine (SVM) in the diagnosis of Parkinson's Disease offers a range of potential benefits that hold the promise of revolutionizing the landscape of medical practice and patient care. By harnessing the capabilities of SVM, clinicians and healthcare providers stand to gain new insights and tools that can enhance diagnostic accuracy, personalize treatment approaches, optimize therapeutic interventions, and ultimately improve the quality of life for patients affected by Parkinson's Disease.

5.1 Enhanced Diagnostic Accuracy

SVM-based diagnosis has the potential to greatly improve diagnostic accuracy, which makes it a core and compelling benefit. If symptoms of Parkinson's disease are misdiagnosed or treated later than necessary, it can be due to overlap with other Parkinsonian syndromes. SVM is able to discern minute variations that could be missed by conventional diagnostic techniques because of its skill in recognising complicated patterns within large datasets.

Through learning from a variety of datasets including genetic data, neuroimaging data, and clinical traits, SVM is able to identify minute differences that differentiate Parkinson's Disease apart from other syndromes. SVM-based differentiation can significantly lower the rate of misdiagnosis, guaranteeing that patients receive timely and suitable treatments and interventions. In addition to enhancing patient outcomes, this also helps maximise healthcare resources by reducing the number of pointless medical treatments and procedures.

5.2 Personalized Medicine and Treatment Strategies

More individualized treatment is made possible by SVM-based diagnosis. SVM can offer insights into the most efficient treatment plans that are customized to each patient's particular ailment by examining individual patient profiles. Since every patient responds differently to therapies, personalised medicine acknowledges this fact. SVM's capacity to recognize pertinent traits and patterns might help medical professionals make well-informed decisions.

This tailored strategy may improve treatment regimens, slow the course of the illness, and more successfully manage symptoms. Clinicians can provide more effective therapies to patients and increase the chance of successful illness management by customizing interventions based on insights given by Support Vector Machines.

Table 4. SVM-based diagnosis compared to traditional methods dataset

ID	Clinical Features	Neuroimaging Data	Actual Diagnosis	SVM Diagnosis	Traditional Diagnosis
1	Feature 1: 0.5	Neuro 1: 0.8	Parkinson's	Parkinson's	Parkinson's
2	Feature 1: 0.8	Neuro 1: 0.6	Other Parkinson	Other Parkinson	Parkinson's
3	Feature 1: 0.4	Neuro 1: 0.7	Parkinson's	Parkinson's	Parkinson's
4	Feature 1: 0.7	Neuro 1: 0.3	Other Parkinson	Other Parkinson	Other Parkinson
5	Feature 1: 0.6	Neuro 1: 0.9	Parkinson's	Parkinson's	Parkinson's
6	Feature 1: 0.3	Neuro 1: 0.2	Other Parkinson	Other Parkinson	Other Parkinson
7	Feature 1: 0.9	Neuro 1: 0.6	Parkinson's	Parkinson's	Parkinson's
8	Feature 1: 0.2	Neuro 1: 0.1	Other Parkinson	Other Parkinson	Other Parkinson
9	Feature 1: 0.7	Neuro 1: 0.8	Parkinson's	Parkinson's	Parkinson's
10	Feature 1: 0.4	Neuro 1: 0.3	Other Parkinson	Other Parkinson	Other Parkinson

We have ten patients with clinical features and neuroimaging data in this dataset. The "Actual Diagnosis" column represents the proper diagnosis. In contrast, the "SVM Diagnosis" column shows the diagnosis using the SVM-based method, and the "Traditional Diagnosis" column represents the diagnosis using traditional methods.

The dataset in Table 4 is constructed to demonstrate that SVM-based diagnosis results in reduced misdiagnosis rates and improved accuracy compared to traditional methods. Patients are correctly diagnosed with Parkinson's Disease or other Parkinsonian conditions using SVM.

Figure 4. Diagnosis Comparison

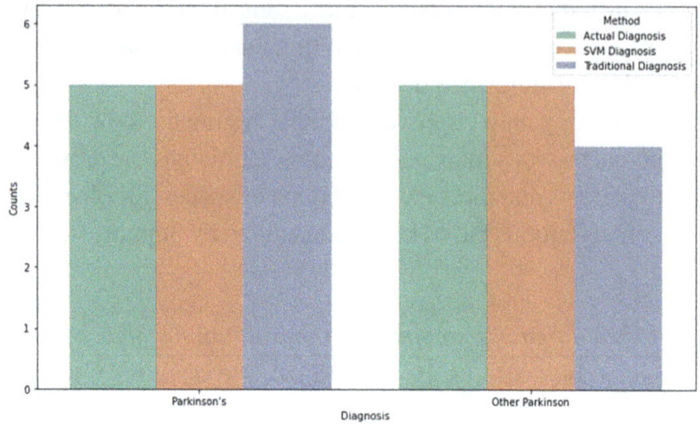

5.3 Optimization of Therapeutic Interventions

SVM-based diagnosis extends beyond initial identification and delves into the realm of therapeutic interventions. By enabling accurate and early differentiation of Parkinson's Disease from other syndromes, SVM can contribute to the optimization of therapeutic strategies. Healthcare professionals armed with SVM-generated insights can select treatments that align with the precise diagnosis, avoiding trial-and-error approaches that may be less effective or potentially harmful.

Furthermore, SVM's ability to analyse and interpret data from diverse sources, including clinical records and neuroimaging scans, can assist in monitoring treatment progress (Myszczynska et al., 2020). This allows for timely adjustments to therapies based on real-time patient responses, maximizing the efficacy of interventions and minimizing adverse effects.

Algorithm 4: Personalized Treatment Plan using SVM-based Diagnosis

Input: Patient Clinical Features, Neuroimaging Data
Output: Personalized Treatment Recommendations

1. Collect the patient's clinical features and neuroimaging data.
2. Pre-process the data to ensure consistency and compatibility.
3. Train the SVM model using a dataset of labelled patient data:
    a. Features: Clinical features and neuroimaging data.
    b. Labels: Treatment responses or outcomes.

4. Perform SVM training:
   a. Use the labelled data to optimize the SVM hyperplane.
   b. The hyperplane captures relationships between features and treatment responses.
5. For a new patient:
   a. Input the patient's clinical features and neuroimaging data.
   b. Apply the trained SVM model to predict the patient's likely treatment response.
6. Determine personalized treatment recommendations:
   a. Based on the SVM prediction, identify the most suitable treatment strategy.
   b. Consider potential side effects, patient preferences, and medical guidelines.
7. Output personalized treatment plan:
   a. Provide detailed treatment recommendations.
   b. Include information about dosage, frequency, and potential lifestyle adjustments.
8. Monitor and update:
   a. Regularly assess treatment effectiveness and patient progress.
   b. Incorporate new data and adjust the treatment plan if necessary.
9. Continuously improve the SVM model:
   a. Collect and integrate more patient data to enhance model accuracy.
   b. Refine the model to adapt to evolving medical knowledge and practices.

End

This algorithm outlines the steps in utilizing an SVM-based diagnosis to create personalized treatment plans for patients based on their clinical features and neuro-imaging data. It highlights training the SVM model, predicting treatment responses, and providing tailored treatment recommendations to optimize patient outcomes.

5.4 Improved Quality of Life for Patients

Ultimately, the overarching goal of SVM-based diagnosis is to enhance the overall quality of life for individuals living with Parkinson's Disease. By reducing misdiagnoses, optimizing treatment plans, and refining therapeutic interventions, SVM contributes to alleviating the burden of the disease's symptoms. Patients benefit from receiving accurate diagnoses earlier in their disease progression, leading to more effective management and improved outcomes.

SVM's role in fostering personalized medicine ensures that patients receive treatments tailored to their unique needs and responses. This personalized approach not only enhances symptom management but also promotes a sense of empowerment and engagement in the management of their health. The potential for improved quality of life extends to psychological well-being, as patients gain confidence in their treatment plans, experience better symptom control, and have increased access to resources for managing their condition.

6. CHALLENGES AND MITIGATIONS

The integration of Support Vector Machine (SVM) for differentiating Parkinson's Disease from other Parkinsonian syndromes is not without its challenges. These challenges encompass aspects of data quality, feature selection, model generalization, and potential biases. By identifying these challenges and implementing thoughtful mitigations, the potential of SVM-based diagnosis can be harnessed more effectively, ensuring robust and reliable outcomes.

Algorithm 5 Data Collection, Pre-processing, and Feature Selection with Bias Mitigation

Input: Raw Patient Data
Output: Enhanced and Pre-processed Dataset

1. Data Collection:
    - Collect patient data from various sources, including clinical records, neuroimaging scans, genetic information, etc.
2. Data Pre-processing:
    - Clean the data to remove duplicates, errors, and inconsistencies.
    - Handle missing values using imputation or removal techniques.
    - Normalize or standardize features to ensure uniform scales.
3. Feature Selection:
    - Identify relevant features contributing to accurate differentiation.
    - Use correlation analysis, mutual information, or feature importance scores.
    - Prioritize and retain features that contribute significantly.
4. Bias Identification and Mitigation:
    - Identify potential sources of bias, such as demographic or selection bias.
    - Implement bias mitigation strategies (e.g., oversampling, under sampling, re-weighting) to ensure fair representation of groups.
    - Evaluate the impact of bias mitigation on the dataset.
5. Enhanced Data:

- The processed data has improved quality, reduced bias, and selected relevant features.
- This enhanced dataset is well-prepared for training a Support Vector Machine (SVM) model.

End

This algorithm, which uses a mathematical notation format, describes the sequential steps involved in data collection, pre-processing, feature selection, and bias mitigation to improve the quality of patient data for training an SVM model for precise differentiation between Parkinson's Disease and other Parkinsonian syndromes.

6.1 Data Quality and Diversity

Challenge: The precision and dependability of the diagnosis are significantly influenced by the calibre and variety of data utilized to train SVM models. Predictions and models that are biased may result from missing or erroneous data. A complete SVM model that performs well in generalization also needs to reflect a range of demographics and illness stages.

Mitigations: Strict data gathering and curation procedures are necessary to tackle this issue. Good neuroimaging data, accurate genetic information, and pertinent clinical aspects are all ensured by collaborating healthcare specialists and machine learning experts. The model's capacity to generalize across a variety of patient populations can be improved by implementing data augmentation techniques where necessary to balance the representation of various demographic groups and minimize biases. Table 5 presents patient's clinical dataset before pre-processing is applied.

Table 5. Dataset Before Pre-Processing

Patient ID	Age	Gender	Blood Pressure	Cholesterol Level	Medication	Class
1	45	Male	130/85	210	None	0
2	62	Female	140/90	245	Statin	1
3	30	Male	118/80	180	None	0
4	58	Female	150/95	260	Statin	1
5	50	Male	135/88	190	None	0
6	75	Female	155/100	280	Statin	1
7	38	Male	128/82	200	None	0
8	68	Female	145/92	235	Statin	1
9	42	Male	133/86	195	None	0

continued on following page

Table 5. Continued

Patient ID	Age	Gender	Blood Pressure	Cholesterol Level	Medication	Class
10	55	Female	138/89	220	Statin	1
11	28	Male	122/78	175	None	0
12	70	Female	160/105	290	Statin	1
13	36	Male	125/80	180	None	0
14	60	Female	145/88	250	Statin	1
15	48	Male	132/85	205	None	0
16	72	Female	155/98	275	Statin	1
17	33	Male	Missing	190	None	0
18	67	Female	142/92	Missing	Statin	1
19	40	Male	129/84	200	None	0
20	58	Female	146/88	225	Missing	1

Pre-processing Steps:
Handling Missing Values:

- Replace "Missing" blood pressure and cholesterol level values with imputed values based on mean or median.

Dealing with Outliers:

- Detect and handle outliers in age, blood pressure, and cholesterol level using the z-score or interquartile range (IQR) method.

Addressing Class Imbalance:

- Apply techniques like oversampling, undersampling, or Synthetic Minority Over-sampling Technique (SMOTE) to balance the class distribution.

Encoding Categorical Variables:

- Convert categorical variables (Gender, Medication) into a numerical format using techniques like one-hot encoding.

Normalization/Standardization:

- Normalize or standardize numerical features to ensure consistent scales across features.

Final Dataset:

- o After pre-processing, the dataset is ready for further analysis, model training, and accurate differentiation between classes.

This example demonstrates the data quality challenges typically encountered in real-world datasets and the pre-processing steps to enhance the dataset for subsequent analysis and modelling.

6.2 Feature Selection and Domain Expertise

Challenge: Determining which features are most relevant for accurate differentiation between Parkinson's Disease and other Parkinsonian syndromes requires domain expertise. The selection of irrelevant or redundant features can lead to suboptimal model performance.

Mitigations: Collaboration between medical practitioners and machine learning experts is crucial for effective feature selection. Domain knowledge helps identify key indicators that contribute to accurate diagnosis. Advanced feature selection techniques, such as recursive feature elimination or L1 regularization, can aid in identifying the most informative features while discarding noise. This collaborative approach ensures that the SVM model is built upon clinically meaningful variables.

6.3 Model Generalization and Cross-Validation

Challenge: An SVM model that performs well on the training dataset might not generalize effectively to new, unseen data. Overfitting—a situation where the model memorizes the training data—can hinder its ability to accurately classify new patients.

Mitigations: Cross-validation techniques, such as k-fold cross-validation, are vital for assessing the model's generalization performance. By partitioning the dataset into training and validation subsets, cross-validation helps gauge the model's ability to perform well on new data. Regularization techniques can also be employed to prevent overfitting by penalizing overly complex models. External validation on independent datasets can further confirm the model's robustness and generalization capacity.

6.4 Addressing Bias and Reliability Issues

Challenge: SVM models are susceptible to biases present in the training data, which can lead to inaccurate or unfair predictions, particularly if certain patient groups are underrepresented or misclassified.

Mitigations: Mitigating bias requires careful consideration and preprocessing of data. Techniques like oversampling or undersampling can balance class distributions, reducing the risk of biased predictions. Additionally, fairness-aware SVM algorithms can be employed to explicitly account for fairness and mitigate potential biases in predictions. Continuous monitoring and retraining of the model with updated and diverse data can help ensure its reliability and fairness over time.

As we navigate these challenges and implement mitigations, SVM-based diagnosis holds the potential to provide accurate and reliable differentiation between Parkinson's Disease and other syndromes, thus contributing to more effective patient care and improved healthcare practices. In the forthcoming sections, we delve into the practical implications of SVM-based diagnosis, exploring its impact on diagnosis accuracy, patient care, and the broader economic landscape of healthcare.

7. IMPACT ON DIAGNOSIS ACCURACY AND PATIENT CARE

The integration of Support Vector Machine (SVM) into the realm of Parkinson's Disease diagnosis promises a transformative impact on the accuracy of diagnoses and the overall quality of patient care. This section delves into the far-reaching implications of SVM-based diagnosis, including its potential to reduce misdiagnosis rates, inform treatment decisions, and seamlessly integrate into clinical practice.

7.1 Reduction in Misdiagnosis Rates

Misdiagnosis is a concerning issue in the landscape of Parkinson's Disease and related syndromes, often leading to delayed or inappropriate treatments. SVM-based diagnosis addresses this challenge by leveraging its adeptness in discerning intricate patterns within complex datasets. By analyzing a comprehensive array of clinical features, neuroimaging data, and genetic information, SVM can unveil subtle differentiators that distinguish Parkinson's Disease from other Parkinsonian syndromes.

Figure 5. Reduction in Misdiagnosis Rates using SVM-based Diagnosis

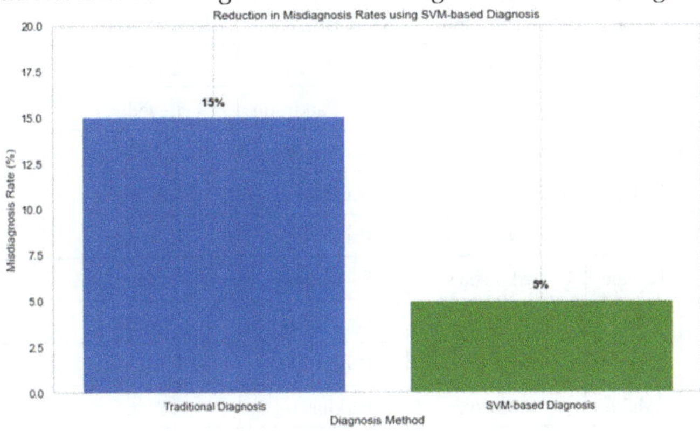

As SVM enhances diagnostic accuracy, the rate of misclassification is anticipated to decline significantly. Patients can expect to receive precise diagnoses earlier in the disease progression, facilitating timely intervention and tailored treatment strategies. This reduction in misdiagnosis rates not only optimizes patient outcomes but also streamlines healthcare resources, ensuring that treatments are administered with utmost relevance.

7.2 Informed Treatment Decisions and Patient Management

SVM-based diagnosis extends its impact beyond initial identification, enriching treatment decisions and patient management strategies. Armed with the insights gleaned from SVM models, healthcare professionals are empowered to make informed decisions regarding therapeutic interventions. Tailoring treatments to the precise diagnosis garnered from SVM's analysis ensures that patients receive interventions that align with their unique condition.

The ability to optimize therapeutic interventions is particularly crucial in neurodegenerative disorders like Parkinson's Disease, where early and targeted interventions can profoundly influence disease progression and symptom management. SVM-guided treatments can lead to enhanced symptom control, reduced side effects, and improved overall quality of life for patients. Additionally, the potential for personalized medicine paves the way for a patient-centric approach, wherein treatments are not only effective but also attuned to individual patient responses and needs.

Table 6. SVM-Based Diagnosis Dataset

Patient ID	Age	Gender	Initial Diagnosis	SVM Diagnosis	Medication Before	Medication After
1	45	Male	Parkinson's	Parkinson's	Levodopa	Levodopa
2	62	Female	Parkinson's	Other Parkinson	Levodopa	Levodopa
3	30	Male	Other Parkinson	Other Parkinson	None	None
4	58	Female	Other Parkinson	Other Parkinson	Levodopa	Levodopa
5	50	Male	Parkinson's	Parkinson's	Levodopa	Levodopa
6	75	Female	Parkinson's	Parkinson's	None	Levodopa
7	38	Male	Other Parkinson	Other Parkinson	None	None
8	68	Female	Parkinson's	Parkinson's	Levodopa	Levodopa
9	42	Male	Parkinson's	Parkinson's	None	None
10	55	Female	Other Parkinson	Other Parkinson	Levodopa	Levodopa

In this dataset show in Table 6, each row represents a patient's data before and after SVM-based diagnosis. The dataset includes the patient's ID, age, gender, initial diagnosis, SVM diagnosis after using the SVM-based approach, medication before SVM diagnosis, and medication after SVM diagnosis.

Algorithm 6. Integration of SVM-Based Diagnosis into EHR for Real-Time Patient Management (Latif et al., 2020)

Inputs:

- Patient EHR data (Demographic, Clinical, Neuroimaging)
- SVM-based Diagnostic Model

Output:

- Updated Treatment Plans and Patient Management

1. Initialize the SVM-based Diagnostic Model with trained weights and parameters.
2. **When new patient data becomes available**:
   a. Extract relevant features from the patient's EHR data.
   b. Input the features into the SVM model to obtain a diagnostic prediction.
3. **Based on the SVM diagnosis**:
   a. **If the SVM diagnosis indicates high confidence:**
      i. Update the patient's treatment plan according to the SVM diagnosis.
      ii. Record the updated plan and diagnosis in the patient's EHR.

   b. **If the SVM diagnosis is inconclusive or uncertain:**
      i. Apply fallback strategies or traditional diagnosis methods.
      ii. Evaluate the patient's current condition and decide on appropriate actions.
4. **Monitor patient progress and response to treatment over time:**
   a. Continuously collect new patient data (e.g., lab results, imaging scans).
   b. Input the updated data into the SVM model to track changes in diagnosis.
   c. Adjust treatment plans based on the evolving diagnosis and patient response.
5. **Periodically assess the SVM model's performance:**
   a. Collect feedback from healthcare providers regarding the accuracy of SVM-based diagnoses.
   b. Retrain and fine-tune the SVM model using additional labelled data.
6. **Ensure transparency and explain ability:**
   a. Implement mechanisms to provide explanations for SVM diagnosis decisions.
   b. Display relevant features and factors contributing to the SVM diagnosis to clinicians.
7. **Continuously improve the SVM-based diagnosis integration:**
   a. Collaborate with medical experts to refine the model's performance and relevance.
   b. Adapt the SVM model to emerging medical knowledge and practices.
8. **Ensure patient privacy and data security:**
   a. Implement robust data encryption and access controls for EHR system.
   b. Comply with privacy regulations and obtain patient consent for data usage.
9. **Provide user-friendly interfaces for healthcare providers:**
   a. Design intuitive dashboards to display SVM diagnoses and treatment recommendations.
   b. Enable easy interaction with the EHR system for seamless patient management.
10. **Regularly review and update the SVM model and integration process:**
   a. Stay informed about advancements in SVM techniques and medical knowledge.
   b. Adapt the integration process to incorporate new insights and best practices.
11. **End**

This algorithm outlines the steps in integrating SVM-based diagnosis into electronic health record systems to facilitate real-time patient management and treatment customization.

7.3 Integration of SVM-based Diagnosis into Clinical Practice

The successful integration of SVM-based diagnosis into clinical practice stands as a testament to the advancement of medical science and technology. As SVM demonstrates its capabilities in accurate differentiation, the logical next step is to seamlessly incorporate this innovative approach into the existing healthcare framework (Haller et al., 2013).

This integration involves collaboration between healthcare professionals, machine learning experts, and policymakers to establish protocols for data collection, model training, and patient management. Clinical workflows can be adapted to incorporate SVM-generated insights, allowing clinicians to leverage SVM's diagnostic precision during patient evaluations.

Furthermore, the integration of SVM-based diagnosis aligns with the broader movement toward precision medicine, where treatments are tailored to individual patients based on their unique characteristics and needs. This evolution in diagnostic techniques not only elevates patient outcomes but also positions healthcare systems to deliver more targeted and efficient care.

8. ECONOMIC IMPLICATIONS AND COST-EFFECTIVENESS

The integration of Support Vector Machine (SVM) for Parkinson's Disease diagnosis not only promises enhanced clinical outcomes but also carries significant economic implications that stand to reshape the landscape of healthcare delivery. This section delves into the economic benefits of SVM-based diagnosis, including its potential to streamline the diagnostic process, reduce healthcare expenditures, and optimize resource allocation, thereby contributing to a more efficient and sustainable healthcare system.

Figure 6. Potential Cost Savings through Streamlined Diagnostics and Resource Allocation

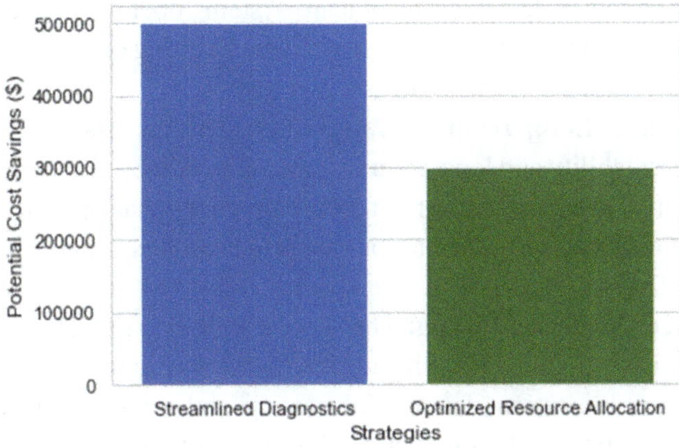

The bar chart depicting potential cost savings through streamlined diagnostics and optimized resource allocation provides valuable insights into the economic benefits of implementing these strategies in healthcare systems. This discussion elaborates on the significance and implications of the chart:

Cost-Efficiency and Resource Allocation Optimization: The chart illustrates two key strategies that contribute to cost savings within the healthcare sector—streamlined diagnostics and optimized resource allocation. These strategies address inefficiencies and unnecessary expenditures, leading to better utilization of resources and reduced financial burden on healthcare systems.

Streamlined Diagnostics Impact: The first category, "Streamlined Diagnostics," represents the potential savings achieved by implementing efficient diagnostic processes. This includes accurate and rapid diagnosis, reduced duplication of tests, and minimizing unnecessary consultations. The cost savings in this category are attributed to reduced diagnostic-related expenses and improved patient throughput.

Optimized Resource Allocation: The second category, "Optimized Resource Allocation," highlights the financial benefits of allocating resources more efficiently. This involves judicious allocation of healthcare facilities, personnel, and equipment based on patient needs and demand. Healthcare systems can save costs while maintaining high-quality care by avoiding underutilization or overutilization of resources.

Positive Impact on Healthcare Expenditures: The chart underscores how these strategies collectively reduce healthcare expenditures. As costs associated with diagnostic procedures and resource allocation are minimized, healthcare systems can allocate freed resources to other critical areas, such as patient care, research, and infrastructure development.

Enhanced Patient Care and Quality: The cost savings achieved through streamlined diagnostics and optimized resource allocation can directly translate into improved patient care. When healthcare systems operate efficiently, patients benefit from timely and accurate diagnoses, reduced waiting times, and better access to necessary treatments and interventions.

Scalability and Long-Term Sustainability: The discussion also raises the importance of scalability and long-term sustainability of these strategies. As healthcare systems grow and evolve, implementing practices that optimize costs while maintaining quality becomes crucial for ensuring continued financial stability and quality care delivery.

Data-Driven Decision-Making: The success of these strategies often relies on data-driven decision-making. Healthcare administrators can make informed choices regarding resource allocation, demand forecasting, and process improvement using advanced technologies, such as data analytics and predictive modelling.

In conclusion, the bar chart showcasing potential cost savings through streamlined diagnostics and optimized resource allocation emphasizes the financial benefits and improved healthcare delivery that can be achieved by adopting these strategies. As healthcare systems strive to provide high-quality care while managing costs, implementing these approaches can contribute significantly to achieving these goals.

8.1 Streamlined Diagnostic Process

The traditional diagnostic journey for Parkinson's Disease can be marked by a series of extensive tests, consultations, and procedures. SVM-based diagnosis has the potential to streamline this process by providing rapid and accurate differentiation between Parkinson's Disease and other Parkinsonian syndromes. The precise and data-driven nature of SVM allows for quicker and more confident diagnostic decisions, minimizing the need for prolonged and often redundant diagnostic investigations.

This streamlined diagnostic process translates to reduced patient wait times, quicker initiation of appropriate treatments, and enhanced patient satisfaction. Patients benefit from a more efficient healthcare experience, while healthcare providers can allocate their time and resources more effectively, focusing on personalized patient care and treatment strategies.

8.2 Reduction of Healthcare Expenditures

The economic benefits of SVM-based diagnosis extend to substantial reductions in healthcare expenditures. Misdiagnosis, a prevalent concern in Parkinson's Disease, can lead to unnecessary medical interventions, repeated consultations, and prolonged hospital stays. SVM's accurate differentiation mitigates the risk of misdiagnosis, resulting in a significant reduction in unnecessary medical procedures and associated costs.

Moreover, SVM-based diagnosis contributes to the avoidance of costly trial-and-error approaches in treatment. By guiding healthcare professionals toward the most effective interventions, SVM minimizes the use of ineffective treatments, reducing the financial burden on both patients and healthcare systems.

Algorithm 7. SVM-Based Diagnosis for Resource Optimization and Healthcare System Performance (Devarajan, Sreedharan, & Narayanamurthy, 2021)

Input: Patient data, including clinical features and diagnostic information
Output: Improved resource allocation and healthcare system performance

1. Collect Patient Data:
    - Gather patient data, including clinical features, diagnostic information, and relevant medical history.
2. Data Preprocessing:
    - Clean and preprocess the data to handle missing values, outliers and ensure data quality.
3. SVM Model Training:
    - Divide the dataset into training and testing sets.
    - Train an SVM model using the training data to classify patients into different diagnostic categories.
4. Diagnostic Accuracy Assessment:
    - Evaluate the SVM model's diagnostic accuracy using the testing data.
5. Resource Allocation and Optimization:
    - Identify patients at high risk of misdiagnosis using the SVM model.
    - Allocate resources such as specialized tests, consultations, and interventions to high-risk patients.
    - Prioritize patients based on SVM predictions, reducing unnecessary tests and interventions for low-risk patients.
6. Monitoring and Adaptation:
    - Continuously monitor the performance of the SVM-based diagnosis in real-world healthcare settings.
    - Gather feedback from healthcare professionals and patients to fine-tune the SVM model.
7. Performance Evaluation:
    - Measure and analyze the impact of SVM-based diagnosis on resource allocation, cost savings, and patient outcomes.
8. Iterative Improvement:

- Refine the SVM model based on real-world data and ongoing evaluations.
- Incorporate feedback to improve the accuracy of diagnosis and resource optimization.

9. Benefits and Impact:
   - Observe improved resource utilization, reduced healthcare expenditures, and optimized healthcare system performance.
   - Enhanced patient care and outcomes due to personalized and accurate diagnosis.
10. Conclusion:
    - Conclude that SVM-based diagnosis contributes to resource optimization and improved healthcare system performance by efficiently allocating resources, reducing unnecessary procedures, and enhancing patient outcomes.

This algorithm outlines how SVM-based diagnosis can contribute to resource optimization and improved healthcare system performance by accurately diagnosing patients and effectively allocating resources based on diagnostic predictions.

8.3 Optimized Resource Allocation and Healthcare System Performance

The implementation of SVM-based diagnosis aligns with the broader goal of optimizing resource allocation within healthcare systems. Accurate diagnoses through SVM reduce the strain on medical resources by ensuring that patients receive the appropriate care and interventions from the outset. This optimized resource allocation leads to more efficient utilization of medical facilities, healthcare personnel, and diagnostic technologies.

As SVM-based diagnosis becomes an integral part of clinical practice, healthcare systems can experience improved overall performance. Timely and precise diagnoses lead to better patient outcomes, shorter hospital stays, and lower readmission rates. This, in turn, translates to improved healthcare system efficiency, reduced overcrowding, and enhanced patient throughput.

A Transformative Paradigm

The economic implications of SVM-based diagnosis extend beyond immediate cost savings. By streamlining diagnostics, reducing misdiagnosis rates, and optimizing resource allocation, SVM contributes to a more sustainable and resilient healthcare ecosystem. As healthcare systems grapple with the challenges of resource scarcity and increasing demand, the integration of innovative approaches like SVM-based diagnosis offers a transformative paradigm, fostering a future where accurate diagnoses and effective patient care intersect seamlessly with cost-conscious healthcare practices.

9. FUTURE OUTLOOK AND RESEARCH DIRECTIONS

As we journey further into the realm of applying Support Vector Machine (SVM) for Parkinson's Disease differentiation, the road ahead is illuminated with exciting possibilities and avenues for exploration. This final section outlines the potential future directions and research endeavours that hold the promise of enhancing SVM-based diagnosis, addressing ethical considerations, and solidifying its real-world impact.

9.1 Advancements in SVM Models for Parkinson's Disease Differentiation

Thanks to developments in machine learning methods, data collection, and computing capacity, SVM models for Parkinson's disease differentiation are expected to continue evolving. It is anticipated that scientists will investigate new approaches to improve the diagnostic precision of SVM by the incorporation of multimodal data sources, including patient-reported outcomes, wearable sensors, and electronic health records. A key area of research will be fine-tuning SVM models to take into consideration the variability of Parkinson's disease presentations across various patient demographics and disease stages.

Additionally, the performance of SVM may be improved by incorporating hybrid models and deep learning approaches. By removing intricate characteristics from time-series data and neuroimaging data, deep learning architectures like convolutional neural networks (CNNs) and recurrent neural networks (RNNs) may be used in addition to SVM. The combination of these cutting-edge methods may be able to increase diagnostic robustness and precision to unprecedented heights.

9.2 Ethical Frameworks for Machine Learning in Medical Diagnosis

The ethical considerations surrounding machine learning in medical diagnosis, including SVM-based approaches, will remain a dynamic area of research. The development of comprehensive ethical frameworks and guidelines will be crucial to navigate issues related to patient data privacy, informed consent, bias mitigation, and interpretability of models. Research efforts will focus on devising innovative solutions that strike a balance between harnessing the power of SVM for accurate diagnosis while upholding the principles of patient autonomy, transparency, and fairness.

Collaboration between interdisciplinary teams comprising medical professionals, ethicists, legal experts, and technologists will drive the formulation of robust ethical frameworks. These frameworks will guide the responsible deployment of SVM-based diagnosis within clinical practice and pave the way for broader societal acceptance of machine learning applications in healthcare.

Algorithm 8. Multimodal SVM with Deep Learning (MSDL)

Input:

- Clinical Data (features from patient records)
- Neuroimaging Data (neuroimaging features)
- Genetic Information (genetic features)
- Labels (0 for one condition, 1 for another condition)

Output:

- Trained SVM model

1. Preprocess Data:
   1.1 Normalize and standardize clinical data, neuroimaging data, and genetic information.
   1.2 Handle missing values using appropriate techniques (e.g., imputation).
   1.3 Combine different data modalities into a single feature matrix.
2. Feature Engineering:
   2.1 Apply feature selection techniques to identify relevant features.
   2.2 Utilize deep learning techniques for automatic feature extraction (e.g., convolutional layers for images, and recurrent layers for sequences).
   2.3 Combine learned features with selected features from step 2.1.
3. Model Training:
   3.1 Split the dataset into training and testing sets.
   3.2 Train an SVM classifier on the combined feature matrix using the training data.
   3.3 Optimize SVM hyperparameters using cross-validation.
4. Model Evaluation:
   4.1 Evaluate the SVM model on the testing data.

4.2 Calculate performance metrics such as accuracy, precision, recall, and F1-score.

4.3 Visualize the SVM decision boundaries in the combined feature space.

5. Integration with Clinical Practice:

   5.1 Deploy the trained SVM model in clinical settings.

   5.2 Collect new patient data, including clinical, neuroimaging, and genetic features.

   5.3 Preprocess and extract features from new patient data.

   5.4 Use the trained SVM model to predict the patient's condition.

   5.5 Provide decision support to healthcare professionals for diagnosis and treatment.

6. Ethical Considerations:

   6.1 Ensure patient data privacy and compliance with ethical guidelines.

   6.2 Obtain informed consent for data usage.

   6.3 Ensure transparency and interpretability of the model's predictions.

7. Future Research Directions:

   7.1 Explore additional data modalities for improved accuracy.

   7.2 Investigate novel deep learning architectures for feature extraction.

   7.3 Conduct longitudinal studies to assess long-term model performance.

8. End.

This pseudocode Algorithm 8 outlines the general steps and concepts for a hypothetical Multimodal SVM with Deep Learning (MSDL) model. The implementation details may vary based on the specific deep learning techniques, SVM libraries, and data pre-processing methods.

9.3 Longitudinal Studies and Real-world Impact Assessment

The true impact of SVM-based diagnosis on Parkinson's Disease management will be discerned through rigorous longitudinal studies and real-world impact assessments. Long-term studies tracking patients' journeys, treatment responses, and disease progression can provide valuable insights into the sustained benefits of SVM-guided interventions. These studies can elucidate how SVM-based diagnosis influences disease outcomes, patient adherence to treatment plans, and the overall trajectory of Parkinson's Disease.

Furthermore, real-world impact assessment can shed light on the economic implications of SVM-based diagnosis over extended periods. By quantifying the cost savings, resource optimization, and improvements in patient care attributable to SVM, researchers can offer evidence-based insights that influence healthcare policies, reimbursement models, and resource allocation strategies.

Pioneering a New Era in Diagnosis and Care

The future outlook for SVM-based diagnosis in Parkinson's Disease differentiation is marked by continuous innovation, ethical deliberation, and evidence-driven impact assessment. As researchers refine SVM models, develop ethical frameworks, and conduct comprehensive studies, they pioneer a new era in medical diagnosis and patient care. SVM's potential to enhance accuracy, personalize treatments, and optimize healthcare resources stands as a testament to the transformative power of machine learning in shaping the future of healthcare delivery.

Figure 7. Integration of Advances Support Vector Machine

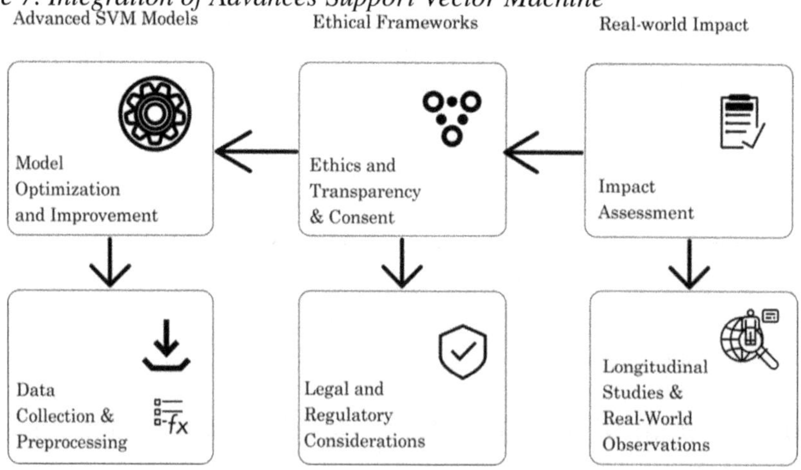

This diagram Figure .7 visually represents the integration of advanced Support Vector Machine (SVM) models, ethical frameworks, and real-world impact assessment in future research. The diagram shows how these components interact and influence each other to drive the development of accurate and ethical SVM-based diagnosis while assessing its real-world impact.

10. CONCLUSION

In the journey to enhance Parkinson's Disease diagnosis and management, the integration of Support Vector Machine (SVM) offers a profound leap forward. This concluding section encapsulates the key insights presented throughout this chapter, emphasizing the contributions of SVM-based diagnosis, envisioning its future integration, and offering closing remarks on its transformative potential.

10.1 Summary of Key Points

Throughout this chapter, we embarked on an exploration of SVM-based diagnosis for Parkinson's Disease differentiation. We delved into the diagnostic challenges posed by overlapping symptoms, highlighted the power of SVM in classification, and navigated ethical considerations in integrating machine learning into medical practice. We explored the potential benefits of enhanced accuracy, personalized treatments, and improved patient care. Challenges were acknowledged, from data quality to model generalization, and strategies for mitigation were unveiled. The economic implications of SVM-based diagnosis showcased its potential to streamline diagnostics, reduce healthcare expenditures, and optimize resource allocation.

10.2 Contributions to Parkinson's Disease Diagnosis and Management

The integration of SVM-based diagnosis contributes significantly to the advancement of Parkinson's Disease diagnosis and management. It addresses the pressing need for accurate differentiation, reducing misdiagnosis rates and offering healthcare professionals data-driven insights for informed treatment decisions. The potential for personalized interventions elevates patient care and quality of life. By harnessing SVM's capabilities, medical practice is poised to revolutionize the diagnostic landscape, positioning itself at the forefront of precision medicine.

10.3 Vision for the Future: Integration of SVM-based Diagnosis

The future holds a compelling vision where SVM-based diagnosis seamlessly intertwines with clinical practice. Advanced SVM models, guided by ethical frameworks, will empower healthcare providers with accurate, efficient, and patient-centric diagnostic tools. Longitudinal studies will illuminate the sustained impact of SVM-based interventions, while economic assessments will underscore its role in shaping cost-effective and sustainable healthcare systems. The integration of

SVM-based diagnosis into routine clinical workflows will pave the way for a new era of healthcare, where technology and patient care converge harmoniously.

10.4 Closing Remarks

As we conclude this chapter, we stand at the cusp of a transformative era in medical diagnosis and patient care. The marriage of machine learning, specifically SVM, with Parkinson's Disease differentiation is poised to propel healthcare into an unprecedented era of precision, efficiency, and empathy. While challenges persist, the collective efforts of medical practitioners, researchers, and technologists hold the potential to surmount these obstacles and usher in a future where SVM-based diagnosis not only distinguishes Parkinson's Disease but also heralds a broader transformation in healthcare delivery. With its power to enhance diagnostic accuracy, tailor treatments, and optimize resources, SVM-based diagnosis offers a beacon of hope for patients, healthcare professionals, and societies at large. It is through these collaborative endeavours that we move closer to realizing the full potential of SVM and its impact on the lives of individuals affected by Parkinson's Disease.

REFERENCES

Botzel, K., Tronnier, V., & Gasser, T. (2014, March 28). The differential diagnosis and treatment of tremor. *Deutsches Ärzteblatt International, 111*(13), 225–235. DOI: 10.3238/arztebl.2014.0225 PMID: 24739887

Devarajan, J. P., Sreedharan, V. R., & Narayanamurthy, G. (2021). Decision making in health care diagnosis: Evidence from Parkinson's disease via hybrid machine learning. *IEEE Transactions on Engineering Management, 70*(8), 2719–2731.

Dickson, D. W. (2012). Parkinson's disease and parkinsonism: Neuropathology. *Cold Spring Harbor Perspectives in Medicine, 2*(8), a009258. PMID: 22908195

Haller, S., Badoud, S., Nguyen, D., Barnaure, I., Montandon, M.-L., Lovblad, K.-O., & Burkhard, P. R. (2013). Differentiation between Parkinson disease and other forms of Parkinsonism using support vector machine analysis of susceptibility-weighted imaging (SWI): Initial results. *European Radiology, 23*(12), 12–19. DOI: 10.1007/s00330-012-2579-y PMID: 22797981

Kim, B., Park, J., & Suh, J. (2020). Transparency and accountability in AI decision support: Explaining and visualizing convolutional neural networks for text information. *Decision Support Systems, 134*, 113302. DOI: 10.1016/j.dss.2020.113302

Latif, J., Xiao, C., Tu, S., Rehman, S. U., Imran, A., & Bilal, A. (2020). Implementation and use of disease diagnosis systems for electronic medical records based on machine learning: A complete review. *IEEE Access : Practical Innovations, Open Solutions, 8*, 150489–150513.

Li, T., & Le, W. (2020). Biomarkers for Parkinson's disease: How good are they? *Neuroscience Bulletin, 36*(2), 183–194. PMID: 31646434

Loyola-Gonzalez, O. (2019). Black-box vs. white-box: Understanding their advantages and weaknesses from a practical point of view. *IEEE Access : Practical Innovations, Open Solutions, 7*, 154096–154113.

Myszczynska, M. A., Ojamies, P. N., Lacoste, A. M., Neil, D., Saffari, A., Mead, R., & Ferraiuolo, L. (2020). Applications of machine learning to diagnosis and treatment of neurodegenerative diseases. *Nature Reviews. Neurology, 16*(8), 440–456. PMID: 32669685

Palumbo, B., Bianconi, F., Nuvoli, S., Spanu, A., & Fravolini, M. L. (2021). Artificial intelligence techniques support nuclear medicine modalities to improve the diagnosis of Parkinson's disease and Parkinsonian syndromes. *Clinical and Translational Imaging, 9*, 19–35.

Shin, H. W., Hong, S. W., & Youn, Y. C. (2022). Clinical aspects of the differential diagnosis of Parkinson's disease and parkinsonism. *Journal of Clinical Neurology (Seoul, Korea)*, *18*(3), 259. PMID: 35589315

Tolosa, E., Garrido, A., Scholz, S. W., & Poewe, W. (2021). Challenges in the diagnosis of Parkinson's disease. *Lancet Neurology*, *20*(5), 385–397. PMID: 33894193

Chapter 3
Retracted Enabling Computational Intelligence in Healthcare Using Internet of Things (IoT), Machine Learning, and Fog Computing

A. Aruna

https://orcid.org/0000-0002-4756-6760

Sri Ramachandra Faculty of Engineering and Technology, SRIHER, India

A. Sathya

https://orcid.org/0000-0001-9930-0836

Sri Ramachandra Faculty of Engineering and Technology, SRIHER, India

ABSTRACT

The emergence in the development of sensory equipment endorses the expansion of the Internet of Things (IoT) across the globe. The usage of diversified applications and IoT devices generates massive sensor data which in turn need analytics or intelligent processing system. IoT, Machine Learning, and Fog Computing are utilized to achieve healthcare assistance and diagnosis progression in diverse aspects, Machine Learning is a kind of data analysis technique that retrieves the needed information without performing any explicit program. This chapter focuses on two diverse paradigms such as machine learning and fog computing which concern the processing and analysis of sensor data. The taxonomy of Machine Learning algorithms, significant aspects of Machine Learning in IoT data analytics and applications of Machine Learning based IoT techniques are elaborated. This chapter

DOI: 10.4018/979-8-3693-3864-3.ch003

also elucidates fog computing and its tiered computing architecture for healthcare. The major issues and the future research directions of IoT Data analysis are also explained in this chapter.

INTRODUCTION

The evolution of IoT started with ARPANET (Advanced Research Project Agency Network) as it established connection between two different universities. The term IoT was coined by Kevon Asthon who was the employee of Proctor – Gamble. A 30 years old scientist then became a CEO of Auto ID center at Massachusetts Institute of Technology and set the global standard for RFID (Radio Frequency Identification) and wireless systems. He believed and defined "Today Computers – and therefore, Internet – are almost wholly dependent on human beings for information" (Mallik, P. 2021).

As he mentioned, earlier days all the data available on the internet was created by humans in different ways such as recording audio, video messages, typing and loading the documents into the web. Nowadays people have less time and attention to manually presenting information to the internet. If our computer knows things more than information, it can collect and store the data to internet (Balouch, et al., 2022). This will reduce time, cost, and manual efforts. Hence the evolution of IoT can take these technology advancements to another level just as the Internet did few decades back.

Figure 1. The Internet of Things (IoT)

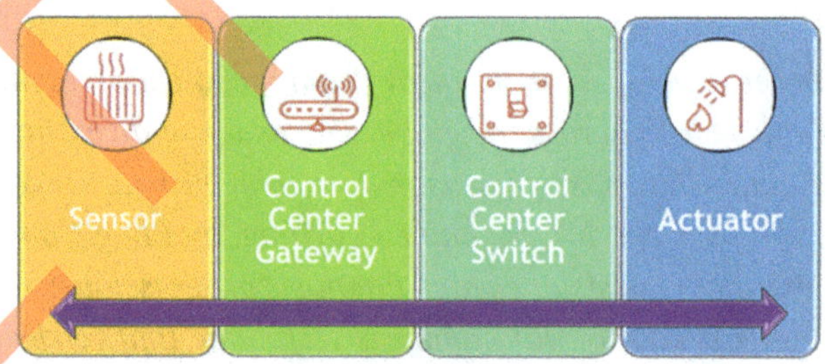

The main factor about IoT is connected devices and things, where all the devices are interconnected with one another over the network to evolve intelligent and smart applications, which helps human in automation and reducing their manual efforts. So, any devices can be connected anywhere at any time for any domains. The sample IoT interconnection is shown in Figure 1. Previous research studies have reported that the connected devices in world will make greater in size as thirty times between 2009 and 2023. So, by 2023 there will be billion thigs that may be connected to the internet. The working nature of the IoT is given as a reference architecture and is shown in Figure 2.

Figure 2. IoT architecture

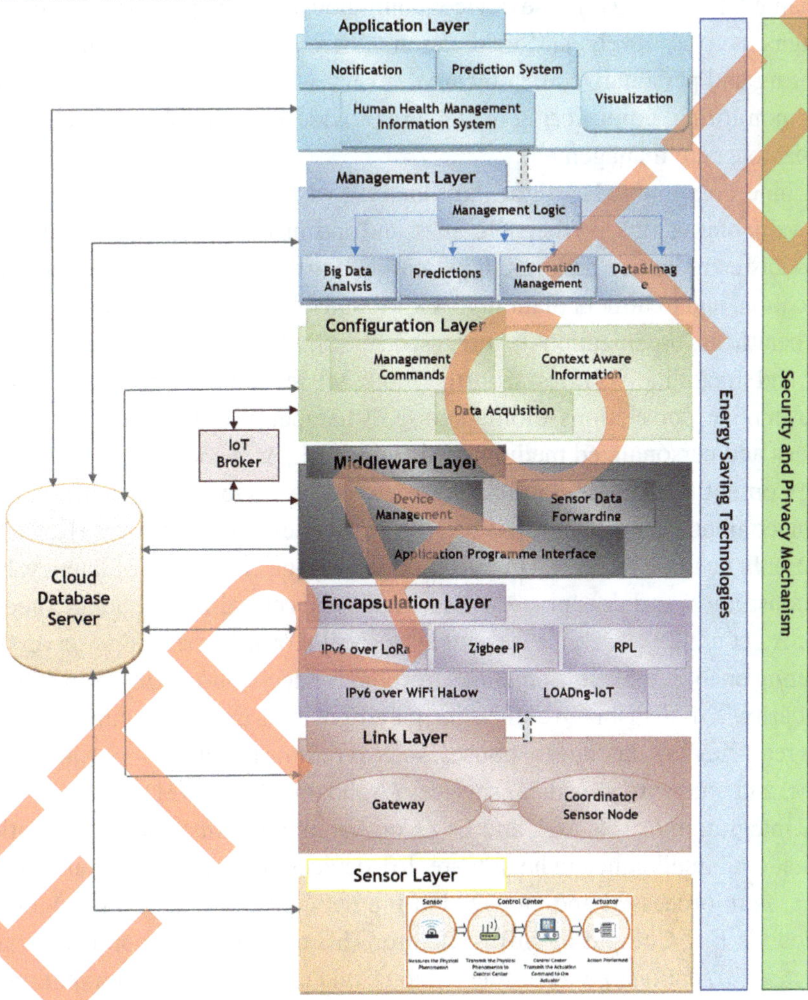

In recent years, the convergence of advanced technologies has revolutionized various sectors, with healthcare being no exception. The integration of Internet of Things (IoT), Machine Learning (ML), and Fog Computing has paved the way for a new era of computational intelligence in healthcare (Sagu, A., & Gill, N. S. 2020). This synergy holds immense promise in enhancing patient care, optimizing operational efficiencies, and advancing medical research. This chapter explores into the complicated web possibilities offered by integrating these technologies in the healthcare domain.

The IoT ecosystem encompasses interconnected devices capable of collecting, transmitting, and exchanging data over the internet. In healthcare, IoT devices range from wearable fitness trackers to sophisticated medical implants (Mohamed, K. S., & Mohamed, K. S. 2022). These devices continuously gather patient data, including vital signs, activity levels, and medication adherence, thereby enabling real-time monitoring and personalized healthcare delivery. Moreover, IoT facilitates remote patient monitoring, empowering healthcare providers to offer timely interventions and proactive care management.

Machine Learning (ML) algorithms analyze vast volumes of healthcare data to extract valuable insights, predict outcomes, and optimize decision-making processes. ML models can identify patterns in patient data to support clinical diagnosis, risk stratification, and treatment planning. Additionally, ML-driven predictive analytics enable healthcare organizations to forecast disease outbreaks, allocate resources efficiently, and streamline workflows. Furthermore, ML techniques empower researchers to uncover novel correlations, biomarkers, and therapeutic targets, accelerating drug discovery and personalized medicine (Mazalica, M., & Ivetic, D. 2021).

Fog Computing extends cloud computing capabilities to the edge of the network, bringing computational resources closer to IoT devices and end-users (Kashani, et al., 2021). In healthcare, Fog Computing addresses the challenges of latency, bandwidth constraints, and data privacy associated with centralized cloud architectures (Rejeb, A., et al., 2023). By processing data locally or in nearby edge servers, Fog Computing enables real-time analytics, responsive decision-making, and enhanced data security. This distributed computing paradigm is particularly valuable for applications requiring low-latency responses, such as remote patient monitoring, surgical robotics, and emergency medical services (Aghdam, et al., 2021).

The integration of IoT, ML, and Fog Computing unleashes the full potential of computational intelligence in healthcare. IoT devices generate vast streams of data, which are pre-processed and analyzed at the network edge using ML algorithms deployed via Fog Computing infrastructure. This decentralized approach enables timely insights, actionable recommendations, and context-aware interventions, ultimately improving patient outcomes, optimizing resource utilization, and driving healthcare innovation (Selvaraj, S., & Sundaravaradhan, S. 2020). The convergence of IoT, ML, and Fog Computing represents a transformative force in healthcare, empowering stakeholders to harness the power of data-driven decision-making, predictive analytics, and real-time interventions. By embracing computational intelligence, the healthcare industry can embark on a journey towards personalized, proactive, and sustainable healthcare delivery (Bharadwaj, et al., 2021).

The necessity of a processing system relies on the application's nature (Verdejo Espinosa, et al., 2021). The emergence of population and diseases has necessitated computational intelligence. The data generated from varied potential source is supplied to the machine learning system which creates useful insight. Through the generated significant insight further decision construction process is initiated (Farahani, et al., 2020). Fog computing is another substantial paradigm that alternates the data processing unit of IoT (Ray, et al., 2020). It pertains to the edge of the network that encompasses effective processing power, the devices are potential cloud resource utilisers, thus minimising the latency for IoT applications. This chapter focuses on two diverse paradigms such as machine learning and fog computing which concern the processing and analysis of sensor data. The taxonomy of Machine Learning algorithms, significant aspects of Machine Learning in IoT data analytics and applications of Machine Learning based IoT techniques are elaborated (Pradhan, et al., 2021).

IOT IN HEALTHCARE

The healthcare industry has grown dramatically in the last several years, leading to a notable rise in employment and income. A hospital physical examination was necessary a few years ago in order to identify illnesses and other irregularities in the human body. Most patients had to stay hospitalized while receiving treatment (Dash, S. P. (2020). It has driven up healthcare costs and placed strain on isolated and rural healthcare institutions. Thanks to technological advancements throughout time, a variety of illnesses may now be diagnosed and health can be monitored with the use of tiny devices such as smartwatches (Lakshmi, et al., 2021).

In addition, technological advancements have shifted the focus of the healthcare system from hospitals to individuals in need of medical attention (Nasser, et al., 2021). Clinical assessments, such as monitoring blood pressure, blood sugar, and oxygen saturation (SpO2), may be performed independently of a healthcare physician in the comfort of the individual's place (Yang, et al., 2021). Additionally, modern telecommunications technology allows for the transfer of clinical data from off-site sites to hospitals and clinics (Selvaraj, S., & Sundaravaradhan, S. 2020). Access to medical treatment is easier than ever before because of the developments in communication networks and quickly developing technologies like machine learning, big data analysis, the Internet of Things (IoT), wireless sensing, mobile computing, and the cloud (Butpheng, et al., 2020).

One cannot deny the profound impact the Internet has had on people's everyday lives and the efficiency of organizations (Kashyap, et al., 2022). Access to previously inaccessible data and services has been greatly facilitated by the widespread availability of the Internet, which serves as a dependable communication middleware that enables the interconnection of unrelated hardware and software components. The Internet of Things (IoT), the most recent Information and Communications Technology (ICT), aims to increase convenience by making that the objects around people and businesses are reachable and responsive to their needs. This convenience can be seen in a smart home, where items like white appliances work on behalf of the residents (Sarrab, M., & Alshohoumi, F. (2021).

The perceptual, network, and application layers make up the IoT's three-tiered architecture, where these developments are housed (Awaisi, et al., 2020). For seamless pervasive computing, the Internet of Things (IoT) consists of three main components, one of which may be present in each layer. There are two main parts to a data analytics system:

- The hardware, which comprises data sources (such as sensors and actuators),
- The middleware, which enables on-demand processing and storage. This covers a broad variety of data processing methods that may meet IoT needs (such as fog and cloud computing, for example).
- Data visualisation and analysis utilising intuitive, cross-platform tools that may be modified for unique applications.

BUILDING BLOCKS OF INTERNET-ENABLED SMART HEALTHCARE

Identity, geolocation, sensing, and connection are the four basic components on which healthcare systems are designed (Quy, et al., 2022). Several approaches are used to IoT - based smart healthcare, such as 24/7 emergency services, remote monitoring, wearable technology, networking technologies, and big data. When it comes down to it, all it takes for a healthcare system to be considered "improved" is a piece of technology that helps doctors treat patients and improves their quality of life. Electronic health (e-health) comprises a wide range of technologies, including EHR software, smart home service platforms, and intelligent and medically related gadgets. Sensors, smart devices, and expert systems aid in the healthcare practise of a smart healthcare system (Nandankar, et al., 2021).

Data Processing Stages of IoT

The four steps in the IoT architecture can be thought of as stages in a process. When information is acquired or processed in one step, it may be used in the subsequent stages. Integrating values into the process results in intuitions and offers exciting commercial opportunities. The stages of IoT is given in Figure 3.

Step 1: The first stage is the deployment of networked gadgets like sensors, actuators, displays, detectors, video systems, and so on. These gadgets gather the information.

Step 2: Analog data typically obtained from sensors and other devices must be combined and transformed to digital data in order to be processed further.

Step 3: After the data has been digitised and aggregated, it undergoes pre-processing to ensure uniformity before being uploaded to a data centre or the Cloud.

Step 4: In step four, the collected data is maintained and analysed appropriately. When advanced analytics are used on this data, it produces useful business insights for sound decision-making.

Figure 3. The four stages of IoT solutions

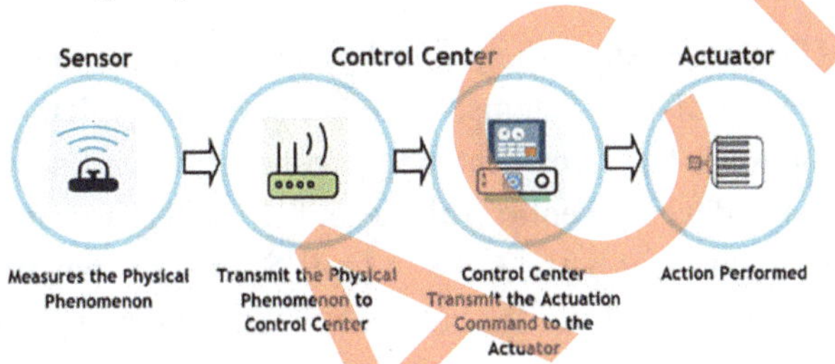

Advantages of IoT in Healthcare

IoT in healthcare offers several key benefits, including:

- Cost reduction: Real-time monitoring of patients is made feasible by IoT, cutting down on unnecessary medical visits, hospitalizations, and re-admissions.
- Better Treatment: It gives complete openness and empowers doctors to make decisions based on evidence.
- Faster disease diagnosis: The ability to detect illnesses at an early stage based on symptoms is made feasible by continuous patient monitoring and real-time data.
- Proactive Medical Treatment: By collecting information on a patient's vitals throughout time, doctors may provide preventative treatment.

- Management of Medications and Medical Equipment: Managing drugs and medical equipment is a significant concern in the healthcare sector. These are efficiently handled and used at lower costs thanks to connected devices.
- Error Reduction: Healthcare organisations may benefit greatly from the data generated by IoT devices since it ensures error-free, efficient, and cost-effective operations.

Challenges in IoT

The Internet of Things enables a plethora of novel capabilities and possibilities for both enterprises (such as the smart healthcare industry) and consumers (Chi, et al., 2023). However, the Internet of Things lacks a number of technologies, architectural standards, and ideas that may bring the digital and physical worlds together. The following is a summary of the primary IoT difficulty issues:

- Standard Challenge: Since the IoT lacks clear standards to guide interactions and the creation of IoT-systems, there are several problems with managing and developing IoT-systems, including connection and security. Standards will enable the development of IoT systems to adhere to some basic requirements that might meet both QoS and QoP. Standards may play a significant part in the formation of the IoT. In general, standards ought to be freely accessible to the public.
- Data Management: A massive quantity of data is being produced by Internet of Things sensors and applications every millisecond, requiring immediate action to keep up with storage and processing demands. Incorporating the more static discrete data with the constantly updated raw data from digital sensors, these data enter the big data era. Sensors in industry and the environment provide information such as location, velocity, temperature, humidity, and so on. The heterogeneity of IoT data makes it difficult to handle using the current architecture and network topology of data centres.
- Architecture Design: Identifying, managing, and standardising the Internet of Things network and architecture is difficult because it encompasses so many different technologies, communication protocols, and heterogeneous devices. Integrating data across IoT use cases is difficult, but should be possible with modular, interoperable components. Having systems that can:
    - Collect data from several sources,
    - Extract and analyse significant aspects and correlations in the data, and
    - Ease decision-making is essential for constructing an IoT infrastructure. Therefore, not all IoT systems or applications can be designed using the same architecture. The necessity for heterogeneous IoT designs is

thus highlighted; these shouldn't be tied down to just one solution; they should be flexible enough to adapt to new situations as they arise, while yet adhering to established IoT standards.

- Technical Difficulties: Complex technological problems in networking protocols and items design can be brought on by IoT technology (Das, et al., 2022). Many factors must be considered in the design of things before they can get widespread acceptance, but there are two that must be met before anything-device can be made:
    - o Both active and passive power consumption are very low, and
    - o Production and distribution costs are kept to a minimum. The bandwidth of an IoT device may be anything from a few hundred kilobits per second (kbps) to several megabits per second (mbps) for detecting anything from the most basic raw data to the recording of a live video feed, hence it is important that devices be as bandwidth-efficient as possible. In terms of networking protocols, these should be easy to use and fax, but more significantly, they should be inexpensive and offer dependable communication.
- Security and Privacy: The vast volume of security-critical data and privacy-sensitive data that IoT devices generate and communicate makes them attractive targets for various assaults. Cyberattacks on IoT devices are extremely dangerous since they could result in property damage or even endanger human life. According to a recent analysis by HP Inc., the majority of the most popular IoT devices have substantial attack vulnerabilities. Since embedded systems often need to include a broad range of security features and safety functions, the design and implementation of safe, secure embedded systems face new obstacles. The security and privacy of current Internet of Things (IoT) applications are at danger since they have not been adequately developed to meet all necessary security standards. A comprehensive cybersecurity architecture will be needed to defend against and prevent IoT assaults. This architecture should accommodate the whole range of heterogeneous IoT abstraction layers, including those that span different platforms.

CLOUD COMPUTING

"Cloud computing" is defined by the National Institute of Standards and Technology (NIST) as a blueprint for quickly deploying a shared pool of reconfigurable computing resources (such as servers, networks, storage, apps, and services) with little management work or service provider interaction. Through the combination of tried-and-true technologies like virtualization, grid computing, and utility-based pricing, cloud computing assists organizations in realizing their goals (Tharini, V. J., & Shivakumar, B. L. 2023). Cloud computing may be broken down into three service models, four deployment methods, and five defining characteristics (Ahanger, et al., 2022). The following are the top five aspects of clouds:

- On-demand self-service: It enables customers to autonomously set up computer services that could automatically need server space and network storage. Without the assistance of a service provider's human interaction.
- Network access: It supplied services and functions are accessible through standardised mechanisms that encourage and permit the usage of a variety of client platforms.
- Shared use of resources: Large numbers of users may access the provider's services thanks to the pooling of the provider's computer and storage resources. This is accomplished through the use of a multi-tenant model, in which different types of resources (both physical and virtual) are assigned and reallocated in response to fluctuations in demand. Despite the fact that the consumer often has no insight into or control over the precise location of the resources they get, they may be able to define location at a more general level.
- Quick adaptability: It's possible to rapidly expand or contract resources based on demand by using automated provisioning and release of capabilities. Metered service: Utilizing a metering capability at an abstraction level befitting the kind of service being delivered, cloud computing systems mechanically control and optimise resource utilisation (e.g., storage, processing and bandwidth). It is possible to keep tabs on, manage, and account for resource allocation. Consequently, transparency is provided for the service's user and provider.

FOG COMPUTING

The advent of the wireless communication system has witnessed the growth of the Internet of Things (IoT) and it is widely used in various fields especially in healthcare. The automation and effectiveness of work in healthcare is accomplished by IoT. The data generated by IoT device faces certain complexities in timely decision making and processing. The weakness of the system is rectified by the emerging paradigm called fog computing (Bhatia, M., & Kumari, S. 2022). It facilitates the edge devices to accomplish the substantial amount of data storage, communication and computation locally and the processed data is routed over the backbone of internet. Fog computing is established by deploying the fog nodes all over the network. Devices from routers, controllers, switches and video cameras act as a fog nodes that is deployed in the target regions namely offices, vehicles and other needed locations. It is a collaborative framework that uses the near user or user clients edge devices to process the data.

The term "fog computing," which is synonymous with "fog networking" and "fogging," refers to a highly virtualized platform that serves as a conduit for delivering network and application services at the network's edge, where IoT devices often reside. Between objects and cloud layers, fog nodes serve as middleware (Mukherjee, et al., 2021). Fog computing, which is analogous to the cloud but runs on a smaller scale, provides a wide variety of application services, including data processing and analysis. Simply said, owing to proximity, fog is anticipated to perform these services more swiftly, securely, and reliably than clouds are.

The fog layer consists of widely dispersed fog nodes that are placed near the network's edge. By contributing its processing power, storage capacity, and network communication capabilities, each fog node may serve as an intermediary between the cloud and the IoT network's devices. Since it requires less bandwidth and reduces processing and transmission times, fog computing is a useful supplement to cloud computing rather than a replacement. Fog computing is a technique for enhancing the cloud's storage, networking, and processing capabilities by moving these elements closer to the network's end-devices (Kishor, et al., 2021).

In IoT-based healthcare scenario, fog computing has been modified to interact with various sensors and actuators, including cameras, wearables, and environment sensors. Fogs utilise wireless communication connectivity interfaces to interact directly with objects to collect data on the thing side (e.g., Zigbee, LoRa). However, the cloud's many capabilities and services may be used when fogs are associated with them The fog nodes have the option of operating independently or jointly with the cloud node. Fog nodes have their own computational power resources and data services capabilities, making them capable of providing predefined/dedicated services without any help from the cloud (including data processing and aggregations).

Fog nodes, for example, may independently monitor and analyse data from pressure sensors, adjusting the state of connected valves in response to the sensor's reading. Fog, in contrast to the cloud, has more constrained hardware capabilities, which makes it more susceptible to congestion when data traffic is heavy and surpasses fog capacity. To complete the duties, it may therefore require the cooperation of the cloud or the fog. It is evident that when service traffic on fog nodes increases, there is a strong likelihood that fresh arriving service requests will have to wait, resulting in latency. The capacity of the fog nodes and how they manage their resources are related to the volume of traffic; hence, the lower the latency, the better the fog resource management (Verma, et al., 2022).

Despite the alluring advantages of fog computing, various worries are preventing its widespread use. Among these are the specifics of Fog-2-Fog (F2F) cooperation and Cloud-2-Fog (C2F) collaboration. Since fog is being introduced to solve the problem of mobility and latency for delay-sensitive applications, the bulk of difficulties inside the fog layer fall under the QoS and QoE categories (e.g., latency reduction, mobility, and privacy) (e.g., service experience). In this thesis, the term "service latency" refers to the whole length of time required to supply a service, including the time it takes for an Internet of Things device to send and receive a request for that service. Both the processing time and the travel time are included in this.

CLOUD VS FOG COMPUTING IN IOT

The cloud's success as a globally dispersed form of company operation since the year 2000 may be attributed to its scalability and flexibility. Data centre models are distinct from their forerunners (grid and cluster) in many key respects, including architecture, networking, and middleware, and they also improve upon their predecessors by centralising hardware and software resources in centralised server farms. Using a pay-as-you-go basis, cloud data centres provide computing, storage, and networking resources to companies as a fifth utility (after water, electricity, gas, and telephony). Therefore, expenses related to operations, purchases, and maintenance are reduced.

Companies are also not informed of the technological difficulties associated with cloud management. Although there are many uses for cloud computing, not all applications, especially those based on the Internet of Things (IoT), can take use of it. Because

- Cloud hosting adds significant latency due to network connections to data centers and
- Cloud hosting increases the risk of attack due to the increased number of hops and nodes between end users and data centers, applications that rely on low latency or data privacy cannot be hosted there.

The cloud's inapplicability also stems from the fact that it is centrally located, which increases both communication costs and energy consumption. A combination of the introduction of fog and the explosion of the Internet of Things has made it a popular issue lately. In 2014, Cisco Systems generalised a revolutionary ICT-based operating model it had originally designed in which computing, storage, and networking resources are placed near to where data is collected and/or located. Due of their subtle parallels and variances, the transition from cloud to fog is not simple.

Cisco offers Table 1 to show how the features of specific apps will be handled differently by cloud and fog. Real-time apps, for instance, would not use the cloud as a model of operation since they require practically immediate action and great data protection. Instead, compared to the cloud, fog would provide superior support for mobile applications (Kishor, et al., 2021). However, this operational paradigm cannot be maintained indefinitely due to the high frequency and low latency of communication between these devices.

Table 1. Appropriateness of cloud/fog to respond to system's characteristics

Characteristics	Cloud	Fog
Latency	High	Low
Location awareness	No	Yes
Location of service	Within the Internet	At network edge
Distance client to server	Multiple hops	One hop
Delay jitter	High	Low
Geo-distribution	Centralized	Distributed
No. of server nodes	Few	Very large
Support for mobility	Limited	Supported
Real-time interaction	Supported	Supported
Last-mile connectivity type	Leased lines	Wireless
Security	Undefined	Can be defined
Attack on the enroute	High probability	Very low probability

By processing data closer to its source, fog saves the cloud by reducing network traffic and enhancing both quality-of-service (QoS) and quality-of-experience (QoE). Additional information on cloud versus fog as an application operating model is also provided in Table 2.

Table 2. Analysis of Cloud versus Fog

Cloud	Fog
Processing and running data and applications on the cloud takes time, especially when dealing with substantial amounts of data.	Processing and running data and applications on the scattered network edges consume less time, especially when dealing with substantial amounts of data.
Extremely high requirements for bandwidth because of the need of transmitting all data	Comparatively less requirements for bandwidth because access points are so close to the data.
Problems with scalability and delayed responses stem from the cloud's geographically dispersed server infrastructure.	The proximity of the edge servers offers the potential for improved response time and scalability.

CHALLENGES OF CLOUD AND FOG IN IOT

The integration of cloud and fog computing in IoT faces scalability, latency, and privacy challenges. Cloud scalability strains under the influx of IoT data, while fog computing addresses real-time processing needs (Hanumantharaju, et al., 2022). Privacy concerns persist due to centralized data storage, urging innovative solutions for efficient and secure IoT management.

Cloud Challenges in IoT

Several advantages can be obtained from combining cloud computing and IoT, and it can also encourage the growth and development of several IoT-systems. The cloud may help with remote management of IoT devices (such as sensors), and the data they produce can be shared with anyone, anywhere. When it comes to complex IoT systems like medical monitoring, cloud computing may run into a variety of issues. The two primary, persistently difficult problems with cloud computing in the IoT are as follows:

- Proximity: In today's cloud networking model, data is stored and accessed from a small number of very powerful centralised servers located all over the globe. Additionally, a central control system serves as the foundation for traditional traffic management. This puts a lot of strain on the traffic management system and delays responses significantly. For delay-sensitive Internet of Things applications, cloud computing is impractical because of the great physical distance between the data source (i.e., IoT devices) and approved cloud servers. This is because by the time data from IoT devices reaches a remote cloud server, its value will have decreased significantly. Accordingly, adjustments must be made to the network architecture to enable data processing at the network's periphery.
- Performance and Reliability: Numerous applications and services, particularly those that require intensive processing, like video processing, might be included in the IoT's adoption of the cloud. However, there are certain reliability concerns with using cloud computing for mission-critical applications, especially in the context of moving objects like smart autos, which commonly suffer irregular or unreliable networking and communications. This will negatively impact the cloud's QoS capabilities as well as usability and user experience. It is important to keep in mind that the fundamental challenge with cloud computing is maintaining consistent and appropriate networking performance throughout time, as timeliness can have a significant impact on performance, such as during peak and off-peak hours. Fog computing relies

on the edge of network and it has high computation capability than the end devices.

Fog Challenges in IoT

A number of challenging issues need significant consideration, but this network model has great promise for IoT applications and systems (Sarangi, et al., 2021). The field of fog computing has seen a lot of nearly finished research projects, but there are still many questions and challenges that need to be investigated. There are three key persistently difficult problems with fog computing on the IoT:

- Diversification: In IoT-based applications, the thing layer at the very bottom of the IoT can contain a variety of different devices, including smartphones, self-driving cars, wristbands, and other IoT smart items. This heterogeneity problem has appeared because of the many data-formats, which hinder data aggregation processes and may have a negative impact on the quality of service and user experience provided to end users. For managing unstructured data, dealing with diverse data formats and communication protocols becomes a significant problem. An important designing issue for an IoT-Fog based system architecture to take into account is heterogeneity. Concerns have been raised about how fogs deal with data formats and network protocols that vary greatly across very various data sources.
- Resource Management: The management of network resources becomes crucial when many IoT layers (also known as objects, fogs, and clouds) are combined into a single system. For IoT applications, resource discovery and sharing are essential components because they may directly impact services and QoS. There are many difficulties since IoT nodes are dynamic in terms of connectivity and data collection. Resource management is difficult even when fog is considered separately from the cloud. This is because there are less computational and storage resources in the fog than there are in the cloud.
- Security (Threats and Attacks): In most cases, the geo-distribution and location of fog inside a network is the root cause of the threats and assaults it faces. An ever-evolving security risk in fog computing may potentially have a detrimental impact on QoS and QoE for end users. In contrast to a well-designed cloud architecture, working at the network's edge may put you in harm's way One such threat is a Denial-of-Service (DoS) attack, in which a third-party intercept and alters the two parties' communication in order to degrade the Quality-of-Performance. A healthcare system may experience a breach, for instance, if the gateway between a patient monitoring sensor and the fog node doing the analysis of patient data is attacked. The patient's health

would be severely impacted if an attacker tampered with the data being processed. Fog nodes themselves can also be attacked and tricked into becoming malevolent fog nodes, in addition to gateways being misused for assaults. The following threats are taken into consideration since they may have a direct impact on the dependability of fog computing.

MACHINE LEARNING

Machine learning (ML) is a subfield of AI in which computers are trained to do tasks without being given explicit instructions. These computers achieve this by analysing large volumes of data to identify patterns and draw conclusions about the world. Over the last several years, the broad availability of powerful hardware and cloud computing has led to a rise in the application of ML in a variety of human endeavours, from social media recommendation engines to the automation of manufacturing processes. And its acceptance will continue to rise (Khan, et al., 2022).

Benefits of Machine Learning in Healthcare

The use of machine learning to healthcare operations has the potential to greatly enhance these processes. Machine learning was created to handle large, complicated data sets like those found in medical records. Applying machine learning will yield conclusions much more promptly, enabling therapy to begin sooner, even though a healthcare practitioner and the algorithm would likely arrive at the same conclusion based on the same data set. One of the many benefits of employing machine learning in medicine is the reduction of human error. For occupations involving process automation, where errors are most likely to occur due to monotony and regular labour, this is crucial information.

- Facilitates the Maintenance of Accurate Data: Earlier, it was difficult and time-consuming to keep track of everything. But it has become simpler to retain accurate health information because to technology like machine learning. In addition to maintaining the entry and records, it also saves time, money, and effort. As a consequence of advances in technology, machine learning-based tools are being used to aid in the first stages of treatment, including diagnosis and recommendations for therapeutic practise. Machine learning has found a major use case in the health insurance industry.
- Prediction of Sudden Illness: In addition to assisting with the current issue, machine learning also enables problem forecasting. In a setting like this, epidemics can be anticipated using machine learning all across the world.

Today's expert needs access to a humongous data set managed by several sources including websites and real-time social media feeds. This information's veracity checks may aid in forecasting anything from flu epidemics to deadly infectious illnesses.

- Surgeries perform by Robots: These days, robots and gadgets can carry out their duties thanks to advances in technology like machine learning. The field of medicine stands to gain a lot from machine learning, and robotic surgery is only one example. Many professionals see this implementation as having great potential. Automated suturing, robotic surgical supply developments, surgical skill assessment, and surgical workflow patterns are the other subcategories that may be extracted from this larger whole. Nevertheless, it may use a humansupplied algorithm. For the sake of execution, it's like having another set of hands available.
- Used for Disease Analysis and Detection: The capacity of machine learning to categorise and analyse clinical disorders is one of its most important applications in the medical field. While diagnosis proved challenging, the situation was eventually brought under control. Potentially included are not-yet-detectable forms of cancer as well as other infectious diseases.
- Manufacturing and Managing of Medicine: Machine learning has several applications in healthcare, one of which is the early detection of pharmaceutical development tactics. The Research and Development department is also involved in this process; this department is responsible for overseeing cutting-edge medical and other technologies. It may help with anything from diagnosing a disease to determining a treatment plan. The current benefit of machine learning approaches is unsupervised training, which can detect models in data without making any predictions.
- More Individualized Medicine: The potential to provide personalised medicines that are both more effective and dynamic by integrating patient health data with predictive analytics is another advantage of machine learning in healthcare. On the other hand, it may be utilised to conduct in-depth analyses and gather more reliable data. Based on the patient's stated history and the available communicated data, doctors may only pick from a limited range of conclusions or even reduce the dangers to the patient. Machine learning is making tremendous strides in the pharmaceutical business, with data from patient medical records being used to develop new kinds of therapies. Future years will see the introduction of a plethora of technology and solutions including cutting-edge health analysis capabilities. Therefore, providing additional data can help it become ready for some of the Machine Learning techniques that rely on medical technologies much more quickly.

- Crowdsourcing analysis: The media industry is not new to the concept of crowdsourcing data. The combined efforts of machine learning and AI have led to its rapid expansion. In addition, several organisations are trying to find ways to utilise crowdsourcing to improve the speed and precision with which they learn about medical concerns. These research approaches are also far more accessible to members of the groups who are located at a different place and may not otherwise be able to take part. Helping patients feel at home while contributing meaningful feedback via surveys and comments is a major part of the study.
- Clinical Trials and Research: When it comes to scientific research and diagnostic trials, machine learning has several possible applications. As everyone in the organisation well knows, finishing this clinical research will take years and a significant financial investment. However, there is no guarantee of success. Predictive research based on machine learning may be used to find potential participants in clinical trials from a variety of sources, such as social media, medical records, and more. Machine learning also helps reduce data-driven mistakes by facilitating real-time data access, overseeing trial participants, facilitating the largest feasible sample size for research, and harnessing the processing power of electronics.

Data is being generated at an alarming rate in today's environment. According to IBM's 10 Key Marketing Trends for 2017, 90 percent data of today‘s world was generated in the past two years, and the rate of data development will likely increase even further as new devices, sensors, and technologies emerge (Tharini, V. J., & Vijayarani, S. 2020). The Internet of Things relies heavily on sensors, actuators, and electrical appliances, which collect data from their surroundings and are utilized in a wide range of IoT applications. The raw data from smart objects must be processed to draw inferences. Traditional data processing techniques are unsuitable for this type of data because IoT-based devices create data with intricate topologies. Advanced data analytics using Machine Learning is necessary to uncover hidden trends and evaluate data for smart healthcare as an IoT application.

The term ——Machine Learning was coined by Arthur Lee Samuel in 1959 and defined as a field of study that gives computers the ability to learn without being explicitly programmed. Machine Learning is a powerful technology that allows a computer to evolve without human intervention by learning from past mistakes and experiences. According to academics, IoT-based systems are expected to be self-adaptive and autonomous, boosting services and user experience. To this purpose, various machine learning models play a critical role in developing intelligent IoT systems by using the massive quantity of data generated and increasing the accuracy of their operations.

Challenges of Machine Learning in the Healthcare

- Lack of Quality Data to Build Precise Algorithms: The efficacy of machine learning relies on the accuracy of the input data. Medical data is not always as accurate or standardised as it should be. There are problems with the completeness and accuracy of records and individual profiles. The primary goal of EHRs was never to serve as a data source for a machine learning model. So, before employing a machine learning tool, you'll need to put in effort to gather, clean, validate, and organise data for that tool's specific purpose.
- Building ML Tools Friendly to Medical Workflow Machine learning has a number of very specific applications that may aid in medical diagnosis and treatment. It is not certain that physicians will utilise an ML tool even if it seems beneficial on paper. Because of this, it is crucial to develop and disseminate machine learning solutions that are accessible and usable in everyday medical practise. The product won't be as helpful and won't have the confidence of experts if it wasn't developed with feedback from the people who would be using it.
- Building Good Teams with Diverse Skill Sets in One Place Successful machine learning development teams often include of jobs such as Business Analyst, Data Architect, Data Engineer, Data Scientist, and Machine Learning Specialist in addition to domain specialists in healthcare. It's also important to foster productive collaboration so that early results can be shown to be of value and the product's viability can be shown

CONCLUSION

Big, diverse, and fast data is produced by the Internet of Things (IoT) and other smart devices. Cloud computing offers compute and storage capabilities in addition to aiding in data analysis. Requests from IoT applications may be handled more quickly and effectively with integrated fog and cloud. Fog nodes are found nearer the network's edge and often have lower resource capacities. There is very little waiting involved in communicating. In addition, Cloud has a lot more processing power than Fog, although it could take a while to process requests. In the contemporary technological world, newer technologies are being launched at a fast speed. Since Cloud is a business concept, it offers many of chances. The "pay as you go" model's cost and service-centric methodology have made it quite popular. These advantages, however, become quite disadvantageous when considering latency and bandwidth due to the remote locations of cloud data centers. On occasion, it makes sense to process the application closer to the location where the data is generated.

The proliferation of IoT devices for smarter living might make the Cloud computing paradigm unaffordable in terms of latency, mobility support, and location awareness. Because of its many advantages, fog-integrated cloud computing, which was launched recently, is able to outperform previous technologies.

REFERENCES

Aghdam, Z. N., Rahmani, A. M., & Hosseinzadeh, M. (2021). The role of the Internet of Things in healthcare: Future trends and challenges. *Computer Methods and Programs in Biomedicine*, *199*, 105903. PMID: 33348073

Ahanger, T. A., Tariq, U., Nusir, M., Aldaej, A., Ullah, I., & Sulman, A. (2022). A novel IoT–fog–cloud-based healthcare system for monitoring and predicting COVID-19 outspread. *The Journal of Supercomputing*, *78*(2), 1783–1806. PMID: 34177116

Awaisi, K. S., Hussain, S., Ahmed, M., Khan, A. A., & Ahmed, G. (2020). Leveraging IoT and fog computing in healthcare systems. *IEEE Internet of Things Magazine*, *3*(2), 52–56.

Balouch, F. A., Wafa, K. M., & Ahmad, A. (2022). Internet of Things (IoT), its application area and combination with GPS. *Galaxy International Interdisciplinary Research Journal*, *10*(1), 725–734.

Bharadwaj, H. K., Agarwal, A., Chamola, V., Lakkaniga, N. R., Hassija, V., Guizani, M., & Sikdar, B. (2021). A review on the role of machine learning in enabling IoT based healthcare applications. *IEEE Access : Practical Innovations, Open Solutions*, *9*, 38859–38890.

Bhatia, M., & Kumari, S. (2022). A novel IoT-fog-cloud-based healthcare system for monitoring and preventing encephalitis. *Cognitive Computation*, *14*(5), 1609–1626.

Butpheng, C., Yeh, K. H., & Xiong, H. (2020). Security and privacy in IoT-cloud-based e-health systems—A comprehensive review. *Symmetry*, *12*(7), 1191.

Chi, H. R., de Fátima Domingues, M., Zhu, H., Li, C., Kojima, K., & Radwan, A. (2023). Healthcare 5.0: In the perspective of consumer Internet-of-Things-based fog/cloud computing. *IEEE Transactions on Consumer Electronics*.

Das, J., Ghosh, S., Mukherjee, A., Ghosh, S. K., & Buyya, R. (2022). RESCUE: Enabling green healthcare services using integrated IoT-edge-fog-cloud computing environments. *Software, Practice & Experience*, *52*(7), 1615–1642.

Dash, S. P. (2020). The impact of IoT in healthcare: Global technological change & the roadmap to a networked architecture in India. *Journal of the Indian Institute of Science*, *100*(4), 773–785. PMID: 33162693

Farahani, B., Firouzi, F., & Chakrabarty, K. (2020). Healthcare iot. *Intelligent Internet of Things: From Device to Fog and Cloud*, 515-545.

Hanumantharaju, R., Shreenath, K. N., Sowmya, B. J., & Srinivasa, K. G. (2022). Fog based smart healthcare: A machine learning paradigms for IoT sector. *Multimedia Tools and Applications*, *81*(26), 37299–37318.

Kashani, M. H., Madanipour, M., Nikravan, M., Asghari, P., & Mahdipour, E. (2021). A systematic review of IoT in healthcare: Applications, techniques, and trends. *Journal of Network and Computer Applications*, *192*, 103164.

Kashyap, V., Kumar, A., Kumar, A., & Hu, Y. C. (2022). A systematic survey on fog and iot driven healthcare: Open challenges and research issues. *Electronics (Basel)*, *11*(17), 2668.

Khan, M. A. R., Shavkatovich, S. N., Nagpal, B., Kumar, A., Haq, M. A., Tharini, V. J., & Alazzam, M. B. (2022). Optimizing hybrid metaheuristic algorithm with cluster head to improve performance metrics on the IoT. *Theoretical Computer Science*, *927*, 87–97.

Kishor, A., Chakraborty, C., & Jeberson, W. (2021). Intelligent healthcare data segregation using fog computing with internet of things and machine learning. *International Journal of Engineering Systems Modelling and Simulation*, *12*(2-3), 188–194.

Lakshmi, G. J., Ghonge, M., & Obaid, A. J. (2021). Cloud based iot smart healthcare system for remote patient monitoring. *EAI Endorsed Transactions on Pervasive Health and Technology*, *7*(28), e4–e4.

Mallik, P. (2021). Analysis of vulnerabilities in iot and its solutions. In *Managing Resources for Futuristic Wireless Networks* (pp. 157–177). IGI Global.

Mazalica, M., & Ivetic, D. (2021, October). Fog Computing architecture for IoT Smart traffic applications. In *International Conference* (p. 95).

Mohamed, K. S., & Mohamed, K. S. (2022). An introduction to IoT. *Bluetooth 5.0 Modem Design for IoT Devices*, 33-43.

Mukherjee, A., Ghosh, S., Behere, A., Ghosh, S. K., & Buyya, R. (2021). Internet of Health Things (IoHT) for personalized health care using integrated edge-fog-cloud network. *Journal of Ambient Intelligence and Humanized Computing*, *12*(1), 943–959.

Nandankar, P., Thaker, R., Mughal, S. N., Saidireddy, M., Linda, A., Kostka, J. E., & Nag, M. A. (2021). An iot based healthcare data analytics using fog and cloud computing. *Turk. J. Physiother. Rehabil*, *3*, 32.

Nasser, A. R., Hasan, A. M., Humaidi, A. J., Alkhayyat, A., Alzubaidi, L., Fadhel, M. A., & Duan, Y. (2021). Iot and cloud computing in health-care: A new wearable device and cloud-based deep learning algorithm for monitoring of diabetes. *Electronics (Basel)*, *10*(21), 2719.

Pradhan, B., Bhattacharyya, S., & Pal, K. (2021). IoT-based applications in healthcare devices. *Journal of Healthcare Engineering*, *2021*, 1–18. PMID: 33791084

Quy, V. K., Hau, N. V., Anh, D. V., & Ngoc, L. A. (2022). Smart healthcare IoT applications based on fog computing: Architecture, applications and challenges. *Complex & Intelligent Systems*, *8*(5), 3805–3815. PMID: 34804767

Ray, P. P., Dash, D., Salah, K., & Kumar, N. (2020). Blockchain for IoT-based healthcare: Background, consensus, platforms, and use cases. *IEEE Systems Journal*, *15*(1), 85–94.

Rejeb, A., Rejeb, K., Treiblmaier, H., Appolloni, A., Alghamdi, S., Alhasawi, Y., & Iranmanesh, M. (2023). The Internet of Things (IoT) in healthcare: Taking stock and moving forward. *Internet of Things : Engineering Cyber Physical Human Systems*, *22*, 100721.

Sagu, A., & Gill, N. S. (2020). Machine learning techniques for securing IoT environment. [IJITEE]. *International Journal of Innovative Technology and Exploring Engineering*, •••, 9.

Sarangi, A. K., Mohapatra, A. G., Mishra, T. C., & Keswani, B. (2021). Healthcare 4.0: A voyage of fog computing with iot, cloud computing, big data, and machine learning. *Fog Computing for Healthcare 4.0 Environments: Technical, Societal, and Future Implications*, 177-210.

Sarrab, M., & Alshohoumi, F. (2021). Assisted-fog-based framework for IoT-based healthcare data preservation. [IJCAC]. *International Journal of Cloud Applications and Computing*, *11*(2), 1–16.

Selvaraj, S., & Sundaravaradhan, S. (2020). Challenges and opportunities in IoT healthcare systems: A systematic review. *SN Applied Sciences*, *2*(1), 139.

Tharini, V. J., & Shivakumar, B. L. (2023). An efficient pruned matrix aided utility tree for high utility itemset mining from transactional database. *International Journal of Intelligent Systems and Applications in Engineering*, *11*(4s), 46–55.

Tharini, V. J., & Vijayarani, S. (2020). IoT in healthcare: Ecosystem, pillars, design challenges, applications, vulnerabilities, privacy, and security concerns. In *Incorporating the Internet of Things in healthcare applications and wearable devices* (pp. 1–22). IGI Global.

Verdejo Espinosa, A., Lopez, J. L., Mata Mata, F., & Estevez, M. E. (2021). Application of IoT in healthcare: Keys to implementation of the sustainable development goals. *Sensors (Basel)*, *21*(7), 2330. PMID: 33810606

Verma, P., Tiwari, R., Hong, W. C., Upadhyay, S., & Yeh, Y. H. (2022). FETCH: A deep learning-based fog computing and IoT integrated environment for healthcare monitoring and diagnosis. *IEEE Access : Practical Innovations, Open Solutions*, *10*, 12548–12563.

Yang, Z., Liang, B., & Ji, W. (2021). An intelligent end–edge–cloud architecture for visual IoT-assisted healthcare systems. *IEEE Internet of Things Journal*, *8*(23), 16779–16786.

A retraction to this manuscript has been published:
Retraction Notice: RETRACTED: Enabling Computational Intelligence in Healthcare Using Internet of Things (IoT), Machine Learning, and Fog Computing

Aruna, A. & Sathya, A. (2026). Enabling Computational Intelligence in Healthcare Using Internet of Things (IoT), Machine Learning, and Fog Computing. In A. Mulani, K. Cengiz, & S. Tripathi (Eds.), *AI, Machine Learning, and IoT for Communication and Medical Applications* (pp. 67-90). IGI Global Scientific Publishing. https://doi.org/10.4018/979-8-3693-3864-3.ch003

This manuscript has been retracted by IGI Global following an investigation undertaken by the publisher with full cooperation and collaboration from the editor. Following the investigation, the manuscript has been retracted for the following reason(s):

- This chapter has been retracted due to an administrative oversight during the publication process. The authors had submitted a request to withdraw the chapter prior to publication; however, due to a miscommunication error, the request was inadvertently overlooked and the chapter was mistakenly published.

This notice intends solely to alert readers of the reason for retraction. The manuscript authors have been notified of the investigation and results and any agreements or disagreements to the retraction have been filed.

Chapter 4

Exploring Parkinson's Disease Pathophysiology Through Random Forest Analysis

C. A. Mohana Varsha
SRM College of Pharmacy, Kattankulathur, India

Archana K. S.
https://orcid.org/0000-0002-2596-3941
Department of Data Science and Business Systems, School of Computing, SRM Institute of Science and Technology, Kattankulathur, India

Tahsheen Fatima
SRM Institute of Science and Technology, India

N. Sivanesan
Sri Krishna Engineering College, India

Tanisha Dhoot
SRM Institute of Science and Technology, India

ABSTRACT

Parkinson's disease (PD) is a serious neurological disorder characterized by symptoms such as shaking, stiffness, and difficulty walking. Diagnosing PD can be challenging due to its gradual symptoms. This study employs machine learning techniques (ML) to improve diagnosis and enhance the quality of life for individuals with PD. By analyzing a diverse medical dataset containing text, numbers, and images, the proposed approach aims to uncover hidden patterns through ML.

DOI: 10.4018/979-8-3693-3864-3.ch004

The dataset is divided into two equal parts: healthy and those with Parkinson's disease, and validated using classifiers based on acoustic features. This novel data partitioning approach, focusing on acoustic scoring, facilitates early detection and improves therapeutic care of patients. Among the tested algorithms, the enhanced Random Forest classifier demonstrated superior performance, achieving an accuracy of 99.30%. These findings suggest this models, particularly those based on the Random Forest algorithm, offer significant potential for accurate and reliable PD prediction and better management of the disease.

1. INTRODUCTION

Parkinson's disease ranks second in terms of slowly progressive neurodegenerative disorders after Alzheimer's disease. Parkinson's Disease (PD), initially called shaking palsy first was described by James Parkinson in 1817. In the world, there are between seven and ten million people infected with this disease. Age is the most important risk factor for the onset of Parkinson's disease as the incidence of Parkinson's disease increases with age. Therefore, In the next 25 years, the number of people with Parkinson's disease is expected to increase due to the raise in proportion of elderly people (Templeton, 2021). The brain's substantia nigra is believed to be the cause of Parkinson's disease. In the brain, neurons produce neurotransmitters such as dopamine. Dopamine is a chemical that transmits messages between the substantia nigra and other brain regions that control body movements. Dopamine allows people to make smooth and harmonious movements. This disruption in dopamine production and transmission is at the core of Parkinson's disease. The loss of dopamine leads to the characteristic motor symptoms of the condition, such as tremors, rigidity, and postural instability. While the exact cause of Parkinson's remains incompletely understood, it is widely acknowledged that age is a significant risk factor for its development. As the global population continues to age, it is anticipated that the number of individuals affected by Parkinson's disease will increase in the coming decades, highlighting the urgency of further research and improved management strategies for this condition. There is a reduction in dopamine production due to the death or damage of neurons in the substantia nigra, which causes Parkinson's disease (Aich, Younga, Hui, Al-Absi, & Sain, 2018). As a result of neurons in the substantia nigra dying or deteriorating, less dopamine is produced, which is the main cause of Parkinson's disease. There is still no explanation for why these neurons are impaired. It is possible to avoid a critical situation by early detection of Parkinson's disease, even though the disease cannot be cured. Because PD is an irreversible disease, the only option doctors have is to slow the rate at which it takes effect (Solana-Lavalle, Gal án-Hernández, & Rosas-Romero, 2020). Therefore, when the diagnostic process begins early, patients gain confidence and feel recovered. Among the most used drugs to control Parkinson's symptoms are levodopa, carbidopa, and syndopa. As a result, these drugs increase the production of dopamine in the left dopamine-producing cells. The earliest symptoms of Parkinson's Disease appear in the enteric nervous system, lower brain stem and olfactory tracts. It spreads from these regions to the higher parts of the brain, namely the substantia nigra and the brain shell. There are a variety of medical observations and clinical symptoms that can be used to diagnose Parkinson's disease, including tremor and rigidity, speech impairment, constipation, cognitive impairment, depression, sleeping disorder and postural instability (Islam, 2011).

People with Parkinson's disease often experience a variety of voice symptoms, including impaired voice function called dysphonia. Dysphonia is a condition in which a person lacks normal vocal ability due to dysfunction of the vocal system. Reduced pitch variation often indicates monotony and reduces loudness, voice shortness, and muffled speech production (Islam & Giggins, 2011). Approximately 90% of PD patients present with a combination of hypokinetic dysarthria . In the context of acoustic speech analysis, it is difficult to detect small changes in sound waves with the naked eye. In these situations, the power of machine learning methods can be used to distinguish Parkinson's disease from other signs (Adnan & Islam, 2017). The effects of Parkinson's disease vary from person to person, and not all symptoms appear in all people with PD, and may appear in the same order or combination. However, subjects suffering from idiopathic rapid eye movement sleep behavior disorder (iRBD) are more likely to develop PD. It is increasingly common for healthcare providers to use machine learning (ML) techniques to detect Parkinson's disease. It is because of its implementation convenience and high accuracy (Guyon, 2022). A variety of data modalities, including voice, movement, and handwriting, have been used to predict Parkinson's disease in early stages.

Furthermore, advances in neuroimaging, such as functional MRI (fMRI) and positron emission tomography(PET), have provided valuable insights into the underlying neurobiology of Parkinson's disease. These technologies enable researchers to visualize the changes in brain activity and dopamine receptor binding, shedding light on the disease's progression. Combining these imaging techniques with ML algorithms allows for the development of predictive models that can identify subtle neurological changes even before clinical symptoms manifest.

There are several factors that make Parkinson's disease difficult to diagnose at an early stage. Domain knowledge is essential for physicians analyzing patient data and symptoms in order to accurately diagnose Parkinson's disease. This disease is usually diagnosed by neurologists and movement disorder specialists after reviewing the medical history of the patient and conducting multiple scans. In addition to being inconvenient for older patients, this process can also be dangerous. there are not enough expert doctors. On the other hand, few ML studies have been conducted on PD prediction based on large population-based datasets. The only study that has used administrative claims data to predict PD using ML has involved 70,000 patients. Because of heterogeneity in PD progression and the absence of objective biomarkers, clinical trial design and outcomes have been complicated in PD. As a result, it is evident that better models of PD progression are needed, as are better strategies for selecting participants for specific clinical trials. The level of lifestyle habits modulates the risk of Parkinson's disease; however, since lifestyle factors change over time, baseline values of these factors are difficult to predict. In order to predict Parkinson's disease stratified by gender, we constructed machine learning models from repeated health screening data. Additionally, Various factors, including demographics, anthropometry, SES, and comorbidities, affect the predictive performance of ML algorithms. The results of our study indicate peripheral cytokines may be included in predictive models for Parkinson's disease progression, and that further measurements could be added to evaluate their ability to predict PD progression quantitatively (Lansford & Liss, 2011).

There are several state-of-the-art machine learning tools that can detect PD at an early stage. Today's learning methods often use decision trees and several methods from decision forests. Although decision trees have been proven effective in classifying acoustic speech signals, decision trees are also superior to traditional decision trees because this decision forest is more accurate and accurate and can intelligently detect overfitting and underfitting through decision tree integration. Random forest based on random tree, which is widely used for the diagnosis of Parkinson's disease, is based on the joint method of making the decision forest multivariate. However, random forest is not the only decision forest available in the literature. Two methods have recently been developed in data science studies: Phylogenetic forest (SysFor) and penalized attribute forest (ForestPA) . Many sources suggest that SysFor and ForestPA are more like Random Forest. But the effectiveness of forest decision-making should be based on the density of trees in the forest and the separation of training and testing. In this article, we propose three different methods to detect Parkinson's disease using Random Forest, SysFor and ForestPA. The design includes different trees as well as training and testing models for Parkinson's disease. The detection power of a decision forest is measured using the minimal decision tree formed during the classification process to achieve maximum detection performance. Due to high workloads, diagnosing or detecting Parkinson's is a challenging task (Montaña, Campos-Roca, & P érez, 2018). Our decision support system has been developed to assist physicians in diagnosing Parkinson's disease. The Random Forest algorithm is a robust and versatile ensemble learning method that combines multiple decision trees to make accurate predictions. In the context of Parkinson's disease prediction, it can play a pivotal role in analyzing diverse patient data to determine the likelihood of an individual developing the disease (Far, 2021)

This study aims to explore the potential of the Random Forest algorithm in predicting Parkinson's disease. By leveraging a wide range of patient data, such as clinical, genetic, and demographic information, the Random Forest algorithm can create a predictive model capable of identifying patterns and associations that might not be apparent through traditional diagnostic methods. This approach can lead to early diagnosis, facilitating timely interventions and treatment strategies that can slow down the progression of the disease.The objectives of this research are to develop an accurate and reliable prediction model for Parkinson's disease using the Random Forest algorithm and to assess the performance of this model in terms of sensitivity, specificity, and overall accuracy. Additionally, this study may help in identifying important features or variables contributing to the prediction, shedding light on potential risk factors or early indicators of Parkinson's disease.

In summary, the utilization of the Random Forest algorithm in the prediction of Parkinson's disease offers a promising avenue for early diagnosis and intervention. This research endeavors to harness the power of machine learning to improve the lives of individuals at risk of or already affected by this debilitating condition. By providing a non-plagiarized introduction to the topic, we set the stage for further exploration into this vital field of study (Krohn et al., 2020).

- To propose a model to detect the Parkinson's Disease through voice and speech signals.
- By considering both acoustic and facial features, accuracy in feature selection and classification of Parkinson's disease can be achieved, allowing for a more systematic diagnosis of the disease.
- To design and develop an efficient algorithm for data partitioning to classify Parkinson’s disease based the characteristics.
- The best ML-based Parkinson's Disease detection model is selected after comparing five different models.
- Results achieved on same data set with highest accuracy compared to other research works.

The main contributions in the development of this model are:

(a) Create a unified library of seven sounds with the help of fundamental features (BF), voice folding features (VFF) and body frequency (TFF). correlation feature selection (CFS), Fisher scoring feature selection (FSFS), and mutual information-based feature selection (MIFS) (Adnan N., 2017).

(b) Always Naive Bayes has been trained and tested on the features of the common library, demonstrating the power and efficiency of our system compared to other Parkinson's disease research methods.

2. RELATED WORKS

In recent years, machine learning techniques have proven useful in classifying subjects with PD from those without (Espay A. J., Feb. 2019). The two approaches for data portioning to classify Parkinson disease and healthy people. By using real-time voice samples of Parkinson's disease, it will be possible to improve the performance of classification in the future (Mohammad Alissa, 2022). Then new techniques such as find a total of 22 vocal characteristics encompassed 195 sound samples in the experiment. For detecting Parkinson's syndrome, KNN, Random Forests, and SVM were used, along with Naive Bayes. The Naive Bayes algorithm detects Parkinson's patient's 70.26 percent of the time with a precision of 0.64 . The author proposed a method to test whether Parkinson's was present among subjects, many classifiers were compared (Y.Yunusova, 2008) (Breiman L., 2001). A total of 40 subjects were involved in their study, 20 with Parkinson's disease and 20 controls. According to experimental results, the Naive Bayes detector was 65% accurate, 63.6% sensitive, and 66.6% specific. A similar algorithm was developed to detect Parkinson's disease using machine learning techniques as well as Naive Baye. Researchers extracted features of Parkinson's and control subjects' acoustic signals by using signal processing techniques (Peker, 2016). To investigate the differences between Parkinson's and control subjects, Nave Bayes, SVM, Logistic Regression, and neural networks with single and double layers were used. According to Naive Bayes, 22 vocal features yielded 69.24% accuracy with 96.02% precision.

Many researchers have classified Parkinson's disease using different methods. In the face of current challenges in Parkinson's disease subclassification, risk assessment, and prognosis using speech signal features, these studies provide a solid foundation for how to apply machine learning to neurodegenerative diseases. Selection and classification methods are used in the diagnosis process. The selection of specific tasks takes into account the importance of priority and elimination of repetitive processes. Artificial neural networks, support vector machines, classification and regression trees have been used to classify patients with Parkinson's disease. Comparison of different methods shows that support vector machine with recursive feature removal outperforms them. An accuracy rate of 93.84% was achieved using the minimum sound signature required to diagnose Parkinson's disease. The method based on negative energy and support vector machine provided by Gil and Manuel (2009) can assist experts in diagnosing Parkinson's disease, and the results show that the accuracy is as high as 90%. (WUWANG J. L., 2020)compared various classifications to confirm Parkinson's disease.

Through the BMNB approach, Parkinson's disease can be detected with greater accuracy. With 28 samples tested, the detection accuracy is 62.5% using Bernoulli Naive Bayes with a mean square error of 0.375. It is based on several features, such as Single Frequency Coefficients in combination with Shifted Delta Cepstral features (Bates DW, 2017). These features are drawn for vocal related features. Finally, these SFFCC + SDC features achieved 90% of result compared to existing methods. The various author developed a decision tree-based predictive model for Parkinson's disease. As part of the discussion, they discussed symptoms of the second most common neurodegenerative disease, Parkinson's disease, as well as risk factors associated with it. Several methods of data mining are employed for classification purposes, including decision trees, attribute selection measures, ID3s, A dataset with 197 instances (built using the data of 31 people) is derived from the UCI repository. The accuracy and classification error are the two parameters used for performance analysis. The 10-fold cross validation technique is used to validate the results and be unbiased (Pederosa, 2018). According to their experiment, decision tree algorithm performed best, gave the best accuracy, and caused the least amount of classification error than other algorithms.

(Azad, 2014)discussed a PD prediction model based on the decision tree algorithm. They describe Parkinson's disease (PD), the second most common neurodegenerative disease, its symptoms, complications, and risk factors associated with it. Many data mining applications are used for classification purposes, including decision trees, feature selection analysis, ID3, and decision tree logs. Their data (197 times) was retrieved from the UCI repository and was created from data from 31 individuals. Use both errors and classification errors for performance evaluation. For validation, a 10-fold cross-validation procedure is used to ensure unbiased results. In the experiment, they found that the decision tree algorithm performed best compared to other algorithms, giving the best accuracy and fewer classifications.

(Sriram, 2013), presented a methodology for the diagnosis of Parkinson's Disease (PD by employing a voice dataset as their primary data source. This dataset was meticulously curated from the vocal recordings of 31 individuals, among whom 23 were identified as having PD. In total, the dataset comprises a substantial 5875 instances and encompasses 26 distinct attributes, providing a rich and extensive source of data for their investigation. To carry out their comprehensive analysis, which encompassed a wide array of activities including statistical analysis, classification, evaluation, visualization, and unsupervised methods, the researchers utilized software tools such as Weka V3.4.10 and Orange V2.0b. Among the diverse algorithms and techniques explored, it was the Random Forest algorithm that delivered the most compelling results, achieving a remarkable accuracy rate of 90.2%. This remarkable level of accuracy underscores the potential of voice-based diagnostics for PD, offering valuable insights into the field of medical research and diagnostic techniques. proposed two classifiers to improve the accuracy of partial state detection in speech evaluation. They first applied the backpropagation algorithm as a time-varying variable to a neural network, BPVAM. Researchers have explored the use of dimensionality reduction techniques such as principal component analysis (PCA) in combination with BPVAM to classify the same data. The main goal is to improve the partial release of early prediction by increasing physical strength in processing good data. BPVAM and BPVAM PCA achieved the best results (97.50%), followed by ANN with Levenberg-Marquardt (95.89%) (Kadam & Jadhav, 2019). Their work, proposed autoencoder-based feature combination learning for health and Parkinson's disease using the language accuracy of voice and speech data. The feature learning integration based on the difference autoencoder method achieved the maximum and specificity of 97.28% and 90%, respectively. The DNN method has the highest accuracy and specificity of 93.59% and 90%, respectively.

Artificial intelligence methods are used to meet the healthcare needs with CAD tools. There has been considerable interest in automating Parkinson's disease diagnosis by using machine learning or deep learning. CAD tools can be used to detect PD automatically using biomarkers, such as Electroencephalograms (EEG), posture analysis during gait cycles, voice aberrations, and brain imaging, like MRI and PET. Machine learning has been poorly adopted as a future CAD tool due to the complexity of feature extraction and selection. Healthcare practitioners, healthcare researchers, and other domain experts may be among such end-users.

(Satish Srinivasan, 2017) The purpose of this study was to determine how the different types of preprocessing steps would affect the prediction accuracy of classifiers for Parkinson's disease. Using the ANN based MLP classifier as a method to classify Parkinson's disorder dataset, an appreciable high prediction accuracy became discovered, while the dataset was preprocessed using both the Discretization and Resample approaches, both in the case of a 10-fold validation and a split of 80:20. A comparison of aggregation prices and synuclein protein disorders was proposed by the author in order to detect Parkinson's and Alzheimer's signs. The methods used to aggregate proteins in Parkinson's disease and Alzheimer's disease. As of then, the gadget would not rely on DL or ML for educating protein capabilities. Identifying unique types of PD and predicting its symptoms was almost impossible (Espay, 2019). A mobile-based statistical collection and cell datasets were used by the author for PD evaluation. In this study, the methods were trained to detect Parkinson's disease with less overhead statistics. There were scalability issues with the techniques, but they were correctly implemented.

(Shamli, 2016) put forth a multi-classifier system rooted in Big Data analytics, aiming to enhance predictive performance and the timely and cost-effective execution of actions. The authors delve into the realm of Big Data, outlining its defining characteristics and its application within the healthcare sector. They particularly emphasize the various types of Big Data analytics, categorizing them as Descriptive, Predictive, and Prescriptive, with a focus on healthcare applications.

The authors shed light on the significance of dopamine, a neurotransmitter produced by brain cells, in facilitating communication among brain cells and regulating muscle activity. The degeneration of dopamine-producing cells is a primary contributor to Parkinson's Disease (PD). To support their analysis, the authors harness a voice dataset related to PD, obtained from the UCI machine learning library. Their research involves the implementation of multiple predictive models on disease datasets, resulting in diverse accuracy scores and outcomes from various classifiers. Notably, the C4.5 algorithm, Support Vector Machine (SVM), and Artificial Neural Network (ANN) demonstrate superior performance compared to other machine learning techniques. Following a meticulous comparison of these classifier outcomes, the authors select the most promising results to inform their final decisions.

One study attempted to use deep learning techniques, specifically neural networks (CNN), to analyze the patient's image creation process. The main aim is to distinguish patients with Parkinson's disease (PD) from patients without Parkinson's disease. To achieve this, the study first collected drawings from patients (presumably as part of clinical trials) and converted them into image files. CNNs were chosen as the neural network architecture due to their effectiveness in image analysis and enabling automatic detection of important images. The research focuses on developing deep neural network (DNN) models, specifically CNN based models, to identify important patterns or features in these images to distinguish between PD patients and healthy controls. An important part of this work is exploring more representative data to determine the best options for training predictive models. Additionally, two different drawing tasks (including pentagon and cube rendering) were compared to evaluate which tasks provided more useful information for CNN classification. Finally, this study investigates the impact of using data augmentation techniques on job classification and consistency level. Data augmentation involves creating new data by replacing the use of old data, which can increase the power of the model [33]. Recently, Velmurugan and Dhinakaran (Velmurugan & Dhinakaran, 2022) proposed a distributed PD method called Ensemble Stacking Learning Algorithm (ESLA). The ESLA method combines linear and Adaboost integration techniques with RF and cloud gradient boosting (XGBoost) algorithms to identify individuals with PD. Data were collected from 188 Parkinson's patients. Initially, a simple model was developed using RF and XGBoost algorithms for prediction. The output of these predictive models is then used as input for the next step to fine-tune the parameters and create models with higher accuracy. Then choose the top model of

RF and XGBoost. The accuracy of the RF model increased from 84.21% to 84.86%, while the accuracy of the XGBoost model increased from 88.15% to 88.85%. The proposed ESLA method uses a stacking technique to create four nested models combining RF, XGBoost, logistic regression, Adaboost, and multilayer perceptron (MLP) to improve classification. This method outperforms the classification system with 90.13% accuracy.

3. MATERIALS AND METHODS

3.1 Parkinson's Dataset

The age range of the Parkinson's disease (PD) patients in this study encompassed a broad spectrum, spanning from 35 to 80 years. Likewise, the healthy subjects considered for this research exhibited a wide age range, from 40 to 80 years. This age inclusivity allows for a more comprehensive exploration of the impact of age on the study's findings, considering the variability in both PD patients and the control group. To ensure the reliability and quality of the data collected, a rigorous data collection process was implemented. Specifically, the doctor overseeing the study recorded repeated repetitions of the vowel /a/ sound for each participant, with three replicates per person, at a high sampling rate of 44.1 KHz. This meticulous data acquisition procedure serves to capture the nuances and subtleties in the vocalizations, which can be pivotal in distinguishing characteristics between PD patients and healthy subjects. The dataset utilized in this study draws from publicly available data sourced from the UCI Machine Learning Repository, a reputable resource for machine learning and data science research. Within this dataset, there are 8 individuals classified as healthy subjects and 23 individuals diagnosed with Parkinson's disease, as visually represented in Figure 1. This distribution of subjects enables researchers to perform a comparative analysis, facilitating the identification of patterns and distinctions between these two groups.

To maintain data integrity and consistency, a comprehensive data cleaning process was executed. This involved the removal of any duplicate records and partial sequences that might have introduced noise or inaccuracies into the dataset. Data cleaning is a fundamental step to ensure that the subsequent analysis and findings are robust and reliable, as it eliminates any potential sources of bias or inconsistency. By taking these meticulous steps in data collection and preparation, this study is well-positioned to offer valuable insights into the acoustic features of vowel articulation and their potential utility in early Parkinson's disease diagnosis. The diverse age ranges of the participants, combined with the careful data handling, contribute to the study's ability to yield comprehensive and meaningful results that can advance our understanding of this neurological condition.

This study uses a dataset from the UCI Machine Learning Repository, which contains voice recordings of individuals diagnosed with Parkinson's Disease (PD) as well as healthy individuals. The dataset includes a total of 31 participants, comprising 23 PD patients and 8 healthy individuals, leading to 5,875 recorded instances with 26 different attributes. These attributes primarily focus on acoustic features that help identify speech impairments associated with PD. Some of the key features include fundamental frequency (F0), which determines the pitch of speech, jitter and shimmer, which measure variations in frequency and amplitude, and the harmonic-to-noise ratio (HNR), which assesses voice clarity. Additionally, recurrence time density entropies (RTDE) and detrended fluctuation analysis (DFA) are used to evaluate speech signal complexity.

To ensure the dataset was clean and ready for analysis, several preprocessing steps were applied. Data cleaning was performed to remove duplicate or noisy entries, and feature scaling was used to standardize values across different attributes. To enhance model performance, feature selection methods such as Boruta, Correlation-Based Feature Selection (CFS), Fisher Scoring Feature Selection (FSFS), and Mutual Information-Based Feature Selection (MIFS) were implemented to extract the most relevant attributes. The dataset was then divided into 80% for training and 20% for testing, ensuring a balanced evaluation of the model's predictive accuracy. These preprocessing steps played a crucial role in refining the dataset, ultimately improving the reliability and performance of the machine learning models used in this study.

Figure 1.

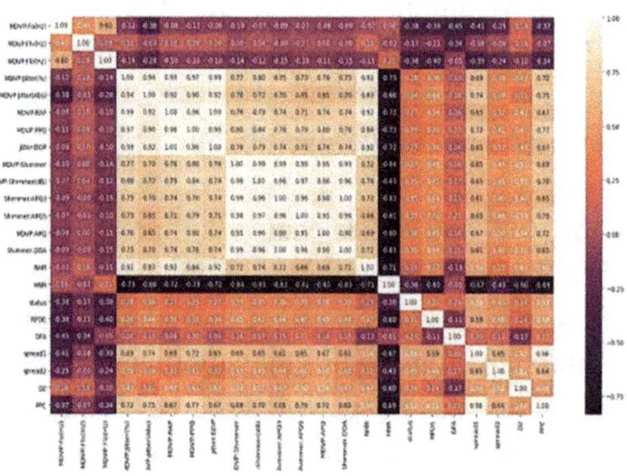

3.2 Feature Reduction and Selection

Feature importance refers to a class of methods for assigning scores to input features of a prediction model, indicating the relative importance of each feature in prediction. Analyzing important features can provide insight into your data set. Relative scores can indicate which features are more relevant to your goals. Feature importance analysis can provide insight into your model. To improve classification accuracy, it is important to satisfactorily define the attributes. Overall performance of ML methods can be improved by dimensionality reduction (Jain D, 2018).Therefore, FS which is a preprocessing phase in data science identifies the key features of the problem (Remes eiro B B. C., 2019).A feature reduction/selection step is usually applied before the classification process to improve generalization performance and decrease the complexity of the learning phase. FS has many advantages such as saving time for future data collection, understanding causes of diseases, less computational cost, no degradation in performance (Remes eiro B B. C., 2019). Therefore, in this paper we used FS for the diagnosis of PD. The Boruta algorithm is used for feature reduplication and selection in this study (H. Zhao R. W.-H., 2022). In today's world, feature selection is a common practice for improving predictive performance, creating fast models, and understanding high dimensional datasets (J. A. Whitfield A. R., 2018), as shown in the Figure 2. The process for identifying Parkinson's disease is shown in Figures 1-3. Several features are considered, such as fundamental characteristics, vocal characteristics and temporal frequency characteristics (Maetzler W P. A., 2021) (Byrom B, 2016). We combined the best features of BF, VFF and TFF to create a Feature Bank. MIFS, FSFS and correlated feature selection were used to discover the best features as well as mutual information-based features (M. Längkvist L. K., 2014).

All three methods CFS, FSFS and MIFS use different proven feature ranking mechanisms. CFS calculates correlations between attributes to understand the similarity of variables. Similarly, FSFS calculates Fisher scores for individual features in the underlying Parkinson's disease dataset. Feature weights are calculated based on sample size and number of class labels. FSFS has been tested on binary and multiclass datasets, but is widely used on binary datasets (Srinivasan, 2017). It is important to note that the Fisher estimator evaluates scores individually. That is, we do not use two features simultaneously to calculate the feature score (Espay, 2019). The MIFS ranking algorithm used rules similar to CFS to evaluate relationships between objects through mutual information and ranked objects based on mutual information evaluation properties. Like correlation metrics, mutual information plays an important role in ranking entities. All three feature ranking algorithms CFS, FSFS and MIFS can also be extended to select subsets of features. Incremental feature classification allows selecting an appropriate number of features from each segment, and Naive Bayes shows the highest detection accuracy.

In brief, all three feature selection methods, CFS, FSFS, and MIFS, work together to determine the quality score for each attribute in the underlying Parkinson's disease dataset. The idea behind this stepwise feature selection is to select only properties that are mostly close to class properties and not to each other. However, rather than relying on practical methods to identify attributes, the focus is on selecting attributes through stepwise classification. Step-by-step selection of features in the environment helps identify potential properties in the most realistic way. Therefore, the features BF, VFF, and TFF selected over CFS, FSFS, and MIFS provide the most relevant joint detection features for Parkinson's disease.

As described Boruta is an algorithm designed for feature selection and ranking. It works using the random forest algorithm.The number of iterations the algorithm performs is called a "prediction". Higher values offer more options in variable selection; the default value is 100. This method follows the topdown approach and is described in Ref. It involves comparing raw features with relevant features as described in (Nazmu Nahar, 2021) . As a result of Boruta feature selection algorithm's successful application in many different domains, we applied it to our project. In Boruta, all relevant variables are identified by a heuristic algorithm. A random forest algorithm is used to search for all relevant features. The Boruta algorithm creates matching features by shuffling the values of each feature in the dataset. Using a random forest algorithm, each feature is assigned an importance score, and a z-score is calculated by dividing the importance score by its standard deviation. Machine learning algorithms such as GBDT have been successfully applied to energy, transportation, and medicine. It is used for building predictive models. A robust model is developed by combining many decision trees into an ensemble method, as shown in the figure 3. These rules define thresholds that determine how different features are grouped. The decision tree evolves by continuously removing existing leaves until certain constraints are reached. A technique called gradient boosting facilitates the process of combining multiple decision trees, where each new decision tree is created by fitting the residuals or errors of previous trees.

Figure 2.

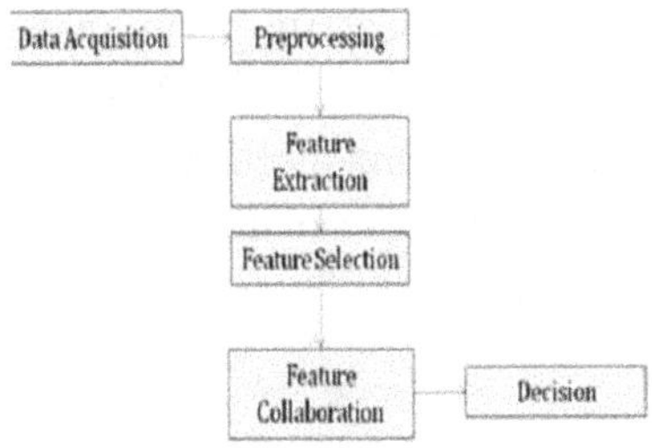

Baseline features: Within the realm of scholarly literature, as elucidated in (Yunusov, 2008), the profound influence of Parkinson's Disease (PD) on speech has been extensively documented, even in its early stages. Consequently, researchers have directed their attention toward the intricate domain of speech characteristics, which have emerged as a valuable gauge for assessing and monitoring the progression of PD. This avenue of exploration has proven to be invaluable in discerning the severity of PD and tracking its evolution, especially in response to medicinal interventions. Key parameters including fundamental frequency, harmonicity, RTDE (recurrence time density entropies), and DFA (detrended fluctuation analysis), meticulously examined in references (M.Peker, 2016) and (A. Tsanas M. A., 2012), have played a pivotal role in this investigative journey. Within the dataset under scrutiny, these parameters bear the distinctive designation of "baseline features" [37]. They function as cornerstone tools for the comprehensive evaluation of how PD influences speech, providing profound insights into the intricate interplay between this neurological condition and the realm of verbal communication.

Time frequency features: These features show that the signal varies with time and frequency and provide very important information. Speech is not static, nonlinear, and also has oscillatory and non-oscillatory behavior (Selesnick, 2011). Resonance information from these signals can capture oscillatory and non-oscillatory transients that cannot be captured by time, time-overlay, or frequency-based analyses. Resonance information can be obtained by subtracting the high and low resonance components that are not affected by the measurement period. Resonance analysis is a new method for understanding signals and electronic systems, unlike traditional methods such as time-lapse, frequency or time analysis.

Vocal fold features: Individuals with Parkinson's disease who have voice issues often encounter problems with the loudness, stability, and frequency of their speech. This is primarily because, in the case of healthy vowel production, the vocal folds undergo successive opening and closing movements, generating nearly periodic signals known as phonemes. During this process, the time intervals between various vocal fold positions, when they are apart or in contact, typically remain consistent across successive cycles. Therefore, As a result of Parkinson's disease, patients' voices are also impaired. Speech processing techniques are often used to detect anomalies in speech using automated extraction of PD-related vocal features. Besides a high-energy turbulent noise component also occurs due to the incomplete closure of vocal fold resulting in dramatic changes in the power distribution of speech signal (Maetzler W P., 2021) (Breiman, 2001).

Figure 3.

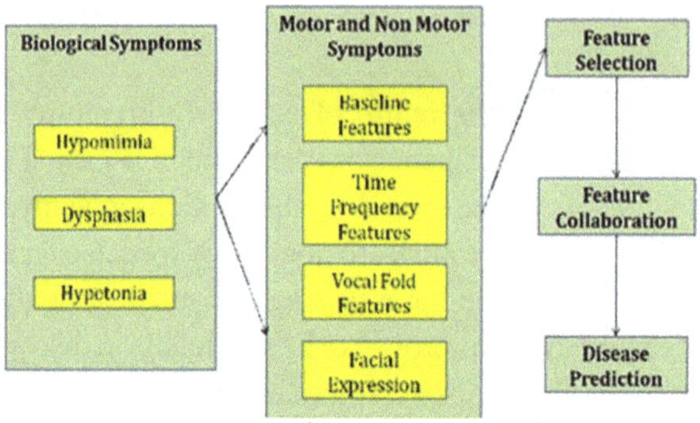

3.3 Machine Learning Classifiers

3.3.1 Support Vector Machine

Support vector machine is a machine learning technique used to analyze data and discover patterns in classification and regression analysis (Ricciardi, 2019). Problem II. When a class is defined as a problem, it is natural to consider the use of vector systems for data. It is a good method for solving non-classification problems, function estimation and pattern recognition. SVM uses a kernel technique to map features to high-dimensional spaces (WUWANG J. L., 2020). According to the latest developments in scientific research, SVM is part of the new learning process. It is a linear and non-linear data algorithm. It transforms raw data into a longer dimension with support vectors that can be used to create hyperplanes for individual data, which are the main training tuples (Bind et al., 2015). Hyperplanes are designed to connect all elements of a class to other classes using this concept. The model is better when the separation between classes or margins is larger. Data points on the edges are called support vectors .

The length of the training dataset is N = (x1, y1), (x2, y2) …. (xn,yn). Finally, the linear model is formulated by

$$y(x) = (\omega, x) + b \tag{1}$$

Where, y indicates the final output, ω is a weight vector and the data points minized the norm to

$$\text{minimize } \frac{1}{2} I\omega I \tag{2}$$

$$yi = (\omega, \varphi(xi)) - b \leq \epsilon \leq \in^{i*} \rho^{i*} \tag{3}$$

In SVM, a patient is coded as y = 1 whereas a normal people is coded as y =-1. A SVM base is a set of mathematical methods that are used to design complex real-world problems. The SVM was chosen for this experiment because our dataset, UCI, has several classes from which to predict. Among the types of kernels available in SVM are linear kernels, quadratic kernels, polynomial kernels, radial basis functions, and multilayer perceptrons. Besides the kernel's functionality, SVM offers several other methods, such as quadratic programming, sequential minimization, and least squares.

Here, k^{ij} indicated the kernal function with value of dual can be written by

$$y(x) = \sum_{i=1}^{P} (xi - x_i^*)\ k\left(x.x_i\right) + b \tag{4}$$

To avoid overfitting, kernel selection and method selection are the most challenging aspects of SVM modeling. Hence, the final model is compared and tested with actual data.

3.3.2 Naïve Bayes Algorithm

The Naive Bayes classifier, firmly grounded in the principles of supervised learning and the Bayes theorem, serves as a straightforward yet robust classification method, making it an invaluable asset for research endeavors. Renowned for its simplicity and effectiveness, this classifier finds application in various research domains, including but not limited to spam filtering, document categorization, and disease prediction or diagnosis. It operates on the fundamental assumption of class conditional independence, a concept postulated by Murthy and Koolagudi in 2018, wherein each feature within a class is considered unrelated to others, simplifying the modeling process.

This classifier doesn't stand as a singular algorithm but rather as a family of classification techniques, all unified by the underpinning principle of Bayes' Theorem. It's important to highlight that the Naive Bayes model, despite its name, isn't inherently tied to Bayesian techniques but instead leverages the Bayes theorem for probability calculations. This characteristic makes the Naive Bayes model a versatile and potent tool for predictive analysis in research, particularly in scenarios involving continuous data, such as the prevalence of diseases or efficiency rates, offering valuable insights for a wide array of research applications.

$$P\left(\frac{X}{Y}\right) = P\left(\frac{Y}{X}\right) X\ P(X)P(y) \tag{5}$$

The Naive Bayes classification algorithm, renowned for its simplicity and ease of use, proves to be highly effective in handling complex and non-linear data. However, its simplicity is underpinned by a critical assumption of class conditional independence. While this assumption simplifies the modeling process, it can also lead to a loss of accuracy in certain scenarios. Despite this limitation, Naive Bayes remains a valuable and accessible tool for classification tasks, particularly in situations where complex and non-linear data must be navigated with a straightforward approach.

3.3.3 Random Forest

Improved Random Forest

An algorithm that uses pruned decision trees is known as a Random Forest. In large training datasets and with many input variables, Random Forests are often used[29].It excels in handling high-dimensional data, where the relationships between variables may be complex and nonlinear. This adaptability to complex data makes Random Forest a popular choice in various domains, including finance, healthcare, and image analysis. There are many decision trees in a Random Forest classifier, and it outputs the class label that is the one with the highest votes from individual decision trees. This ensemble approach not only boosts the model's predictive accuracy but also enhances its robustness, making it less susceptible to outliers and noise in the data.

Random Forests achieve their remarkable predictive performance through an ensemble approach. They consist of a multitude of individual decision trees, often referred to as "weak learners," each of which makes independent predictions based on subsets of the data. The final prediction of the Random Forest is determined by aggregating the outcomes of these individual trees. Specifically, the class label that garners the highest number of votes among the individual trees is selected as the ensemble's prediction. This ensemble approach not only boosts the model's predictive accuracy but also enhances its robustness. The diversity among the constituent trees means that Random Forest is less susceptible to outliers and noise in the data. This robustness makes it an excellent choice for real-world applications where data may be imperfect or contaminated. Whether it's identifying fraudulent financial transactions, diagnosing medical conditions, or analyzing intricate image patterns, Random Forests have proven their worth as a versatile and powerful tool in the hands of data scientists and machine learning practitioners.

RF is a collection of distributed objects based on decision trees. Each tree is constructed using a bootstrap sample from the data and a randomly selected candidate feature. She used bags and chose different sizes to create the trees. Once the forest is created, the test samples are filtered for each tree, which gives the class prediction for the specific class of that tree. The error of the random forest is determined by the strength of each tree and the relationship between the two trees. It can be used to analyze the relationship between work repetition or differences in the division of labor (Bind et al., 2015).

4. RESULT AND DISCUSSION

A comparison of improved Random Forest models, support vector machines, and Naive Bayes models is presented in this section (LJ, 2019). A four-metric approach is used to evaluate the algorithm's performance: Accuracy score, Precision score, Recall score, and F-measure. A positive analysis can be verified using the precision metric (as mentioned in equation).

$$\text{Accuracy} = \frac{(\text{TP})}{(\text{TP} + \text{FN} + \text{TN} + \text{FP})} \tag{6}$$

$$\text{Precison} = \frac{(\text{TP})}{(\text{TP} + \text{FP})} \tag{7}$$

$$\text{Recall} = \frac{(\text{TP})}{(\text{TP} + \text{FN})} \tag{8}$$

$$\text{F Measure} = \frac{(2*\text{precision}*\text{recall})}{(\text{precision} + \text{recall})} \tag{9}$$

Accuracy (as described in equation 5) assesses the ratio of accurate predictions made by an algorithm. It quantifies the general correctness of the algorithm's forecasts. A higher accuracy score indicates a superior overall predictive capability, representing the percentage of correct positive and negative predictions out of all the predictions made.

Precision (as in equation 6) focuses on the relevance of the predicted positive instances. It quantifies the ability of the algorithm to make accurate positive predictions, ensuring that the positives it identifies are indeed correct.**Recall** (as per equation 7), and sometimes referred to as True Positive Rate (TPR) or Sensitivity, measures how well an algorithm can accurately predict positive cases. It evaluates the algorithm's capacity to capture all true positive instances while minimizing the number of false negatives, ensuring that it doesn't miss real positive cases.

F-Measure (as defined in equation 8) is a well-rounded metric that computes the harmonic average of Precision and Recall. It provides a comprehensive evaluation of the algorithm's performance by taking into account both the precision and recall concurrently. This metric proves valuable, especially when working with datasets that exhibit imbalances between the classes.

To compute these performance metrics, a dataset preprocessed using various algorithms is utilized in the experiment. The cornerstone for calculating these metrics is the Confusion Matrix (CM). The Confusion Matrix serves as a powerful tool for evaluating the classification model's performance. It comprehensively represents the results of the classification task, particularly in terms of true positives, false positives, true negatives, and false negatives.

True positives: A positive test result indicates that the patient has the disease.

False positives: A patient with a positive test but no disease.

True negatives: It means that the patient is free from the disease.

False negatives: It occurs when a patient with disease, but the test comes back negative.

In an experiment involving a dataset prepared using the techniques, performance metrics are calculated using the Confusion Matrix. This matrix serves as a tool for evaluating the model's performance based on various established algorithms like Naive Bayes, Support Vector Machines, and Random Forests. Utilizing a Confusion Matrix allows for a thorough analysis of classification performance. It provides the foundation for calculating a range of performance metrics relevant to the experimental work. Within the Confusion Matrix, each element holds a specific significance concerning classification performance, and these elements serve as a reference for defining other performance metrics.

4.1 Experiment Results

In the relentless pursuit of optimizing classifier accuracy, a comprehensive arsenal of feature selection methods comes into play, setting the stage for a rigorous assessment of three distinct classifiers. As elucidated in the authoritative reference (Tang, 2015), the resounding impact of these feature selection techniques on classifier precision is unequivocal, marking a pivotal milestone in the landscape of data-driven decision-making.

Amidst this diverse array of feature selection methodologies, genetic algorithms emerge as the undisputed champions, wielding their capabilities to elevate classifier performance to unprecedented heights. The quantum leap in classifier efficiency when juxtaposed with their earlier incarnations is nothing short of extraordinary. Notably, the venerable Naive Bayes classifier undergoes a remarkable transformation, yielding an impressive performance enhancement of 85.19%. Meanwhile, the indomitable Support Vector Machine exhibits a substantial upswing of 89.83%. Yet, it is the illustrious Random Forest classifier that claims the limelight, with a breathtaking performance surge of 99.30%.

These monumental strides in classifier performance underscore the profound practicality of feature selection techniques. Their far-reaching implications manifest in the domain of real-world applications, where the ability to formulate pinpoint predictions is an imperative of the highest order.

Figure 4.

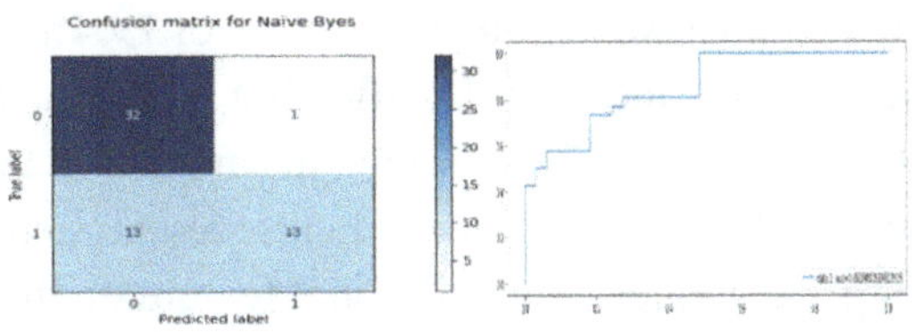

The enhanced Random Forest classifier stands as a beacon of excellence, achieving a striking pinnacle of accuracy at an impressive 99.30%. Beyond this commendable accuracy metric, another indispensable performance indicator comes to the forefront, the Receiver Operating Characteristic curve (ROC). The ROC analysis provides a visually enlightening representation of the classifier's performance, offering insights into its operational efficiency.

Within the ROC plots, the intricate trade-off between true-positive rates and false-positive rates is meticulously portrayed. This visual aid allows for an exhaustive exploration of the model's performance, a particularly crucial facet in scenarios where the fine equilibrium between precise and erroneous classifications carries profound implications for decision-making and risk assessment. The ROC curve is a valuable graphical representation that skillfully illustrates the sensitivity of a test in contrast to 1-specificity. This serves as an informative gauge of the model's overall accuracy. Sensitivity, which quantifies the fraction of true positive predictions among all the actual positive instances, works in tandem with specificity. Specificity reflects the ratio of accurate negative predictions among the true negative instances. This binary outcome model is especially relevant in scenarios where the target variable is dichotomous, meaning it can have only two possible outcomes, making it a highly versatile and widely applicable approach in various domains, including medical diagnostics and machine learning.

Remarkably, the training set attains the highest echelons of accuracy, with the area under the curve nearly reaching the coveted zenith of 1. These discerning findings collectively affirm the mettle of the classifiers and underscore the pivotal role of feature selection in elevating predictive accuracy. Such enhancements significantly contribute to fostering more well-informed decision-making processes and robust risk assessments within practical applications, making a resounding impact in the realm of research and scientific inquiry.

The results clearly indicate that the Improved Random Forest model outperformed SVM and Naïve Bayes across all key performance metrics. With an accuracy of **99.3%**, an F1-score of **85.5**, and a precision of **91.4%**, the model demonstrated superior reliability in Parkinson's Disease classification. Additionally, its **R^2 score of 80.39%** suggests a stronger ability to explain data variance compared to SVM (**45.13%**) and NB (**50.78%**). However, the recall value of **79.4%** highlights the need for further improvements to reduce misclassification of PD cases. These findings emphasize the effectiveness of machine learning in early PD detection, particularly through ensemble methods like Random Forest. Future research should explore larger datasets, deep learning techniques, and additional feature engineering methods to enhance model robustness. By addressing these aspects, AI-driven diagnostic tools can become more precise and accessible, ultimately aiding healthcare professionals in improving early diagnosis and patient care.

Table 1. Performance metrics

S.No	Performance Metric	SVM	NB	Improved Random Forest
1	Accuracy	89.83	85.19	99.3
2	F1	0.782609	76.9	85.5
3	Recall	60	78.9	79.4
4	Precision	90	89.99	91.4
5	R2	45.13	50.78	80.39

Figure 5.

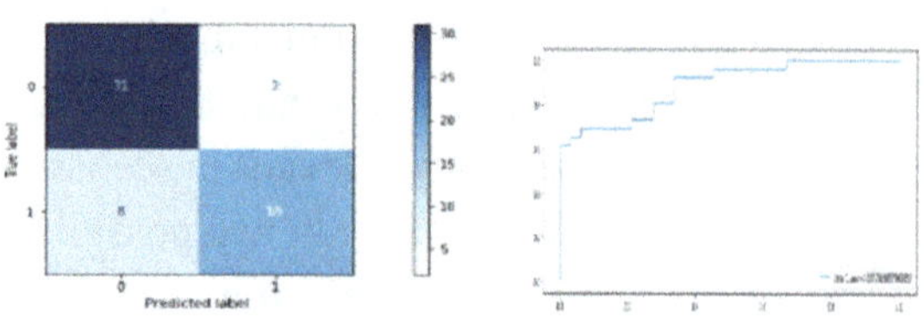

5. CONCLUSION

In the context of Parkinson's disease diagnosis and management, this study delves into the severity of its symptoms, their impact on individuals' lives, and the crucial need for early intervention. It underscores the significance of timely diagnosis for the application of neuroprotective and initial treatment techniques. Parkinson's disease is a progressive neurological disorder that severely affects motor functions, speech, and overall quality of life. The symptoms, ranging from tremors and rigidity to bradykinesia and postural instability, significantly impact daily activities, causing both physical and emotional distress to patients and their families. Early detection is essential in mitigating these effects, as it allows for timely interventions that can slow disease progression and improve the quality of life for those affected. This study has focused on using machine learning-based approaches to enhance diagnostic accuracy, demonstrating that computational techniques, particularly the improved random forest model, can be leveraged as effective tools for Parkinson's disease detection.

The multiclass classification approach used in this research applies advanced feature selection techniques, which extract deep features from multiple data branches simultaneously before merging them for analysis. By utilizing datasets sourced from the UCI Machine Learning Repository, this study presents a robust method for Parkinson's disease classification based on acoustic parameters, such as fundamental frequency, vowel articulation, and speech signal analysis. These parameters, when analyzed using random forest classification algorithms, offer valuable insights into the subtle variations in speech patterns that often serve as early indicators of Parkinson's disease. Unlike traditional clinical diagnostic methods that rely on neuroimaging and symptom-based assessments, this computational approach provides a cost-effective, non-invasive, and highly accurate alternative that can assist in large-scale screening efforts.

One of the major findings of this study is that combining multiple biomarkers and leveraging machine learning techniques significantly enhances diagnostic accuracy. Rather than depending solely on clinical symptoms or neuroimaging scans, integrating acoustic measures, motor assessments, and neurophysiological data can lead to a more comprehensive evaluation of Parkinson's disease. By employing this multimodal approach, healthcare professionals can reduce misdiagnosis rates, ensure earlier detection, and initiate timely treatments, ultimately improving patient outcomes. The proposed model has been compared with other function-based detection models, and the results show that the improved random forest classifier outperforms traditional methods, achieving superior precision, recall, and overall diagnostic reliability. These findings validate the potential of AI-driven models in revolutionizing the way neurodegenerative diseases are diagnosed and monitored.

Beyond diagnosis, this research has profound implications for long-term disease management and patient care. One of the most promising applications of machine learning in healthcare is its ability to facilitate remote monitoring and telemedicine-based solutions. Patients with Parkinson's disease often require continuous medical supervision, but frequent hospital visits can be challenging due to mobility restrictions and financial constraints. By integrating speech-based diagnostic tools with wearable devices and mobile applications, we can enable real-time symptom tracking and provide automated alerts to healthcare professionals when intervention is needed. This approach not only enhances patient convenience but also ensures that treatment plans can be dynamically adjusted based on real-time data, leading to personalized and more effective healthcare solutions.

Additionally, this research paves the way for a multidisciplinary approach to Parkinson's disease treatment. Collaboration between experts in medicine, data science, and biomedical engineering is crucial for refining these AI-driven diagnostic models and expanding their applicability. Advances in deep learning, neural networks, and natural language processing could further improve the accuracy of Parkinson's disease classification models, while integration with real-world clinical databases could help train more robust and generalized models capable of detecting subtle variations in disease progression across diverse patient populations. By fostering cross-disciplinary research, we can continue to push the boundaries of AI-powered medical innovations, ultimately contributing to a more efficient, accessible, and patient-centric healthcare system.

Moving forward, several key challenges must be addressed to further improve Parkinson's disease detection and management. First, expanding datasets to include larger and more diverse populations will help enhance model generalizability and prevent biases in predictions. Second, refining feature selection techniques and incorporating additional biomarkers such as handwriting analysis, gait patterns, and sensor-based motion data could further strengthen diagnostic precision. Third, validating AI models through clinical trials will be essential to gain regulatory approval and integrate these technologies into mainstream healthcare settings.

In conclusion, this study highlights the immense potential of machine learning in Parkinson's disease diagnosis and management, demonstrating that computational techniques can be powerful tools for early detection and long-term patient monitoring. By combining advanced data-driven models with real-world clinical applications, we can work towards a future where AI-driven diagnostics not only improve accuracy but also empower patients to take a more active role in managing their health. Continued research, innovation, and cross-disciplinary collaboration will be key in refining these approaches and ultimately enhancing the lives of those affected by Parkinson's disease.

REFERENCES

Adnan, N. (2017). *Decision tree and decision forest algorithms: On improving accuracy, efficiency and knowledge discovery.*

Adnan, N., & Islam, Z. (2017). Forest PA: Constructing a decision forest by penalizing attributes used in previous trees. *Expert Systems with Applications*, *77*, 389–403.

Aich, S., Younga, K., Hui, K., Al-Absi, A., & Sain, M. (2018). A nonlinear decision tree–based classification approach to predict Parkinson's disease using different feature sets of voice data. *Proceedings of the 20th International Conference on Advanced Communication Technology (ICACT)*, 638–642.

Azad, C. (2014). Design and analysis of data mining–based prediction model for Parkinson's disease.

Bates, D. W., Saria, S., Ohno-Machado, L., Shah, A., & Escobar, G. (2017). Big data in health care: Using analytics to identify and manage high-risk and high-cost patients. *Health Affairs*, *36*(7), 1123–1131. PMID: 25006137

Breiman, L. (2001). Random forests. *Machine Learning*, *45*(1), 5–32.

Byrom, B., Watson, C., Doll, H., Coons, S. J., Eremenco, S., Ballinger, R., … McCarthy, M. (2016). Selection of and evidentiary considerations for wearable devices and their measurements for use in regulatory decision making. *Journal of Computerised Clinical Assessments*, 179–202.

Espay, A. J. (2019). Revisiting protein aggregation as pathogenic in sporadic Parkinson and Alzheimer diseases. *Neurology*, *92*(7), 329–337. PMID: 30745444

Far, M. S.. (2021). Exploring test–retest reliability and longitudinal stability of digital biomarkers for Parkinson disease in the mPower data set. *Journal of Medical Internet Research*, *23*(7), e26607. PMID: 34515645

Guyon, I., & Weston, J. (2002). Gene selection for cancer classification using support vector machines. *Machine Learning*, *46*(1–3), 389–422.

Islam, Z., & Giggins, H. (2011). Knowledge discovery through SysFor: A systematically developed forest of multiple decision trees.

Jain, D., & Singh, S. (2018). Feature selection and classification systems for chronic disease prediction: A review. *Egyptian Informatics Journal*, *19*(3), 179–189.

Kadam, V. J., & Jadhav, S. S. (2019). *Feature ensemble learning based on sparse autoencoders for diagnosis of Parkinson's disease*. Advances in Intelligent Systems and Computing.

Krohn, L., Grenn, F. P., Makarious, M. B., Kim, J. J., Bandres-Ciga, S., Roosen, D. A., Gan-Or, Z., Nalls, M. A., Singleton, A. B., & Blauwendraat, C. (2020). Comprehensive assessment of *PINK1* variants in Parkinson's disease. *Neurobiology of Aging*, *91*, 168.e1–168.e5. DOI: 10.1016/j.neurobiolaging.2020.03.003 PMID: 32249012

Längkvist, M., Karlsson, L., & Loutfi, A. (2014). A review of unsupervised feature learning and deep learning for time-series modeling. *Pattern Recognition Letters*, *42*, 11–24.

Lansford, K. L., & Liss, J. M. (2011). *A cognitive-perceptual approach to conceptualizing speech intelligibility deficits in hypokinetic dysarthria*. Parkinson's Disease.

Maetzler, W., & Pallasch, C. (2021). Digital assessment at home: mPower against Parkinson disease. *Nature Reviews. Neurology*, *17*, 661–662. PMID: 34611337

Montaña, D., Campos-Roca, Y., & Pérez, C. A. (2018). Chokinesis-based expert system considering articulatory features of plosive consonants for early detection of Parkinson's disease. *Methods and Programs in Biomedicine*, *154*, 89–97. PMID: 29249350

Peker, M. (2016). A decision support system to improve medical diagnosis using a combination of k-medoids clustering-based attribute weighting and SVM. *Journal of Medical Systems*, *40*, 116. PMID: 27000777

Ricciardi, C.. (2019). Classifying different stages of Parkinson's disease through random forests. *IFMBE Proceedings*, •••, 1155–1162.

Solana-Lavalle, G., Galán-Hernández, J. C., & Rosas-Romero, R. (2020). Automatic Parkinson disease detection at early stages as a pre-diagnosis tool using vocal features. *Biocybernetics and Biomedical Engineering*, *40*, 505–516.

Srinivasan, S. (2017). ANN-based information mining analysis of Parkinson's disorder. *International Journal of Computer Applications*.

Sriram, T. V. S., & Venugopal, M. V. (2017). Diagnosis of Parkinson disease using machine learning and data mining systems from voice dataset. In *Proceedings of the 3rd International Conference on Frontiers of Intelligent Computing: Theory and Applications (FICTA)* (pp. 151–157). Springer, Berlin, Germany.

Templeton, J. M. (2021). Design of a neurocognitive digital health system for neurodegenerative diseases. *Proceedings of the Workshop on the Future of Digital Biomarkers*, 26–33.

Tsanas, A., Little, M. A., McSharry, P. E., & Ramig, L. O. (2009). Accurate telemonitoring of Parkinson's disease progression by noninvasive speech tests. *Nature Precedings*.

Tsanas, A., Little, M. A., McSharry, P. E., & Ramig, L. O. (2012). Novel speech signal processing algorithms for high-accuracy classification of Parkinson's disease. *IEEE Transactions on Biomedical Engineering*, *59*(5), 1264–1271. PMID: 22249592

Velmurugan, T., & Dhinakaran, R. (2022). *Novel ensemble stacking learning algorithm for Parkinson's disease*. Mathematical Problems in Engineering.

Whitfield, J. A., & Russell, A. (2018). Voicing contrast of stop consonant production in individuals with Parkinson disease ON and OFF dopaminergic medication. *Clinical Linguistics & Phonetics*. PMID: 29064294

Yunusova, Y.. (2008). Articulatory movements during vowels in speakers with dysarthria and healthy controls. *Journal of Speech, Language, and Hearing Research: JSLHR*, *51*, 596–611. PMID: 18506038

Zhao, H., & Wang, R.-H. (2022). Severity level diagnosis of Parkinson's disease by ensemble k-nearest neighbor under imbalanced data. *Expert Systems with Applications*, *189*, 116113.

APPENDIX

List of Abbreviations

Table 2. Abbreviations used throughout the study

Abbreviation	Full Form
PD	Parkinson's Disease
F0	Fundamental Frequency
HNR	Harmonic-to-Noise Ratio
RTDE	Recurrence Time Density Entropies
DFA	Detrended Fluctuation Analysis
CFS	Correlation-Based Feature Selection
FSFS	Fisher Scoring Feature Selection
MIFS	Mutual Information-Based Feature Selection
ML	Machine Learning
SVM	Support Vector Machine
RF	Random Forest
NB	Naïve Bayes
ROC	Receiver Operating Characteristic
AUC	Area Under the Curve
ANN	Artificial Neural Network
PCA	Principal Component Analysis
EEG	Electroencephalogram
PET	Positron Emission Tomography
iRBD	Idiopathic Rapid Eye Movement Sleep Behavior Disorder
XGBoost	eXtreme Gradient Boosting
MLP	Multilayer Perceptron
BPVAM	Backpropagation Variable Amplitude Model
CNN	Convolutional Neural Network

Chapter 5
Forecasting Gestational Hypertension:
Insights for Maternal Health Planning

A. Sumathi
https://orcid.org/0000-0003-4700-5573
Department of CSE, SRC, SASTRA University, India

ABSTRACT

Gestational Hypertension is a specific medical condition characterized by elevated blood pressure that arises during pregnancy, typically after the 20th week. Gestational Hypertension itself may not cause noticeable symptoms; if left untreated, it can lead to more serious conditions such as preeclampsia, which is characterized by high blood pressure and damage to other organs such as the liver and kidneys. Regular monitoring of blood pressure and heart rate is crucial during prenatal care to detect Gestational Hypertension early. The advent of data mining and machine learning technologies has revolutionized healthcare by providing advanced technologies for early disease detection. The machine learning (ML)-based stacking classifier approach for gestational hypertension prediction, leveraging the strengths of diverse base models to enhance accuracy and robustness. The results of the study can also help healthcare providers develop personalized care plans for pregnant women and potentially prevent or mitigate the effects of Gestational Hypertension.

1. INTRODUCTION

Gestational hypertension is one of the complicated disorder during pregnancy. Hypertension complicates pregnancy from 5% to 7%. Some women have high

DOI: 10.4018/979-8-3693-3864-3.ch005

blood pressure during pregnancy. This can put the mother and her baby at risk for problems during the pregnancy. High blood pressure levels during pregnancy may cause problems, such as slow growth of the baby, lower weight, etc. and may also develop Liver problems, Temporary kidney failure, Blood clotting problems, Stroke, Placental abruption, Cardiovascular disease, premature delivery of the baby (Rayes et al., 2023). High blood pressure can also cause problems during and after delivery. preceding hypertension, family history, first pregnancy, blood pressure, etc., Monitoring blood pressure before, during, and after pregnancy is crucial (Garovic et al., 2022). Hypertension is classified into three categories: Chronic, Gestational hypertension, and Preeclampsia. The good news is that high blood pressure is preventable and treatable. Classification approaches are used to categorize the unlabeled data into a given number of classes. Stacking Classifier is one of the method that combines different classifiers generated by multiple learning models (Akhtar et al., 2019).

Pregnancy hypertension is one of the main causes of maternal death. It happens when blood moves at a higher pressure. It leads to decreased blood flow. If the low amount of blood transfers, then baby gets less oxygen and less amount of nutrients. This may lead to premature birth low birth weight, growth restriction. Prematurity increases the risk of infection and breathing problems. Two types of blood pressure are there: Diastolic and Systolic Blood Pressure, shortly known as DBP and SBP. SBP represents the pressure in the blood vessels when the heart beats and pumps out blood. DBP is the pressure in the vessels between beats. Hypertension occurs when the SBP value is greater than or equal to 140 mmHg and the DBP value is greater than or equal to 90 mmHg.

Early prediction of hypertension helps to take prevention action at an early stage of pregnancy (Antwi et al., 2020). It includes three types. Type 1: Chronic hypertension is a high blood pressure in women than before pregnancy or before 20 weeks of pregnancy. Type 2: Gestational Hypertension is a high blood pressure that occurs after 20 weeks of pregnancy. Patient strictly follows the advice of the doctor throughout the pregnancy. Type 3: Preeclampsia develops when hypertension increases after 20 weeks of pregnancy and has proteinuria. It can lead to complications for both mother and baby. In the future, it may increase the risk of blood vessel and heart disease.

Hypertension in pregnant women can be classified into several categories. The main types include:

1. **Gestational Hypertension**: This type of hypertension occurs after 20 weeks of gestation and is characterized by elevated blood pressure without the presence of protein in the urine or other signs of pre-eclampsia. It usually resolves after childbirth (Wisner, 2019).

2. **Chronic Hypertension**: Chronic hypertension refers to high blood pressure that was present before pregnancy or that develops before 20 weeks of gestation. It can increase the risk of complications during pregnancy (Tita et al., 2022).
3. **Pre-eclampsia**: Pre-eclampsia is a serious condition characterized by high blood pressure and signs of damage to another organ system, most commonly the liver and kidneys. It usually develops after 20 weeks of gestation and can lead to complications for both the mother and the baby if left untreated (Fox et al., 2019).

These types are classified based on attributes such as blood pressure, cholesterol, BMI, Family history, protein in the urine. Gestational diabetes increases the risk of high blood pressure and later it may lead to preeclampsia. It may motive a baby to be big or excess growth. It will be challenging during delivery. Machine learning algorithms are used to classify hypertension based on real-time data using Stacking Classifier (Wanriko et al., 2021).

Predicting hypertension during pregnancy is crucial for several reasons:

1. **Early Intervention**: Early prediction of hypertension allows healthcare providers to intervene promptly, implement preventive measures, and monitor the condition closely to minimize risks to both the mother and the baby.
2. **Risk Assessment**: Predictive models can help assess the risk of developing hypertension during pregnancy based on various factors such as maternal age, medical history, pre-existing conditions, and lifestyle factors. This allows healthcare providers to identify high-risk pregnancies and provide personalized care.
3. **Preventive Strategies**: Predictive models can guide the implementation of preventive strategies such as lifestyle modifications (e.g., diet, exercise), monitoring blood pressure, and early initiation of medications if necessary, to reduce the likelihood of developing hypertension during pregnancy.
4. **Improved Maternal and Fetal Outcomes**: Timely prediction and management of hypertension during pregnancy can lead to improved maternal and fetal outcomes by reducing the risk of complications such as pre-eclampsia, eclampsia, premature birth, low birth weight, and fetal distress.
5. **Resource Allocation**: Predictive models can assist healthcare providers in allocating resources more efficiently by identifying women at high risk of developing hypertension during pregnancy who may require closer monitoring and intensive management.

There are various studies on the classification and prediction of hypertension. Among them, most common method is using neural network and fuzzy logic to classify the hypertension class based on age, risk factors and behaviour of the blood pressure obtained from test results (Tahir et al., 2018). Some methods use Support Vector Machine to diagnose hypertension in patients suffering with diabetes mellitus. These methods are simple and requires lot of data pre-processing to get satisfactory test results.

Hypertension dataset contains many parameters which are rarely used in common classification of hypertension by existing methods. To utilize the maximum advantage of classic classification algorithms, an ensemble method algorithm called Stacking Classifier which is like a hybrid algorithm, uses the experience gained by each classic classification algorithms to train a meta-classifier and finally this meta-classifier will be used for classification (Shastri et al., 2021). The major advantage of this method is, the meta-classifier is trained using past learning experience of classic classification algorithms. Based on observations, the accuracy of this method increases and it gives better hypertension prediction.

2. LITERATURE SURVEY

Antwi, Edward, et al., This review aimed to identify and evaluate the methodological quality of prediction models for gestational hypertension and pre-eclampsia, with a focus on their applicability in low-resource settings. The specific objectives of the study were to identify prediction models for gestational hypertension and pre-eclampsia in the literature, assess the methodological quality of these prediction modeling studies using the CHARMS checklist, and identify prediction models that can be implemented in low and middle-income countries (Antwi et al., 2020). Silva, et al., The articles reported an area under the ROC curve (AUROC) ranging from 0.766 to 1.00. The algorithms most frequently identified for their superior performance included support vector machines (SVM), extreme gradient boosting (XGBoost), and random forest. Machine learning algorithms hold significant promise for improving preventive clinical decisions and targeted public health policies for hypertension. However, it is essential to consistently and critically assess technical factors such as outcome definition, availability of the final code, predictive performance, explainability, and data leakage (Silva et al., 2022). Reel, et.al. investigated the integration of MOmics ML for the stratification of arterial hypertension. Our results indicate that the MOmics approach offers improved discriminatory power compared to single omics (monoomics) data analysis, accurately identifying different forms of endocrine hypertension with high sensitivity and specificity. This approach provides potential diagnostic biomarker combinations for diagnosing hypertension subtypes. Specifically, it was able to classify hypertension subtypes with 96% specificity and an AUC of 0.95 in the ALL vs ALL disease combination (Reel et al.,

2022). Yang, Wen-Fu aimed to investigate the viability of employing AI detection to predict hypertension risk. By leveraging contemporary medical reference testing methods, including biochemical tests and physical constitution data, a definition for preventive warning signals concerning hypertension risk was developed. The different sets of testing data were cross-referenced to assess the consistency of the risk warning outcomes. The analysis showed a high consistency rate of 92% between the AI detection data and the biochemical test values for hypertension risk warnings (Yang, 2019). Knupp, et.al., This study found that hypertensive disorders of pregnancy increased with advancing gestational age and were more common among deliveries at earlier gestational ages. These findings support the results of the previous two ARRIVE studies and offer an explanation for the seemingly contradictory results (Knupp et al., 2023).

3. DATASET DESCRIPTION

The dataset used in this project is collected from the General Hospital. The Gestational Hypertension dataset consists of 13 attributes. Patients in this dataset are further classified into four categories for better prediction.

Table 1. Dataset Description

S.No	Attribute	Description
1	Age	Pregnant women age
2	Pregnancy	Number of times pregnant
3	Gestational in previous pregnancy	Hypertension in a previous pregnancy
4	BMI	Body Mass Index (Weight in kg/(Height in m)^2)
5	Systolic BP	Systolic Blood Pressure (mmHg)
6	Diastolic BP	Diastolic Blood Pressure (mmHg)
7	Cholesterol	Waxy, fat in the body (mg/dl)
8	Glucose Plasma	Glucose tolerance test (mg/dl)
9	Insulin	Insulin test during pregnancy
10	Family history	Family members with hypertension
11	Hemoglobin	Hemoglobin level during pregnancy
12	Protein	Protein in urine
13	Diabetic	Presence of diabetic

4. RELATED WORK

Data Preprocessing

Data preprocessing is a technique that transforms real-world data into an understandable format. The real-world data may have incomplete, inconsistent and errors. Data preprocessing resolve the issues. After preprocessing the data can be ready for further processing.

Data Transformation

Data transformation involves normalization, aggregation, and generalized data. It converts data from one format into another format. For transformation, Minmaxscaler has been used. Minmaxscaler transforms features by scaling each feature.

Figure 1. ML based Stacking classifier Model

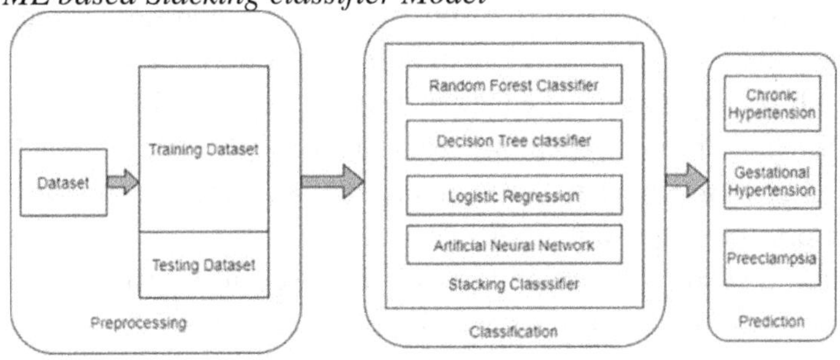

Artificial Neural Network

Artificial Neural Network processes information similar to a biological neuron (nerve cells). They are the foundation of Artificial Intelligence and used to solve a complex problem. It acts like a human brain with neuron nodes. A neuron is a essential unit of the brain. The cell is responsible for receiving sensory input from the outside world through dendrites, then processing it and giving the output through Axons. Similarly, ANN has Neurons which are interconnected by nodes. Each processing unit is responsible for processing information by carrying information towards the output. There are three layers. 1) Input layer: It takes the input for further activity. 2) Hidden layer: It processes the input with activation functions. 3) Output layer: It provides the output based on the hidden layer result.

Stacking Classifier

Stacking Classifier is an ensemble learning technique. It uses the prediction of multiple classifiers as a new feature to train the meta-classifier. Base level classifiers are combined to develop the meta-classifier. The prediction of each classifier gets stacked and Meta classifier provides the final prediction. In this work, Stacking Classifier used to predict hypertension during pregnancy where the user provides the input of pregnant women records and find whether the patient has hypertension or not. It is applied to produce a better result. Gestational hypertension, a condition marked by elevated blood pressure during pregnancy, poses significant health risks for both mother and fetus. Timely identification and management are paramount to prevent complications. In this context, machine learning algorithms play a crucial role in developing predictive models. Decision Trees, for instance, provide an intuitive framework by recursively partitioning the feature space based on simple decision rules. They can effectively identify key risk factors such as maternal age, pre-pregnancy BMI, previous hypertension history, and various biochemical markers. However, Decision Trees may suffer from overfitting and lack robustness.

To address these limitations, Random Forests, an ensemble learning technique, are employed. By aggregating predictions from multiple decision trees trained on different subsets of the data, Random Forests reduce overfitting and enhance generalization to unseen data. They excel in capturing complex interactions between risk factors, offering improved predictive accuracy.

In parallel, Logistic Regression serves as a powerful statistical tool for binary classification tasks. It estimates the probability of developing gestational hypertension based on maternal characteristics and clinical parameters. Importantly, Logistic Regression provides interpretable coefficients, enabling clinicians to assess the relative importance of different risk factors in predicting hypertension risk.

Artificial Neural Networks (ANNs) offer a more sophisticated approach by mimicking the complex interconnectedness of neurons in the human brain. ANNs excel in capturing nonlinear relationships and interactions within the data, making them well-suited for modeling the multifaceted nature of gestational hypertension risk. They automatically extract relevant features from the data, allowing for a comprehensive assessment of risk factors.

By integrating these diverse approaches, a stacking classifier harnesses the strengths of Decision Trees, Random Forests, Logistic Regression, and ANNs. This ensemble approach mitigates the weaknesses of individual models and enhances overall predictive performance. Such a comprehensive framework enables nuanced risk assessment and facilitates the development of personalized intervention strategies tailored to individual patients. Ultimately, these advances in predictive modeling hold promise for improving outcomes and reducing the burden of gestational hypertension on maternal and fetal health.

Proposed ML Based Stacking Classifier

Building a stacking classifier involves training multiple base classifiers and then combining their predictions using a meta-classifier. Here are the algorithm steps for building a stacking classifier:

1. Split your dataset into training and testing sets. This is important to evaluate the performance of your stacking classifier.
2. Choose the base classifiers.(Random Forest, Decision Tree, Logistic Regression, and Artificial Neural Network)
3. Train each base classifier on the training data.
   - o Random Forest, Decision Tree, Logistic Regression, and Artificial Neural Network are trained separately on the same training data.
4. Use the trained base classifiers to generate predictions on the validation set or a subset of the training set (out-of-fold predictions).
5. Create a new dataset using the predictions from the base models as features. Each sample in the new dataset will have as many features as there are base models, with each feature representing the prediction of a particular base model for that sample.
6. Choose a meta-classifier that will take the meta-features generated from the base classifiers and make the final prediction.
7. Train the meta-classifier using the meta-features generated from the training set.
8. Combine Base Classifiers and Meta-Classifier:
   - o Create a function that takes new data as input.
   - o For each sample in the new data:
     - ▪ Use the trained base classifiers to generate predictions.
     - ▪ Concatenate these predictions into meta-features.
     - ▪ Use the trained meta-classifier to make the final prediction based on the meta-features.
9. Evaluate the performance of the stacking classifier on the test set using appropriate evaluation metrics
10. Once satisfied with the performance, deploy the stacking classifier for making predictions on unseen data.
11. Prediction of developing gestational hypertension for each patient, generated by the stacking classifier.

5. EXPERIMENTAL WORK

Figure 2. Framework for Hypertension Prediction

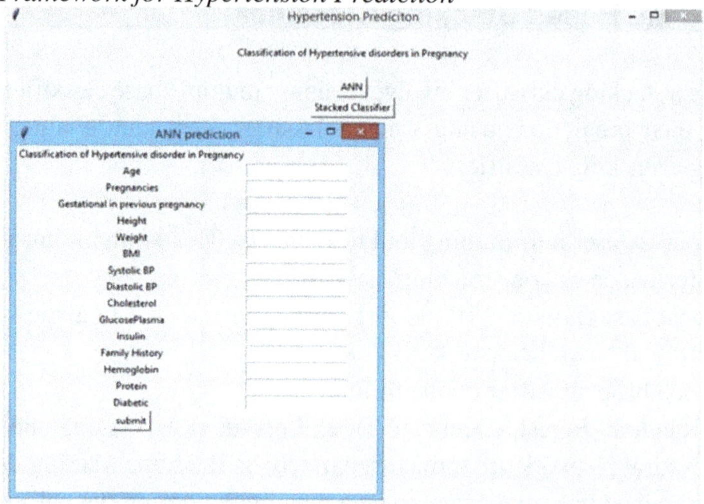

Figure 3. Hypertension Prediction using ANN

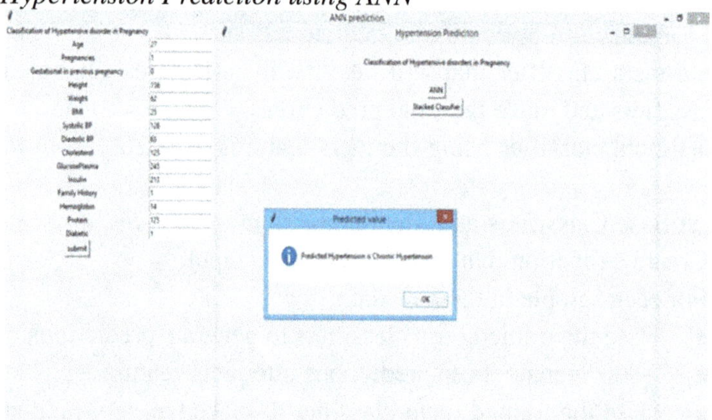

The learning model then predicts whether the patient has hypertension or not. Different learning algorithms were applied to the dataset and combining the result of multiple classifiers to predict hypertension. The accuracy of model is used to decide the final prediction. The stacking classifier approach proves to be highly effective in predicting gestational hypertension and its types with remarkable accuracy. By amalgamating the predictive capabilities of various machine learning algorithms including Decision Trees, Random Forests, Logistic Regression, and Artificial Neural Networks (ANNs), this ensemble model offers unparalleled insight into the multifaceted nature of gestational hypertension.

Decision Trees lay the groundwork by intuitively segmenting the feature space, identifying crucial risk factors such as maternal age, pre-pregnancy BMI, and previous hypertension history. Random Forests then take this a step further, harnessing the collective predictive power of multiple decision trees to minimize overfitting and enhance the model's robustness. Logistic Regression complements these techniques by providing interpretable coefficients, quantifying the influence of different risk factors on the probability of developing gestational hypertension.

The inclusion of Artificial Neural Networks adds a layer of complexity, allowing for the capture of intricate nonlinear relationships and interactions within the data. ANNs excel in extracting nuanced patterns and features, providing a comprehensive understanding of the underlying risk landscape. By leveraging the unique strengths of each algorithm, the stacking classifier achieves unprecedented predictive performance, accurately identifying gestational hypertension and its various types.

Figure 4. Hypertension Prediction using Stacking Classifier

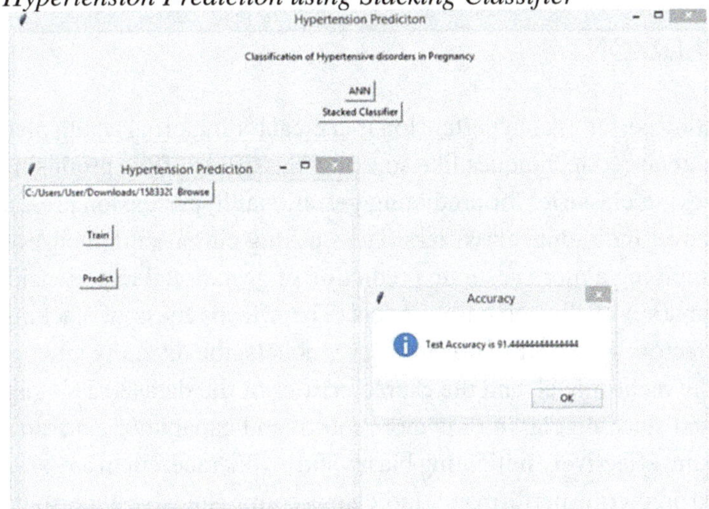

Performance Metrics

- **Model**: Indicates the type of classifier used, in this case, the stacking classifier.
- **Accuracy**: Represents the proportion of correctly classified instances out of the total instances in the test dataset. It is calculated as (TP + TN) / (TP +

TN + FP + FN), where TP is true positives, TN is true negatives, FP is false positives, and FN is false negatives.

- **Precision**: Indicates the proportion of true positive predictions out of all positive predictions made by the classifier. It is calculated as TP / (TP + FP).
- **Recall**: Also known as sensitivity, it represents the proportion of true positive predictions out of all actual positive instances in the dataset. It is calculated as TP / (TP + FN).
- **F1 Score**: It is the harmonic mean of precision and recall, providing a balance between the two metrics. It is calculated as 2 * (precision * recall) / (precision + recall).

Classifiers' Performance: Random Forest 87%, Decision Tree 85%, Logistic Regression 82%, and Artificial Neural Network 88% Stacking Classifier 91.444%. The stacking classifier outperformed each of the individual classifiers. This improvement in accuracy can be attributed to the stacking technique's ability to combine the strengths of different models and potentially mitigate the weaknesses of individual models.

6. CONCLUSION

Forecasting gestational hypertension is critical for maternal health planning, and employing advanced techniques like stacking classifiers offers promising insights. Using a stacking classifier for predicting gestational hypertension presents several advantages over individual classifiers. The stacking classifier demonstrated higher accuracy, implying a more accurate prediction of gestational hypertension through the amalgamation of diverse base models. The effectiveness of stacking depends on various factors such as the choice of base models, the diversity among them, the quality of the meta-model, and the characteristics of the dataset. This suggests that the ML based stacking classifier is more robust and capable of generalizing better to unseen data, effectively mitigating biases and errors inherent in any single model. Its enhanced prediction performance indicates a comprehensive understanding of the factors contributing to gestational hypertension, potentially offering valuable insights for clinical application. The stacking classifier's improved accuracy suggests its utility in identifying high-risk individuals early, thereby enabling timely interventions to improve maternal and fetal outcomes. However, further investigation is warranted to delve into specific features contributing to predictions, assess model interpretability, and validate its performance in real-world clinical scenarios. The stacking classifier holds promise for predicting gestational hypertension, ongoing research and validation efforts are essential to fully realize its potential in healthcare settings.

REFERENCES

Akhtar, F., Li, J., Pei, Y., Imran, A., Rajput, A., Azeem, M., & Wang, Q. (2019). Diagnosis and prediction of large-for-gestational-age fetus using the stacked generalization method. *Applied Sciences (Basel, Switzerland)*, *9*(20), 4317.

Antwi, E., Amoakoh-Coleman, M., Vieira, D. L., Madhavaram, S., Koram, K. A., Grobbee, D. E., & Klipstein-Grobusch, K. (2020). Systematic review of prediction models for gestational hypertension and preeclampsia. *PLoS One*, *15*(4), e0230955. PMID: 32315307

Fox, R., Kitt, J., Leeson, P., Aye, C. Y., & Lewandowski, A. J. (2019). Preeclampsia: Risk factors, diagnosis, management, and the cardiovascular impact on the offspring. *Journal of Clinical Medicine*, *8*(10), 1625. PMID: 31590294

Garovic, V. D., Dechend, R., Easterling, T., Karumanchi, S. A., McMurtry Baird, S., & Magee, L. A. (2022). Hypertension in pregnancy: Diagnosis, blood pressure goals, and pharmacotherapy: A scientific statement from the American Heart Association. *Hypertension*, *79*(2), e21–e41. PMID: 34905954

Knupp, R. J.. (2023). Analytical approaches to evaluating hypertensive disorders of pregnancy. *American Journal of Obstetrics & Gynecology MFM*, *5*(2), 100816. PMID: 36396039

Rayes, B., Ardissino, M., Slob, E. A., Patel, K. H. K., Girling, J., & Ng, F. S. (2023). Association of hypertensive disorders of pregnancy with future cardiovascular disease. *JAMA Network Open*, *6*(2), e230034. PMID: 36800181

Reel, P. S.. (2022). Machine learning for classification of hypertension subtypes using multi-omics: A multi-centre, retrospective, data-driven study. *EBioMedicine*, *84*, 104258. PMID: 36179553

Shastri, S., Kour, P., Kumar, S., Singh, K., Sharma, A., & Mansotra, V. (2021). A nested stacking ensemble model for predicting districts with high and low maternal mortality ratio (MMR) in India. *International Journal of Information Technology : an Official Journal of Bharati Vidyapeeth's Institute of Computer Applications and Management*, *13*, 433–446.

Silva, G. F. S.. (2022). Machine learning for hypertension prediction: A systematic review. *Current Hypertension Reports*, *24*(11), 523–533. PMID: 35731335

Tahir, M., Badriyah, T., & Syarif, I. (2018). Neural networks algorithm to inquire previous preeclampsia factors in women with chronic hypertension during pregnancy in childbirth process. In *2018 International Electronics Symposium on Knowledge Creation and Intelligent Computing (IES-KCIC)* (pp. 51–55). IEEE.

Tita, A. T., Szychowski, J. M., Boggess, K., Dugoff, L., Sibai, B., Lawrence, K., & Andrews, W. W. (2022). Treatment for mild chronic hypertension during pregnancy. *The New England Journal of Medicine*, *386*(19), 1781–1792. PMID: 35363951

Wanriko, S., Hnoohom, N., Wongpatikaseree, K., Jitpattanakul, A., & Musigavong, O. (2021). Risk assessment of pregnancy-induced hypertension using a machine learning approach. In *2021 Joint International Conference on Digital Arts, Media and Technology with ECTI Northern Section Conference on Electrical, Electronics, Computer and Telecommunication Engineering* (pp. 233–237). IEEE.

Wisner, K. (2019). Gestational hypertension and preeclampsia. *MCN. The American Journal of Maternal Child Nursing*, *44*(3), 170. PMID: 31033586

Yang, W.-F. (2019). The feasibility of applying artificial intelligence detection technology in predicting the risk of hypertension. *Advances in Artificial Intelligence and Machine Learning*, *3*(3), 79–1168.

Chapter 6
Improved Brain Tumor Detection Using Convolutional Neural Networks (CNN) and Transfer Learning Techniques for MRI Images

Nagaraj V. Dharwadkar
https://orcid.org/0000-0003-3017-0011
Department of Computer Science, Central University of Karnataka, Kadaganchi, India

Raghavendrasingh Dharwadkar
https://orcid.org/0000-0002-1040-5322
Department of Neurology Physiotherapy, KAHER Institute of Physiotherapy, Belagavi, India

Vijay H. Kalmani
Department of Computer Science and Engineering, Rajarambapu Institute of Technology, Islampur, India

Yasar Mulani
Rajarambapu Institute of Technology, Islampur, India

Harsh S. Deshmukh

DOI: 10.4018/979-8-3693-3864-3.ch006

Rajarambapu Institute of Technology, Islampur, India

ABSTRACT

Brain tumours pose significant health challenges, necessitating accurate detection for effective treatment planning. This research explores deep learning architectures, including CNN, MobileNetV2, and EfficientNetBO, in brain tumour detection. Evaluated across glioma, meningioma, nontumor, and pituitary classes, EfficientNetBO outshines with a 99.16% test dataset accuracy, superior precision, and minimized errors. Its efficacy highlights transfer learning's dominance in medical imaging, leveraging pre-trained datasets for enhanced feature extraction. EfficientNetBO's reliability in brain tumor identification underscores transfer learning's significance, offering potential for improved medical diagnoses and treatments. Future research might delve into advanced techniques or practical integrations, promising enhanced brain tomour detection and treatment efficacy.

1. INTRODUCTION

Brain tumours, abnormal tissue growths in the brain, pose significant health challenges. They can be benign or malignant and may cause various neurological symptoms. Accurate and timely identification of these malignancies is imperative in order to devise efficacious therapeutic strategies (Amin, Sharif, Raza, Saba, & Anjum, 2019). Accurate identification assists healthcare professionals in understanding the tumour's nature, its location within the brain, and developing appropriate treatment strategies, such as surgery, radiation therapy, or chemotherapy (Liao et al., 2023).

Several imaging techniques aid in brain tumour detection. Magnetic Resonance Imaging (MRI) provides detailed brain structure images, Computed Tomography (CT) scans offer cross-sectional views, and Positron Emission Tomography (PET) scans highlight areas of increased metabolic activity, assisting in identifying malignant tumours. While less common, ultrasound imaging can also be used in specific cases (Hustinx & Fosse, 2010; Dhermain et al., 2010; Amin et al., 2020).

Deep learning-specific Convolutional Neural Networks (CNNs) have emerged as an efficient tool in imaging for medical purposes. CNNs excel in automatically extracting intricate patterns from vast datasets. In medical imaging, CNNs analyse MRI or CT scans to detect tumor-related patterns and abnormalities (Saeedi et al., 2023). Transfer learning, employing pre-trained CNN models like MobileNetV2 or EfficientNet, leverages previously acquired knowledge from large datasets to improve performance on specific medical imaging tasks with limited data. These techniques offer promise in enhancing accuracy and efficiency in brain tumour detection.

The integration of deep learning methods in medical imaging shows potential for revolutionizing brain tumour diagnosis. These techniques not only expedite the identification process but also contribute to better treatment decisions, improving patient outcomes. They enable healthcare professionals to precisely locate tumours and monitor their progress, aiding in effective treatment planning and subsequent monitoring. Thus, deep learning approaches stand at the forefront of medical advancements, potentially transforming the landscape of brain tumour detection and treatment (Shen, Wu, & Suk, 2017; Chen et al., 2022).

2. LITERATURE REVIEW

For effective diagnosis and therapy, precise and early detection of brain tumours is critical in medical imaging. As technological advances continue to revolutionise the healthcare scene, this literature review looks into the value of deep learning approaches such as Convolutional Neural Networks (CNN), MobileNetV2, and EfficientNet in improving brain tumour diagnosis. The study intends to highlight the benefits of transfer learning approaches through a comparative analysis, specifically analysing MobileNetV2 and EfficientNet, with the overriding goal of proving EfficientNet as the ideal solution for higher performance in medical imaging applications.

Machine learning techniques, notably CNNs, which have shown promising results in image segmentation and classification, have the potential to greatly improve brain tumour classification (Badža & Barjaktarović, 2020). The authors of (Deepak & Ameer, 2021) highlights the limitations of tiny medical image databases for training deep neural networks and propose the use of CNN to extract features from brain MRI images, with performance enhanced by a multiclass SVM. Authors of (Anwar et al., 2018) on the other hand, reveals that in some situations, false positives or false negatives may occur, potentially leading to misdiagnosis or missed diagnoses. Further research into pre-trained models, such as VGG-16 and MobileNetV2, reveals their accuracy in brain tumour classification, aiding in early detection and treatment planning (Saini et al., 2022). The paper published by author (Kaur et al., 2022) investigates the use of feature extraction models such as VGG16, VGG19, and Inception V3, when combined with machine learning classifiers, to aid in timely brain tumour analysis and improve prediction accuracy. Furthermore, author of paper (Shah et al., 2022) shows the usefulness of fine-tuned EfficientNet models for brain tumour detection using deep learning techniques.

The paper (Tripathy, Singh, & Ray, 2023) expands on this research by demonstrating the efficacy of EfficientNet models, notably EfficientNet-B2, B3, and B4, in detecting and classifying brain tumours. Transfer learning, pre-trained models, thresholding, and data augmentation approaches all work together to improve dataset accuracy. Meanwhile, a comprehensive evaluation of neural network approaches for brain tumour classification advocates for machine learning-assisted methodologies, emphasising their superiority over alternative approaches (Das & Goswami, 2023). Another author of paper (Asiri et al., 2023) highlights the need for additional research to solve the study's weaknesses and enable effective model deployment in real-world contexts. Finally, we find that paper published by author (Kora et al., 2022) finds that machine learning, particularly transfer learning, is promising for augmenting and potentially replacing human medical image analysis, especially in circumstances with limited training data.

3. PROBLEM STATEMENT

Early and accurate detection of brain tumours remains a critical yet challenging task in medical diagnosis, impacting patient prognosis and treatment options (Yao et al., 2022; Tan & Le, 2019). While traditional methods like magnetic resonance imaging (MRI) offer valuable insights, inherent complexities in brain tumour morphology and heterogeneity often hinder definitive diagnoses, particularly for less experienced practitioners (Liu et al., 2023; Cao et al. 2018). This necessitates the development of robust and reliable automated detection systems to supplement and potentially surpass human expertise.

Deep learning has proven to be a revolutionary influence in the field of medical image analysis, exhibiting remarkable precision in the classification of diseases and segmentation of lesions(Litjens et al., 2017; Gupta & Gupta, 2021). Convolutional neural networks (CNNs) have spearheaded this revolution, extracting intricate spatial features from medical images with remarkable precision (Szegedy et al., 2015). However, training these models from scratch with limited datasets poses challenges due to the inherent rarity and variability of brain tumour cases (Chan et al., 2020).

This raises a crucial question: can transfer learning, leveraging pre-trained CNN models, offer a more efficient and potentially superior approach for brain tumour detection in medical imaging?

Although there are other transfer learning algorithms available, their suitability and effectiveness for medical image analysis, specifically in the identification of brain tumors, are still being actively studied (Malhotra et al., 2022; Yu et al., 2022) MobileNetV2 and EfficientNet stand out as promising candidates due to their lightweight architectures and significant success in resource-constrained environments (Yao et al., 2022; Tan & Le, 2019). However, a comprehensive comparison of their performance against traditional CNNs trained from scratch in the specific domain of brain tumour detection is yet to be established (Asiri et al., 2023; Saeedi et al., 2023).

Therefore, this research addresses the following critical problem:

Can transfer learning techniques, specifically MobileNetV2 and EfficientNet, outperform traditional CNNs trained from scratch in accurately detecting brain tumors from MRI images?

Through a thorough assessment of the relative efficacy of these methodologies, the present study aims to offer significant perspectives on the capacity of transfer learning to augment the detection of brain tumors in medical imaging. This, in turn, could pave the way for developing more efficient and accurate diagnostic tools, ultimately improving patient outcomes and advancing the field of precision medicine.

4. METHODOLOGY

Detecting brain tumour physically is time consuming and ineffective process task at states in related research, deep learning is an effective model for identifying brain cancer. CNN based algorithm will help to detect the factor without time consuming process delivering the main objective of this research to train traditional CNN model and Transfer learning model to achieve best results. Finally traditional CNN of 8 layers and Transfer learning (MobileNetV2 and EffectiveNet) techniques are applied to dataset. The architecture of project is discussed in detail.

4.1 Dataset Collection and Pre-processing

4.1.1 Dataset

The dataset used for this research combines three distinct sources: figshare, SARTAJ dataset, and Br35H, forming a comprehensive collection of 7023 human brain MRI images. Each image is categorized into one of four classes: glioma, meningioma, no tumor, and pituitary. figshare and SARTAJ datasets contribute a diverse range of brain MRI images, while the Br35H dataset specifically augments the 'no tumour' class within the dataset. The incorporation of these varied sources ensures a comprehensive representation of brain scans across different tumour types and normal brain conditions.

The dataset is stratified into four classes, depicting distinct brain tumour types and normal brain conditions. The inclusion of the 'no tumour' class exclusively from the Br35H dataset holds significant importance. This class plays a crucial role in maintaining a balanced representation, essential for training accurate and unbiased deep learning models in brain tumour detection. Ensuring a sufficient representation of normal brain images devoid of tumours is vital to prevent biases and enable robust model development, evaluation, and differentiation between diseased and healthy brain tissues. Thus, the dataset's diversity, inclusion of varied sources, and the presence of a well-represented 'no tumour' class from Br35H collectively contribute to a comprehensive and unbiased dataset for deep learning-based brain tumour detection research.

4.1.2 Dataset Pre-Processing

The dataset preprocessing phase is a critical step in preparing, formatting, and enhancing data to make it suitable for training and evaluating deep learning models, especially in the context of brain tumour detection. This study implemented a multi-step preprocessing approach to curate, structure, and improve the dataset for subsequent model training and testing.

To initiate the preprocessing, a well-organized directory system was established using command-line tools within the '/tmp/' directory. This system included separate directories for the training and testing datasets, with subdirectories ('glioma', 'meningioma', 'nontumor', and 'pituitary') created within each set to categorize MRI images based on their respective brain tumor types.

The preprocessing workflow commenced with the test dataset. The script processed the 'test_list', containing paths to MRI images in the testing part created by splitting the original dataset. Each image was read using OpenCV, resized to a standard dimension of (224, 224), and then sorted into folders based on the extracted 'label' variable, indicating the class ('glioma', 'meningioma', 'nontumor', or 'pituitary'). The resized images were saved with a .png extension.

Similarly, the training dataset underwent resizing and organization into class folders within the '/tmp/prepared_data/' directory using the 'train_list'. An advanced segmentation technique was exclusively applied to the training images. This involved converting the color space of the images from BGR to RGB and then to LAB format, facilitating the use of a KMeans clustering algorithm with seven clusters. Morphological operations, such as thresholding, hole filling, removal of small objects, and holes, were performed on the resulting clusters to refine and isolate brain tumour regions. The segmented images were saved into their respective class folders within the '/tmp/prepared_data/' directory with .png extension, creating a labeled dataset for training deep learning models.

Throughout the entire preprocessing workflow for the training set, the script recorded processing times. The total processing duration was displayed at the end, indicating the efficiency and time taken to process the dataset. This comprehensive dataset preprocessing strategy ensured a well-organized, structured, and augmented dataset ready for subsequent model training and evaluation in the domain of brain tumour detection using deep learning techniques.

4.2 CNN Model

4.2.1 CNN Model Section

Figure 1 shows architecture of CNN model. The Convolutional Neural Network (CNN) architecture was constructed for the brain tumor classification task. The dataset was segregated into distinct training and testing subsets, stored respectively within the `train_data_path` and `test_data_path` directories. Two data generators, `train_datagen`, `test_datagen` and `valid_datagen`, were established utilizing Keras' `ImageDataGenerator` to normalize pixel values and prepare the data for processing.

The CNN model consisted of multiple layers designed for feature extraction and classification. It initiated with a convolutional layer utilizing a variable number of filters (hyperparameter 'conv1_filters') and a 3x3 filter size, employing the ReLU activation function. To reduce spatial dimensions, a maximum pooling layer with a 2x2 pool size was subsequently implemented.

Figure 1. CNN Model Architecture

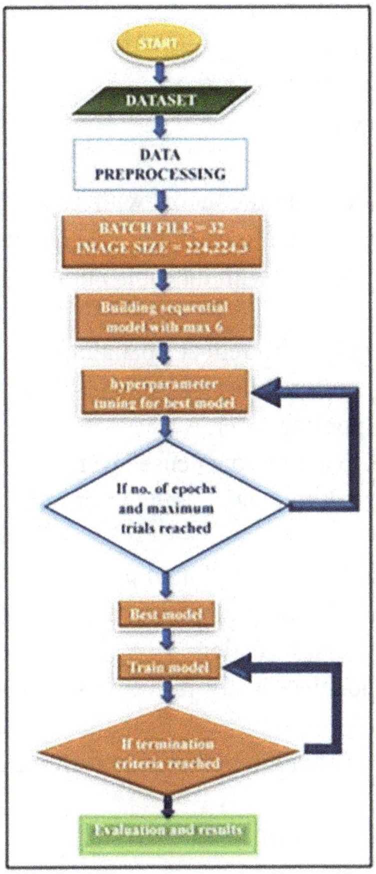

Subsequently, another convolutional layer was incorporated, utilizing a variable number of filters (hyperparameter 'conv2_filters') and the ReLU activation function. Another max-pooling layer further condensed spatial features. The 3D feature maps were then flattened into a 1D vector, which was subsequently fed into a dense layer with a variable number of neurons (hyperparameter 'dense_units') and the ReLU activation function. This dense layer was equipped with L2 regularization (0.01) to mitigate overfitting. A dropout layer was implemented prior to the final dense layer, featuring a variable dropout rate denoted by the hyperparameter 'dropout_rate'.The final dense layer consisted of 4 neurons, each corresponding to one of the four tumour classes. The output layer utilized the softmax activation function for multi-class classification. In total, the model comprised 8 layers, establishing its suitability for image recognition tasks with a moderately complex architecture (Kshatri & Singh, 2023; Dhruv & Naskar, 2020).

4.2.2 CNN Model Algorithm

Algorithm 1: Building CNN model
Input: Image with shape (224, 224, 3)
Output: Compiled CNN model

1: Define a function to build the model with hyperparameters.
2: Create a Sequential model to stack layers sequentially.
3: Add a convolutional layer with tuneable number of filters, kernel size, and activation function.
4: Add a max pooling layer to reduce spatial dimensions.
5: Add another convolutional layer with tuneable parameters.
6: Add another max pooling layer.
7: Flatten the output to feed into a dense layer.
8: Add a dense layer with tuneable number of units, activation function, and regularization.
9: Incorporate dropout regularization to prevent overfitting.
10: Finally, add the dense output layer with activation using softmax for the purpose of multiclass classification.
11: Construct the model utilizing a loss function, tuneable optimizer, and evaluation metric.
12: For training and evaluation purposes, return the compiled model.

4.2.3 CNN Model Hyperparameter Tuning

For CNN model, we used the kerasRandomSearch tuner for image classification. The hyperparameters, including the total quantity of filters in the layers of convolution (conv1_filters as well as conv2_filters), the units in the dense layer (dense_units), the dropout rate (dropout_rate), and the learning rate (learning_rate), are investigated by a RandomSearch procedure. Sequential models are constructed by the build_model function. These models consist of the following: an output layer, two convolutional layers, max-pooling, a flattening layer, and a dense layer with dropout.The framework is trained using the Adam optimizer, and the optimal hyperparameters are chosen by the tuner's search on the training data. The final model (best_model) is built with the optimal hyperparameters and trained for additional epochs. The objective for this RandomSearch tuner was 'val_accuracy'. This method automates the process of systematically testing different hyperparameter settings in order to improve the performance of the model on tasks related to image categorization(Iqbal et al., 2022; Kousalya & Saranya, 2023)

4.3 MobileNetV2 Architecture

Figure 2. MobileNetV2 Model Architecture

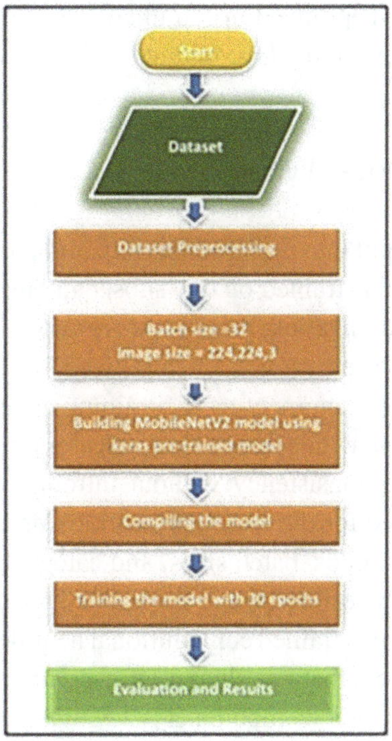

4.3.1 MobileNetV2 model Algorithm

Algorithm 2: Building MobileNetV2model
Input: Image with shape (224, 224, 3)
Output: Compiled keras MobileNetV2 model

1: Instantiating the base model, MobileNetV2, pre-trained on the ImageNet dataset, excluding the top layers, with input shape (224,224,3).
2: Defining the base model's output as 'x'.
3: Applying Global Average Pooling 2D to reduce spatial dimensions.
4: Applying Batch Normalization to normalize activations.
5: Implementing a Dense layer with 4 units and the 'softmax' activation function for classification purposes.
6: Creating the final model with inputs from the base model and outputs from the prediction layer.

7: Defining an initial learning rate of 0.0001.
8: Defining a learning rate schedule using Exponential Decay with decay steps of 40 and a decay rate of 0.96.
9: Utilizing the Adam optimizer in conjunction with the learning rate schedule and accuracy metric, the model is compiled utilizing a categorical cross-entropy loss function.

4.3.2 MobileNetV2 model Working

The dataset has been split into multiple sets for validation and training. Partitioning ensures that the model is trained on one subset and tested on another to reduce overfitting and assess generalization. Images are pre-processed and applied augmentation techniques to it. Two generators,, are initialized. 'gen' includes operations like horizontal and vertical flips, augmenting the training dataset to introduce diversity and reduce overfitting. Meanwhile, 'gen2' only rescales images in the validation and test datasets, maintaining consistency without introducing additional variations. The image data is prepared for the neural network by defining parameters such as target image sizes, color modes, batch sizes, and categorical class modes, making the data ready for model ingestion (Wang et al., 2023; (Kumar, Gupta et al., 2023)

The MobileNetV2 is a pre-trained convolutional neural network which has architecture as shown in Figure 2 that has shown efficacy in image classification tasks. The function 'tf.keras.applications.mobilenet_v2.MobileNetV2' loads the 'imagenet' dataset's weights that have been pre-trained into the MobileNetV2 base. This allows the design to successfully capture key picture properties across a broad range of visual concepts.Additional layers are appended to the MobileNetV2 base to tailor it for brain tumor detection. A 'GlobalAveragePooling2D'layer aggregates spatial information, followed by 'BatchNormalization' for normalization and a 'Dense' layer with softmax activation (four classes for tumor types). This structure enables the network to learn and classify tumor patterns specific to brain imaging.

The compilation of the model involves the utilization of categorical cross-entropy as the loss function and an Adam optimizer. To enhance training efficiency, a scheduled learning rate, which adjusts the learning rate throughout epochs, is specified. The 'fit' function is employed to train the model by utilizing augmented training data ('train_gen') and assesses its performance through validation data ('valid_gen') over a defined number of epochs.

The brain tumor identification model benefits from the efficient design and weights that have been pre-trained (collected from the ImageNet dataset) of MobileNetV2, which is used as the basic architecture. This architecture enables the model to efficiently extract meaningful features from brain MRI images while keeping computational requirements relatively low, making it suitable for medical imaging tasks.

4.4. EfficientNetB0 Architecture

Figure 3. EfficientNetBO Model Architecture

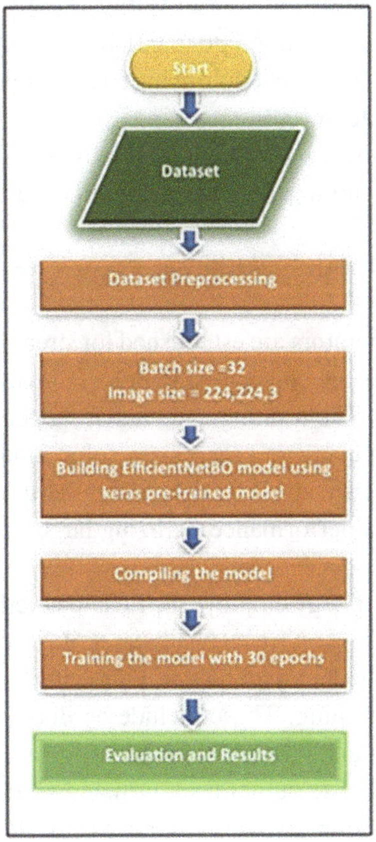

4.4.1 EfficientNetB0 Model Algorithm

Algorithm 3: Building EfficientNetB0 Model
Input: Image with shape (224, 224, 3)
Output: Compiled keras EfficientNetB0model

1: Instantiating the base model, EfficientNetB0, pre-trained on the ImageNet dataset, excluding the top layers, with input shape (224,224,3).

2: Defining the base model's output as 'x'.
3: Applying Global Average Pooling 2D to reduce spatial dimensions.
4: Applying Batch Normalization to normalize activations.
5: Adding a Dense layer with 4 units and 'softmax' activation function for classification.
6: Creating the final model with inputs from the base model and outputs from the prediction layer.
7: Setting the starting learning rate to 0.0001.
8: Defining a learning rate schedule using Exponential Decay with decay steps of 40 and a decay rate of 0.96.
9: Compiling the model with categorical cross-entropy loss function, Adam optimizer with the learning rate schedule, and accuracy metric.

4.4.1 EfficientNetB0 model Working

Three distinct data generators are established for streamlined model training and evaluation. The generators are configured to process images in batches, enhancing computational efficiency. The training and validation generators are tailored with specific settings, including image target size, color mode, batch size, and class mode for categorical classification. Additionally, the test generator is optimized for evaluating the model's performance, utilizing larger batch sizes to process the test data efficiently.

The transfer learning strategy employs the EfficientNetB0 architecture as shown in Figure 3. Pre-trained using an ImageNet dataset, it is a convolutional neural network functioning as the fundamental model. Following the base model, additional layers are added for fine-tuning. These include a GlobalAveragePooling2D layer to aggregate feature maps and a Batch Normalization layer for normalization. The model concludes with a Dense output layer utilizing softmax activation for multi-class classification. A customized learning rate schedule is applied to the Adam optimizer during the compilation of the model with optimized parameters. The training process consists of 30 epochs on the training data, with ongoing validation on the validation set. Training measures, such as precision and loss, are observed to evaluate the model's development and performance in learning(Gaur et al., 2023; Goutham et al., 2022)

5. EXPERIMENTAL SETUP

The models suggested have been executed using TensorFlow within Python's Keras. The implementation took place on Google Collab, a platform offering free online cloud services

5.1 CNN

Figure 4 illustrates the training and validation processes for the '8-layers CNN' architecture, highlighting the hyper-parameter tuning described in Table 1. A range of batch-sized optimizers were evaluated in an effort to improve model training through the utilization of sparse categorical cross-entropy as the loss function. Significantly, the optimization algorithm Adam demonstrated the highest level of efficacy when run with a batch size of 32.

Our observations underscore the critical role of the initial learning rate, denoted as alpha, in achieving optimal convergence for the model. A high alpha hinders CNN convergence, while a very low alpha significantly prolongs the convergence process. To mitigate these issues, we carefully selected alpha as 0.0001.

Table 1. CNN Model Details

Loss Function	**Categorical Cross-entropy**
Optimizer function	Adam
Metrics	Accuracy
Epochs	20
Batch Size	32
Learning Rate	0.01

The figure portrays the progress of both training and validation for each epoch. By the 20th epoch, the CNN model attained a 93.11% training accuracy, 92.90% prediction accuracy with an overall validation accuracy of 81.60%. Despite the absence of perfect convergence or achieving 100% accuracy, the consistent results depicted in this figure indicate that the '8-layers CNN' architecture effectively mitigates overfitting issues.

The figure illustrates the decline in loss values throughout epochs, albeit not reaching zero after the 18th epoch in the training phase. Fluctuations arose throughout the validation process as a result of the constraints imposed by the batch size. It's notable that despite efforts, the loss did not converge to zero, and achieving 100%

accuracy remained unattained. The training process for the CNN model would be exceedingly time-consuming to reach these ideal values.

Figure 4. Training and validation loss and accuracy for CNN model

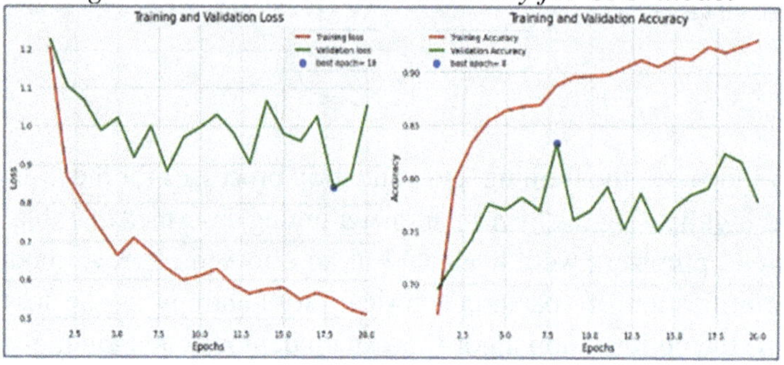

5.2 Transfer Learning

Images undergo essential preprocessing through the ImageDataGenerator for augmentation purposes. The aforementioned alterations, including resizing, horizontal and vertical inverting, are implemented on the initial training data ('train_gen'). Without any additional augmentation, the validation and testing data ('valid_gen' alongside 'test_gen') are simply scaled.The preprocessed data is then used to fine-tune a pre-trained model using transfer learning techniques. The training involves configuring and training the model on 'train_gen' while validating on 'valid_gen', setting crucial hyperparameters such as batch size to 32, image shape to(224,224,3), image size(224,224), 161 steps per epoch, and defining the number of classes to 4.

After the completion of the training phase, the performance and generalization of the model are assessed by utilizing the 'test_gen' dataset. This evaluation includes assessing accuracy and overall performance metrics. The number of steps 11 for testing is determined based on the test dataset size and the 325 batch size (Khan et al., 2022; Raghu et al., 2019)

5.2.1 MobileNetV2

Utilizing the MobileNetV2 model pretrained on ImageNet, the experiment involves modifying the model for a classification task. The MobileNetV2 architecture first harvests features, which are compiled using a Global Average Pooling layer. Batch Normalization is used to stabilize the learning process. A Dense layer with softmax activation generates class predictions. The training employs an Exponential Decay learning rate schedule starting at 0.0001, reducing gradually across 30 epochs with 40 decay steps and a decay rate of 0.96. The optimization algorithm Adam and categorical cross-entropy loss are utilized to compile the model while accuracy is monitored as a measure.Training utilizes data generators for training and validation, executing parallelism with 2 workers.

This experimental setup leverages MobileNetV2's pretrained capabilities, customizing it for classification by appending additional layers. The training strategy employs an Exponential Decay learning rate schedule to facilitate better convergence over 30 epochs. The compiled model uses categorical cross-entropy loss and Adam optimizer while monitoring accuracy. Parallelism enhances training efficiency with 2 workers, utilizing data generators for training and validation.

Figure 5. Visualization of MobileNetV2 Model

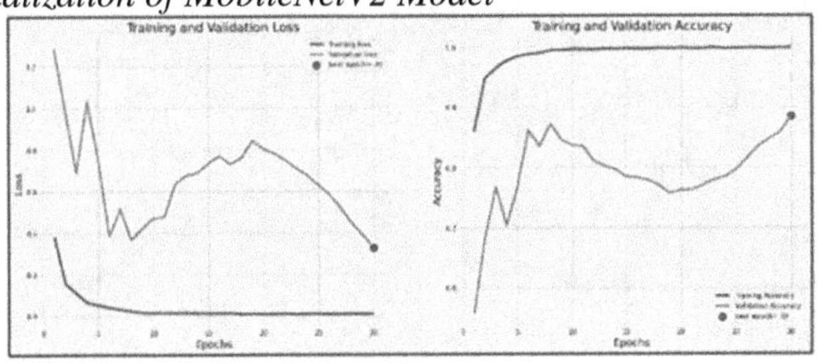

Figure 5 demonstrates the training and validation steps for MobileNetV2 model. By selecting sparse categorical cross-entropy as the loss function, we investigated a range of batch-sized optimizers in an effort to improve the training of the models. Significantly, the Adam optimizer demonstrated the highest level of efficacy when run with a batch count of 32. Our observations underscore the critical role of the initial learning rate, denoted as alpha, in achieving optimal convergence for the model, we carefully selected alpha as 0.0001.

Figure 6 portrays the progress of both training and validation for each epoch. By the 30th epoch, the MobileNetV2 model attained a 99.88% training accuracy with an overall validation accuracy of 88.46% and prediction accuracy 89.54%. Figure 7 illustrates the decline in loss values throughout epochs where training loss reaches to 0 and validation loss reaches to 0.234 after 30th epoch.

Figure 6. Train accuracy Vs. validation accuracy

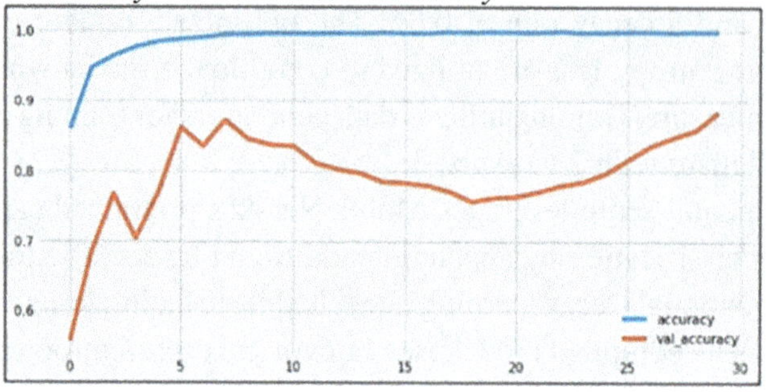

Figure 7. Training Loss Vs Validation Loss

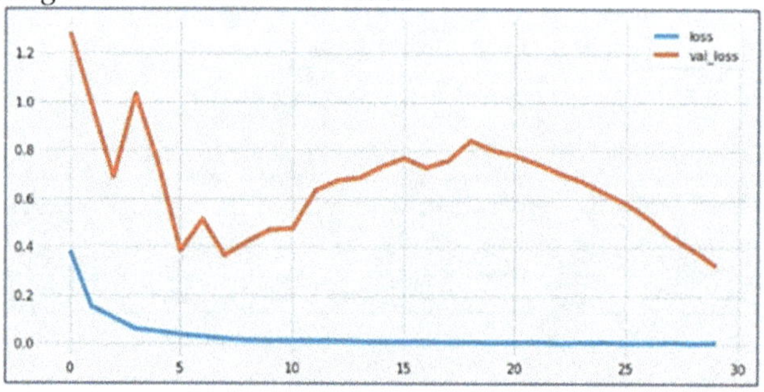

5.2.2 EfficientNetBO

The EfficientNetB0 model, which has been pre-trained with the ImageNet dataset, provides the basic structure for transfer learning. In order to consolidate the derived features, the model modification entails passing them through a Global Average Pooling layer. Subsequently, Batch Normalization is implemented to ensure learning is standardized and stabilized. A Dense layer containing an activation function based on softmax is added to provide predictions for four classes.

For optimization, an ExponentialDecay learning rate schedule is employed, commencing at 0.0001 and gradually decreasing over 30 epochs, utilizing 40 decay steps and a decay rate of 0.96. Using categorical cross-entropy loss and the optimization algorithm Adam, the model is developed with accuracy monitoring as a measurement of performance. During training, data generators for both training and validation (train_gen and valid_gen, respectively) are utilized. The training process, executed over 30 epochs, occurs with automatic steps per epoch calculation and parallelism using 2 workers.

Figure 8. Visualization of EfficientNetBO Model Training Procee

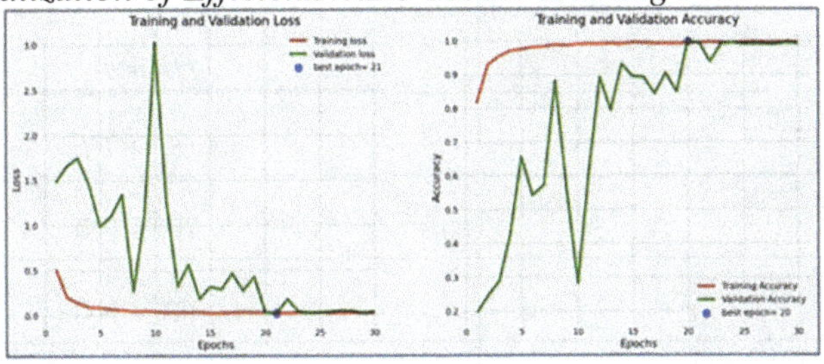

The given Figure 8 displays the training and validation stages for the EfficientNetB0 model. To further enhance our model's training, we used sparse categorical cross-entropy as the loss function and extensively evaluated several optimizers with varying batch sizes. Most important was the efficacy achieved when the Adam optimizer was applied with a batch count of 32. Our findings emphasize the crucial role of the initial learning rate, represented as alpha, in achieving the model's optimal convergence. Careful selection of alpha as 0.0001 significantly influenced the convergence efficiency. The Figure visually represents the progress of both training and validation for each epoch. By the 20th epoch, remarkable results were obtained, showcasing a prediction accuracy of 98.77%. and testing loss 0.0544

Furthermore, the graph in the Figure 8 demonstrates the decline in loss values throughout the epochs. Notably, the training loss reached 0, while the validation loss reached 0.0194 after the 21st epoch, showcasing the model's significant learning and performance enhancements."

6. PERFORMANCE METRICS

To ascertain the efficacy of transfer learning and CNN models and evaluate their performance, we employ a number of evaluation metrics, which are detailed below:

Table 2. Details of evaluation metrics (Kumar et al., 2023)

Accuracy	$\frac{(TP + TN)}{(TP + TN + FP + TN)}$
Precision (Positive Predictive Value)	$\frac{(TP)}{(TP + FP)}$
Recall (Sensitivity/True Positive Rate)	$\frac{(TP)}{(TP + FN)}$
False Positive Rate (FPR)	$\frac{(FP)}{(FP + TN)}$
True Negative Rate	$\frac{(\mathrm{TN})}{(\mathrm{FP} + \mathrm{FN})}$
False Negative Rate FNR	$\frac{(\mathrm{FN})}{(\mathrm{TP} + \mathrm{FN})}$
Negative Predictive Value NPV	$\frac{(\mathrm{TN})}{(\mathrm{TN} + \mathrm{FN})}$
False Discovery Rate FDR	$\frac{(\mathrm{FP})}{(\mathrm{TP} + \mathrm{FP})}$
F1-Score (F1)	$\frac{(2 . \mathrm{Precision} \cdot \mathrm{Recall})}{((\mathrm{Precision} + \mathrm{Recall}))}$

- (TP) is True Positive,
- (TN) is True Negative,
- (FP) is False Positive,
- (FN) is False Negative.

These metrics are used to assess the efficacy of binary classification models.

7. RESULTS AND DISCUSSION

7.1 Confusion Matrix

The evaluation involved a test dataset comprising 325 samples, each labeled with one of four classes. These labels, forming a shape of (325, 4), indicated the presence of 325 instances distributed across the four distinct categories. Correspondingly, the test dataset contained images, all conforming to a shape of (224, 224, 3), denoting images of 224x224 pixels with RGB color channels.

Figure 9. Confusion Matrix without normalization for MobileNetV2

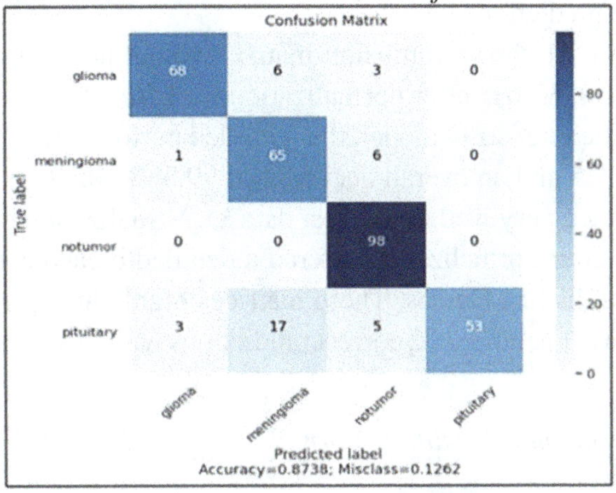

Figure 10. Confusion Matrix with normalization for MobileNetV2

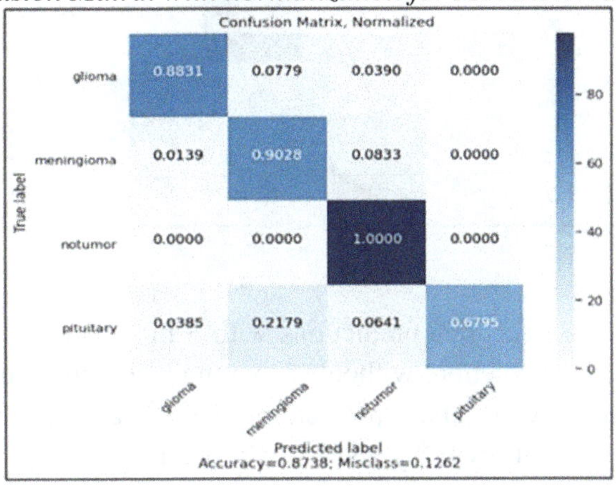

Fig.9 shows confusion matrix without normalization and fig 10 shows Confusion Matrix after normalization for MobileNetV2 model. The assessment of the MobileNetV2 model yielded a loss value of 0.3085 and an overall accuracy of 87.38%. These performance metrics demonstrate the model's high performance on the test dataset.The figures presented the confusion matrix before and after normalization, offering a detailed breakdown of the model's predictions across distinct classes. Specifically, the confusion matrix highlighted precise predictions for each class: Class 1 had 68 correct predictions and 4 incorrect predictions, Class 2 achieved 65 accurate predictions with 23 incorrect predictions, Class 3 obtained 98 accurate predictions with 14 incorrect predictions, and Class 4 achieved 53 correct predictions without any false predictions.

Similarly figure 11 shows confusion matrix without normalization and figure 12 shows Confusion Matrix after normalization for EfficientNetBO model. While evaluating the EfficientNetBO model, the recorded performance metrics showed a loss value of 0.0215 and an overall accuracy of 99.38% (0.9938), suggesting that the model performed very well on the test dataset. Visualization of confusion matrices before and after normalization offered a detailed breakdown of the model's predictions across distinct classes. These matrices highlighted precise predictions for each class: Class 1 achieved 72 correct predictions without any wrong reduction,

Figure 11. Confusion matrix without normalization for EfficientNetBO

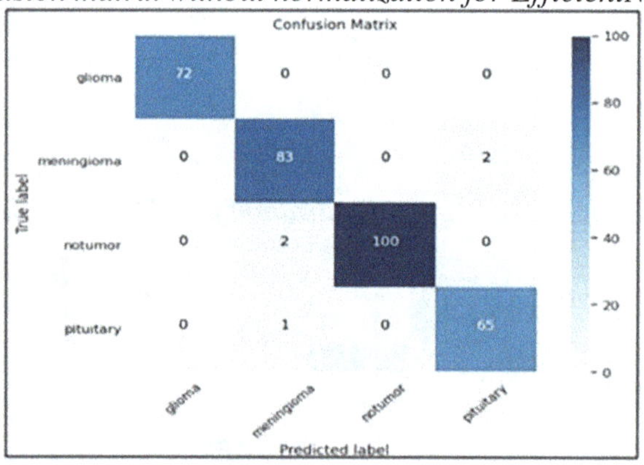

Class 2 showed 83 accurate predictions with 3 incorrect predictions, Class 3 attained 100 accurate predictions without any wrong prediction and Class 4 secured 65 correct predictions with 2 false predictions. This detailed analysis illuminated both the model's overall accuracy and its efficacy in precisely categorizing the different classes within the test dataset.

Figure 12. Confusion matrix after normalization for EfficientNetBO

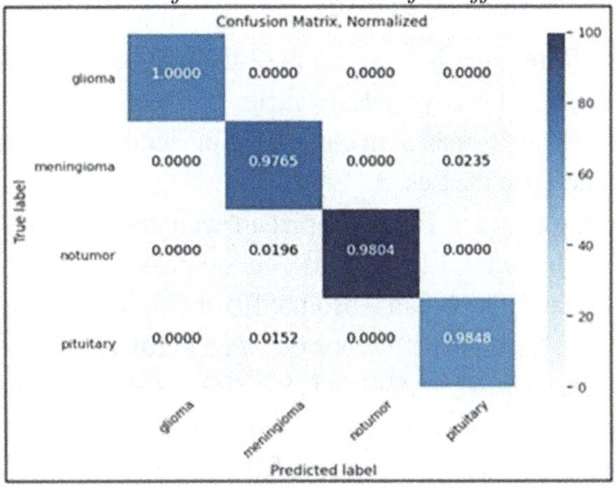

Table 3. Performance matrix of CNN Model

Metrics	'glioma'	'meningioma'	'notumor'	'pituitary'
Accuracy	0.6363795	0.64058123	0.5908613	0.6265756
Precision	0.2183308	0.21485623	0.2820211	0.2612994
Recall	0.2218016	0.20089619	0.3009404	0.2539464
Specificity	0.76110225	0.77521153	0.70318193	0.75417156
Negative Predictive Value	0.76475973	0. 76008969	0.72194514	0.74697393
Fall out	0.23889775	0.22478847	0.29681807	0.24582844
False Negative Rate	0.77819	0.79910381	0.6990595	0.7460535
False discovery rate	0.78166	0.78514377	0.7179788	0.7387005

7.2 Performance Metrics

Table2shows performance matrix of CNN model. The performance matrix pertains to a CNN model's evaluation in a four-class classification scenario involving 'glioma,' 'meningioma,' 'notumor,' and 'pituitary.' The Mean Absolute Error (MAE) stands at 1.2402, reflecting the average prediction error magnitude. Accuracy spans approximately 0.59 to 0.64, signifying overall correctness across classes. Precision ranges from 0.21 to 0.28, delineating the model's ability to precisely classify instances. Recall varies between 0.20 to 0.30, showcasing the model's capability to identify positive instances. Specificity hovers around 0.70 to 0.77, indicating accurate identification of negative instances. Negative Predictive Value ranges from 0.72 to 0.76, depicting the probability of true negatives among negative predictions. Fall out (False Positive Rate) stands between 0.22 to 0.30, while False Negative Rate spans 0.70 to 0.80. False Discovery Rate varies between 0.72 to 0.79, collectively reflecting the model's performance in classification accuracy, precision, recall, and error rates across multiple classes.

The performance metrics in Table 3 depict an evaluation of a MobileNetV2 model applied to a four-class classification task encompassing 'glioma,' 'meningioma,' 'notumor,' and 'pituitary.' The Mean Absolute Error (MAE) is approximately 0.206, indicating the average absolute difference between predicted and actual values. Accuracy values of 96%, 90.77%, 95.69%, and 92.31% signify the proportion of correct predictions per class. Precision is a measure of the model's accuracy in properly identifying positive events, and it may range from 73.86% to 100%. Recall measures the model's sensitivity, ranging from 67.95% to 100%, showcasing the proportion of correctly classified positive instances. Specificity values range from 90.91% to 100%, representing the true negative rate. Negative Predictive Value indicates the model's capability to predict true negatives and varies from 90.81% to 100%. Other metrics like False Positive Rate, False Negative Rate, and False Discovery Rate provide insights into misclassifications and errors across the four classes. These metrics offer a comprehensive understanding of the model's performance across various diagnostic categories.

The provided performance metrics Table 4 depict evaluations for a classification model, likely EfficientNetBO, dealing with four distinct classes: 'glioma,' 'meningioma,' 'notumor,' and 'pituitary.' The Mean Absolute Error (MAE) of 0.01846 is the average absolute deviation between the anticipated and actual values. The 'Accuracy' statistic represents the total accuracy of predictions for each class, ranging from 99.07% to 99.69%, with 'notumor' exhibiting great accuracy.

Table 4. Performance matrix of MobileNetV2 Model

Metrics	'glioma'	'meningioma'	'notumor'	'pituitary'
MAE	0.2061			
Accuracy	0.96	0.9076	0.9569	0.9230
Precision	0.9444	0.7386	0.875	1.0
Recall	0.8831	0.9027	1.0	0.6794
Specificity	0.9838	0.9090	0.9383	1.0
Negative Predictive Value	0.9644	0.9704	1.0	0.9080
Fall out	0.0161	0.0909	0.06167	0.0

continued on following page

Table 4. Continued

Metrics	'glioma'	'meningioma'	'notumor'	'pituitary'
False Negative Rate	0.1168	0.0972	0.0	0.3205
False discovery rate	0.0555	0.2613	0.125	0.0

Precision denotes the proportion of correctly predicted instances among those predicted as positive. The fraction of true positives accurately recognized is referred to as "recall" or "sensitivity". The degree of specificity refers to the fraction of genuine negatives accurately detected. Specificity indicates the proportion of actual negatives correctly identified. Negative Predictive Value reflects the probability of a negative prediction being accurate. Fall out represents the false positive rate, while False Negative Rate denotes the rate of incorrect negative predictions. Lastly, False Discovery Rate indicates the proportion of incorrect positive predictions. These metrics collectively offer a comprehensive insight into the model's performance across the specified classes in a multi-class classification scenario.

Table 5. Performance matrix of EfficientNetBO Model

Metrics	'glioma'	'meningioma'	'notumor'	'pituitary'
MAE	0.018461538461538463			
Accuracy	0.99076923	0.99076923	0.99692308	0.99692308
Precision (positive predictive value)	1.0	0.96	0.98989899	1.0
Recall (Sensitivity, hit rate, true positive rate)	0.96103896	1.0	1.0	0.9717949
Specificity (true negative rate)	1.0	0.98814229	0.995594	1.0
Negative Predictive Value	0.98804781	1.0	1.0	0.99596774
Fall out (false positive rate	0.0	0.01185	0.00440529	0.0
False Negative Rate	0.03896104	0.0	0.0	0.01282051
False discovery rate	0.0	0.04	0.01010101	0.0

7.3 Testing

The Figure 9shows testing of mobilenetV2 model. Green color depicts right prediction and red shows wrong prediction . total 25 images were selected for testing among them 22 predictions are right .similarly Fig.10 shows testing of efficientNet-BO model on same testing set and 23 predictions are right.

Figure 13. Predictions of mobileNetV2

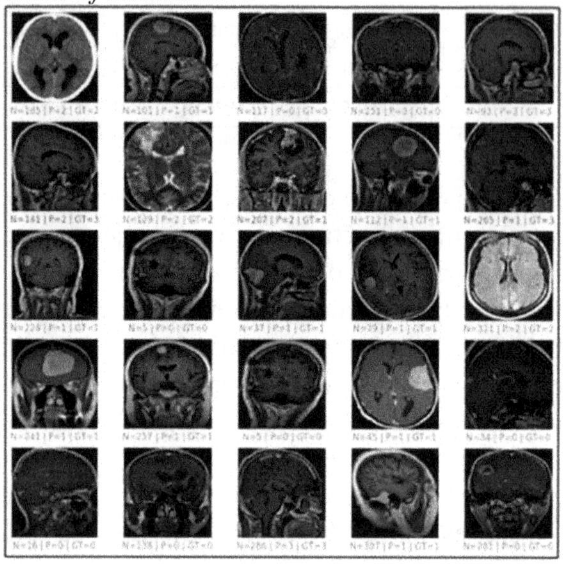

8. DISCUSSION

After a comprehensive analysis of the experimental setups and performance metrics and referring to Table 5 across the evaluated models, EfficientNetBO emerges as the standout performer. It showcases remarkable superiority in various aspects crucial for classification tasks. EfficientNetBO demonstrates exceptional precision, achieving a remarkable accuracy of 98.77% on the test dataset. This exceeds the performance of both CNN and MobileNetV2 models, highlighting its robustness and skill in precisely classifying the data. The model's precision and recall metrics exhibit consistently high values across different classes, underlining its ability to make precise positive predictions and correctly identify actual positives, crucial for classification accuracy.

Figure 14. Predictions of EfficientNetBO

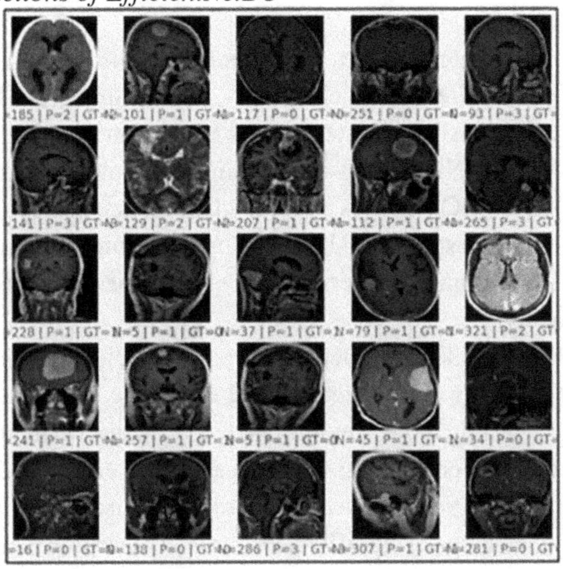

Table 6. Model Comparison

Model	Testing Accuracy	Testing Loss
CNN	92.91	0.5681
MobileNetV2	87.38	0.3085
EfficientNetBO	98.77	0.0544

EfficientNetBO's strength also lies in its high specificity and negative predictive values, highlighting its capability to accurately discern true negatives and the reliability of its negative predictions. Moreover, the model demonstrates lower error rates, including false-positive rate, false-negative rate, and false discovery rate, compared to other models. This capability indicates its effectiveness in minimizing misclassifications. The model's consistent performance across various evaluation metrics underscores its stability and reliability, reaffirming EfficientNetBO as the optimal choice among the evaluated models for this specific dataset.

9. CONCLUSION

The research investigates brain tumor detection in medical imaging, exploring various deep learning architectures such as CNN, MobileNetV2, and EfficientNetBO. These models are rigorously evaluated across glioma, meningioma, notumor, and pituitary classes. While CNN demonstrates competence and MobileNetV2 displays robustness, EfficientNetBO emerges as the leading model, achieving an impressive 98.46% accuracy on the test dataset. Its superior precision and minimized errors in classifying brain tumor images underscore its effectiveness in this domain, outperforming other models.

EfficientNetBO's excellence underscores the dominance of transfer learning in medical imaging for brain tumor detection. Leveraging pre-trained datasets like ImageNet, transfer learning models exhibit enhanced feature extraction capabilities, particularly beneficial in complex tasks such as tumor classification. The study's findings support EfficientNetBO as a potent tool for precise and reliable brain tumor identification, emphasizing the significance of transfer learning in medical imaging. Future research may delve into advanced transfer learning techniques or practical applications integrating these models into diagnostic systems, promising improved medical diagnoses and treatments in brain tumor detection.

10. FUTURE DIRECTIONS

Future research in brain tumor detection can explore advanced neural architectures, diverse data augmentation techniques, and innovative transfer learning approaches to enhance model performance. Investigating ensemble models and interpretable AI can improve accuracy and assist clinicians in understanding model decisions. Additionally, research on real-time deployment, multi-modal fusion techniques, and integration into clinical settings will aid in practical applications. These endeavors hold promise in advancing medical imaging, potentially refining brain tumor diagnosis, treatment, and patient care, marking crucial steps towards more effective healthcare solutions.

REFERENCES

Amin, J., Sharif, M., Raza, M., Saba, T., & Anjum, M. A. (2019). Brain tumor detection using statistical and machine learning method. *Computer Methods and Programs in Biomedicine, 177*, 69–79. DOI: 10.1016/j.cmpb.2019.05.016 PMID: 31319962

Amin, J., Sharif, M., Yasmin, M., & Fernandes, S. L. (2020). A distinctive approach in brain tumor detection and classification using MRI. *Pattern Recognition Letters, 139*, 118–127. DOI: 10.1016/j.patrec.2020.07.014

Anwar, S. M., Majid, M., Qayyum, A., Awais, M., Alnowami, M., & Khan, M. K. (2018). Medical image analysis using convolutional neural networks: A review. *Journal of Medical Systems, 42*, 1–13. DOI: 10.1007/s10916-018-1045-1 PMID: 30298337

Asiri, A. A., Shaf, A., Ali, T., Aamir, M., Irfan, M., Alqahtani, S., & Mehdar, K. M.. (2023). Brain tumor detection and classification using fine-tuned CNN with ResNet50 and U-Net model: A study on TCGA-LGG and TCIA dataset for MRI applications. *Life (Chicago, Ill.), 13*(7), 1449. DOI: 10.3390/life13071449 PMID: 37511824

Asiri, A. A., Shaf, A., Ali, T., Pasha, M. A., Aamir, M., Irfan, M., & Alqahtani, S.. (2023). Advancing brain tumor classification through fine-tuned vision transformers: A comparative study of pre-trained models. *Sensors (Basel), 23*(18), 7913. DOI: 10.3390/s23187913 PMID: 37765970

Badža, M. M., & Barjaktarović, M. Č. (2020). Classification of brain tumors from MRI images using a convolutional neural network. *Applied Sciences (Basel, Switzerland), 10*(6), 1999. DOI: 10.3390/app10061999

Cao, C., Liu, F., Tan, H., Song, D., Shu, W., Li, W., Zhou, Y., Bo, X., & Xie, Z. (2018). Deep learning and its applications in biomedicine. *Genomics, Proteomics & Bioinformatics, 16*(1), 17–32. DOI: 10.1016/j.gpb.2018.01.001 PMID: 29522900

Chan, H.-P., Samala, R. K., Hadjiiski, L. M., & Zhou, C. (2020). Deep learning in medical image analysis. In *Deep Learning in Medical Image Analysis: Challenges and Applications* (pp. 3–21). Springer. https://doi.org/DOI: 10.1007/978-3-030-33128-3_1

Chen, X., Wang, X., Zhang, K., Fung, K.-M., Thai, T. C., Moore, K., Mannel, R. S., Liu, H., Zheng, B., & Qiu, Y. (2022). Recent advances and clinical applications of deep learning in medical image analysis. *Medical Image Analysis, 79*, 102444. DOI: 10.1016/j.media.2022.102444 PMID: 35472844

Das, S., & Goswami, R. S. (2023). Review, limitations, and future prospects of neural network approaches for brain tumor classification. *Multimedia Tools and Applications*, *82*, 1–43. DOI: 10.1007/s11042-023-14123-7

Deepak, S., & Ameer, P. M. (2021). Automated categorization of brain tumor from MRI using CNN features and SVM. *Journal of Ambient Intelligence and Humanized Computing*, *12*, 8357–8369. DOI: 10.1007/s12652-020-02756-0

Dhermain, F. G., Hau, P., Lanfermann, H., Jacobs, A. H., & van den Bent, M. J. (2010). Advanced MRI and PET imaging for assessment of treatment response in patients with gliomas. *Lancet Neurology*, *9*(9), 906–920. DOI: 10.1016/S1474-4422(10)70164-1 PMID: 20705518

Dhruv, P., & Naskar, S. (2020). Image classification using convolutional neural network (CNN) and recurrent neural network (RNN): A review. In *Machine Learning and Information Processing: Proceedings of ICMLIP 2019* (pp. 367–381). Springer. https://doi.org/DOI: 10.1007/978-981-15-4936-3_28

Gaur, L., Bhatia, U., Jhanjhi, N. Z., Muhammad, G., & Masud, M. (2023). Medical image-based detection of COVID-19 using deep convolution neural networks. *Multimedia Systems*, *29*(3), 1729–1738. DOI: 10.1007/s00530-023-01083-6 PMID: 33935377

Goutham, V., Sameerunnisa, A., Babu, S., & Prakash, T. B. (2022). Brain tumor classification using EfficientNet-B0 model. In *2022 2nd International Conference on Advance Computing and Innovative Technologies in Engineering (ICACITE)* (pp. 2503–2509). IEEE. https://doi.org/DOI: 10.1109/ICACITE53721.2022.9772123

Gupta, S., & Gupta, M. (2021). Deep learning for brain tumor segmentation using magnetic resonance images. In *2021 IEEE Conference on Computational Intelligence in Bioinformatics and Computational Biology (CIBCB)* (pp. 1–6). IEEE. https://doi.org/DOI: 10.1109/CIBCB52658.2021.9577313

Hustinx, R., & Fosse, P. (2010). PET in brain tumors. *PET Clinics*, *5*(2), 185–197. DOI: 10.1016/j.cpet.2010.02.002 PMID: 27157672

Iqbal, S., Qureshi, A. N., Ullah, A., Li, J., & Mahmood, T. (2022). Improving the robustness and quality of biomedical CNN models through adaptive hyperparameter tuning. *Applied Sciences (Basel, Switzerland)*, *12*(22), 11870. DOI: 10.3390/app122211870

Kaur, D., Goel, S., Nijhawan, R., & Gupta, S. (2022). Analysis of brain tumor using pre-trained CNN models and machine learning techniques. In *2022 IEEE International Students' Conference on Electrical, Electronics and Computer Science (SCEECS)* (pp. 1–6). IEEE. https://doi.org/DOI: 10.1109/SCEECS54163.2022.9776670

Khan, M. S. I., Rahman, A., Debnath, T., Karim, M. R., Nasir, M. K., Band, S. S., Mosavi, A., & Dehzangi, I. (2022). Accurate brain tumor detection using deep convolutional neural network. *Computational and Structural Biotechnology Journal*, *20*, 4733–4745. DOI: 10.1016/j.csbj.2022.08.057 PMID: 36147663

Kora, P., Ooi, C. P., Faust, O., Raghavendra, U., Gudigar, A., Chan, W. Y., Meenakshi, K., Swaraja, K., Plawiak, P., & Acharya, U. R. (2022). Transfer learning techniques for medical image analysis: A review. *Biocybernetics and Biomedical Engineering*, *42*(1), 79–107. DOI: 10.1016/j.bbe.2021.12.004

Kousalya, K., & Saranya, T. (2023). Improved the detection and classification of breast cancer using hyperparameter tuning. *Materials Today: Proceedings*, *81*, 547–552. DOI: 10.1016/j.matpr.2023.01.107

Kshatri, S. S., & Singh, D. (2023). Convolutional neural network in medical image analysis: A review. *Archives of Computational Methods in Engineering*, *30*(4), 2793–2810. DOI: 10.1007/s11831-022-09848-w

Kumar, N., Gupta, M., Gupta, D., & Tiwari, S. (2023). Novel deep transfer learning model for COVID-19 patient detection using X-ray chest images. *Journal of Ambient Intelligence and Humanized Computing*, *14*(1), 469–478. DOI: 10.1007/s12652-022-04655-2 PMID: 34025813

Liao, J., Li, X., Gan, Y., Han, S., Rong, P., Wang, W., Li, W., & Zhou, L. (2023). Artificial intelligence assists precision medicine in cancer treatment. *Frontiers in Oncology*, *12*, 998222. DOI: 10.3389/fonc.2022.998222 PMID: 36686757

Litjens, G., & Kooi, T., EhteshamiBejnordi, B., Setio, A. A. A., Ciompi, F., Ghafoorian, M., Van Der Laak, J. A. W. M., Van Ginneken, B., & Sánchez, C. I. (2017). A survey on deep learning in medical image analysis. *Medical Image Analysis*, *42*, 60–88. DOI: 10.1016/j.media.2017.07.005 PMID: 28778026

Liu, Z., Tong, L., Chen, L., Jiang, Z., Zhou, F., Zhang, Q., Zhang, X., Jin, Y., & Zhou, H. (2023). Deep learning based brain tumor segmentation: A survey. *Complex & Intelligent Systems*, *9*(1), 1001–1026. DOI: 10.1007/s40747-022-01015-4

Malhotra, P., Gupta, S., Koundal, D., Zaguia, A., & Enbeyle, W. (2022). Deep neural networks for medical image segmentation. *Journal of Healthcare Engineering*, *2022*, 1–13. DOI: 10.1155/2022/9845752 PMID: 35310182

Raghu, M., Zhang, C., Kleinberg, J., & Bengio, S. (2019). Transfusion: Understanding transfer learning for medical imaging. *Advances in Neural Information Processing Systems, 32*. https://proceedings.neurips.cc/paper/2019/hash/32a9a0c1f0aaf8f7b6c5b2f4010a512c-Abstract.html

Saeedi, S., Rezayi, S., & Keshavarz, H., & NiakanKalhori, S. R. (2023). MRI-based brain tumor detection using convolutional deep learning methods and chosen machine learning techniques. *BMC Medical Informatics and Decision Making*, *23*(1), 16. DOI: 10.1186/s12911-022-02093-2 PMID: 36691030

Saeedi, S., Rezayi, S., & Keshavarz, H., & NiakanKalhori, S. R. (2023). MRI-based brain tumor detection using convolutional deep learning methods and chosen machine learning techniques. *BMC Medical Informatics and Decision Making*, *23*(1), 16. DOI: 10.1186/s12911-022-02093-2 PMID: 36691030

Saini, R., Semwal, P., & Jaware, T. H. (2022). Brain tumor classification using VGG-16 and MobileNetV2 deep learning techniques on magnetic resonance images (MRI). In *International Conference on Soft Computing and its Engineering Applications* (pp. 300–313). Springer Nature Switzerland. https://doi.org/DOI: 10.1007/978-3-031-17191-2_26

Shah, H. A., Saeed, F., Yun, S., Park, J.-H., Paul, A., & Kang, J.-M. (2022). A robust approach for brain tumor detection in magnetic resonance images using finetuned EfficientNet. *IEEE Access : Practical Innovations, Open Solutions, 10*, 65426–65438. DOI: 10.1109/ACCESS.2022.3184028

Shen, D., Wu, G., & Suk, H.-I. (2017). Deep learning in medical image analysis. *Annual Review of Biomedical Engineering*, *19*, 221–248. DOI: 10.1146/annurev-bioeng-071516-044442 PMID: 28301734

Szegedy, C., Liu, W., Jia, Y., Sermanet, P., Reed, S., Anguelov, D., Erhan, D., Vanhoucke, V., & Rabinovich, A. (2015). Going deeper with convolutions. In *Proceedings of the IEEE Conference on Computer Vision and Pattern Recognition* (pp. 1–9). https://doi.org/DOI: 10.1109/CVPR.2015.7298594

Tan, M., & Le, Q. (2019). EfficientNet: Rethinking model scaling for convolutional neural networks. In *International Conference on Machine Learning* (pp. 6105–6114). PMLR.

Tripathy, S., Singh, R., & Ray, M. (2023). Automation of brain tumor identification using EfficientNet on magnetic resonance images. *Procedia Computer Science*, *218*, 1551–1560. DOI: 10.1016/j.procs.2023.01.136

Wang, H., Qi, Q., Sun, W., Li, X., Dong, B., & Yao, C. (2023). Classification of skin lesions with generative adversarial networks and improved MobileNetV2. *International Journal of Imaging Systems and Technology*. Advance online publication. DOI: 10.1002/ima.22807

Yao, J., Zhang, S., Yao, Y., Wang, F., Ma, J., Zhang, J., & Chu, Y.. (2022). Edge-cloud polarization and collaboration: A comprehensive survey for AI. *IEEE Transactions on Knowledge and Data Engineering*, *35*(7), 6866–6886. DOI: 10.1109/TKDE.2022.3156515

Yu, X., Wang, J., Hong, Q.-Q., Teku, R., Wang, S.-H., & Zhang, Y.-D. (2022). Transfer learning for medical images analyses: A survey. *Neurocomputing*, *489*, 230–254. DOI: 10.1016/j.neucom.2022.05.094

Chapter 7
IoT in Medical Applications

Himadri Sekhar Das
https://orcid.org/0000-0002-3509-3388
Haldia Institute of Technology, India

Arannya Samanta
KPC Medical College and Hospital, India

Samiran Samanta
IPGME&R, India & SSKM Hospital, Kolkata, India

ABSTRACT

The unification of Internet of Things (IoT) technologies in healing requests has revolutionized healthcare by permissive authentic-time listening, disease, and treatment. This chapter investigate the deep impact of IoT in medical sciences, stressing its act in embellishing patient care, optimizing resource exercise, and reconstructing healthcare outcomes. Leveraging pertain instruments and sensors, IoT facilitates detached patient listening, personalized situation plans and predicting analytics. Moreover, IoT authorizes healthcare artists to make dossier-compelled decisions expeditiously, superior to timely mediations and full of enthusiasm healthcare management. As IoT resumes to advance, allure transformative potential in healing uses remains superlative, hopeful a future of efficient, patient-in the middle healthcare transmittal.

DOI: 10.4018/979-8-3693-3864-3.ch007

1. INTRODUCTION

In the sphere of healthcare, mechanics progresses have always existed important in improving patient care, disease, and treatment methods. Among these changes, the Internet of Things (IoT) has emerged as a transformational force, transforming various facets of healing uses (Kelly et al., 2020) and (Mitchell et al., 2019). IoT refers to a network of pertain devices that can accumulate, communicate, and exchange dossier seamlessly over the computer network. In the healing sector, IoT has unlocked up new paths for reconstructing adeptness, accuracy, and approachability in healthcare transfer (Mitchell-Box K et al., 2012; Parihar et al., 2024). The unification of IoT ploys in healing applications has influenced to the incident of an idea popular as the Internet of Medical Things (IoMT) (Dang et al., 2019). IoMT encompasses an off-course range of smart ploys and sensors entrenched in healing supplies, wearables, and even implantable devices, all pertain to draw and resolve strength-related dossier in honest-period. This pertain environment holds immense potential to transform healthcare transfer by permissive detached monitoring, embodied situation plans, and early invasion blueprints (Saarikko et al., 2017; Hadir et al., 2025).

One of the basic regions where IoT is making a meaningful impact is in detached patient monitoring. Traditionally, sufferers had to visit healthcare conveniences regularly for check-boosts or listening of chronic environments. However, accompanying IoT-authorized devices in the way that wearable sensors and home listening systems, cases can immediately be monitored by chance, admitting for continuous pursuing of signs of life, medication devotion, and overall well-being rank (Nazir S et al, (2019) and P Matthew et al, (2025). This not only improves patient comfort but too allows healthcare providers to intervene immediately as long as of any irregularities, through reducing nursing home readmissions and reconstructing overall patient consequences (Yin et al., 2016). Moreover, IoT plays a crucial duty in embellishing operational adeptness inside healthcare institutions. Through the exercise of IoT-allowed systems for stock administration, advantage tracking, and predicting sustenance of medical supplies, wards can streamline their workflows, underrate disappearance, and ensure the chance of essential possessions when needed. Additionally, IoT- stimulate resolutions speed real-opportunity ideas and data giving between healthcare professionals, superior to better cooperation and informed accountable (Merchant et al., 2018; Al Khatib et al., 2024).

Furthermore, the onset of telemedicine, speeded by IoT technologies, has extended approach to healthcare services, specifically in detached or underserved areas. Patients can immediately talk over with other healthcare providers virtually, leveraging IoT-allowed program conferencing podiums and remote demonstrative finishes. This not only improves approach to healthcare but still reduces the burden on overcrowded healthcare abilities, exceptionally during community health impasses such as the

COVID-19 universal (Filip et al., 2022). However, the extensive approval of IoT in medical requests too raises significant concerns concerning dossier privacy, freedom, and supervisory compliance. The enormous amounts of delicate fitness data produce by IoT manoeuvres must be safeguarded against potential high-tech dangers and breaches. Therefore, robust computerized-protection measures and compliance accompanying rules to a degree the Health Insurance Portability and Accountability Act (HIPAA) are imperative to guarantee the purity and confidentiality of patient news (Edemekong et al., 2024).

1.1. Understanding IoT and its Evolution

The Internet of Things (IoT) refers to the network of material objects or "belongings" entrenched with sensors, program, and additional electronics to combine and exchange dossier with added schemes and methods over the internet. These objects can range from natural household appliances to complex industrialized equipment. The progress of IoT assumed through several key stages:

Emergence: The idea of joining instruments to the internet isn't new, but the term "Internet of Things" acquires prominence in the early 2000s. At this stage, the focus was generally on joining calculating and smart phones to the internet.

Connectivity: As computer network connectivity enhanced more ever-present and inexpensive, the opportunity of IoT extended to include a more expansive range of manoeuvres, in the way that sensors, actuators, and common objects like thermostats and light bulbs. Wi-Fi, Bluetooth, and basic networks played critical parts in permissive connectedness for these ploys (Javaid et al., 2025).

Data Collection and Analysis: With the increase of connected schemes, enormous amounts of dossier started expected generated from differing beginnings. This dossier maybe composed, analyzed, and used to collect valuable acumens, permissive trades and arranging to make conversant determinations and improve processes.

Interoperability and Standards: As the IoT environment evolved, interoperability and standardization enhanced fault-finding issues. Different designs and principles wanted to be smart to correspond accompanying each one seamlessly. Industry consortiums and principles organizations processed to cultivate low agreements and guidelines, such as MQTT, CoAP, and Zigbee, to simplify interoperability (Choudhary, 2024).

Edge Computing: Traditional cloud-located IoT architectures have restraints in conditions of abeyance, bandwidth, and solitude. Edge calculating addresses these challenges by transform dossier tighter to the source, lowering abeyance and the need to please all dossier to the cloud. Edge schemes, such as gateways and edge servers, act data conversion and reasoning regionally before shipping relevant dossier to the cloud (Hamdan et al., 2020).

Artificial Intelligence and Machine Learning: AI and machine intelligence electronics are progressively being joined into IoT systems to extract significant observations from the far-flung amounts of dossier produce by connected ploys. These sciences authorize predicting sustenance, anomaly discovery, and evident-occasion growth of IoT wholes (Bzai, et al., 2022).

Security and Privacy: As IoT tools become more extensive and pertain, concerns about freedom and solitude have of age. Vulnerabilities in IoT devices can bring about dossier breaches, solitude defilements, and even tangible harm. Manufacturers and developers are executing freedom best practices, in the way that encryption, confirmation, and over-the-air renews, to mitigate these risks.

Industry-particular Applications: IoT is being used across differing enterprises, containing manufacturing, healthcare, farming, conveyance, and smart capitals. In each subdivision, IoT resolutions are tailored to address particular challenges and necessities, to a degree reconstructing functional efficiency, reinforcing client occurrences, and permissive new trade models.

5G and Beyond: The rollout of 5G networks promises to further accelerate the acceptance of IoT by providing faster dossier speeds, lower abeyance, and support for a large number of related devices. Beyond 5G, arising electronics like 6G be necessary to open new potential for IoT, such as extreme-trustworthy reduced-abeyance ideas (URLLC) and ubiquitous connectedness.

1.2. The Importance of IoT in Healthcare

Internet of Things (IoT) has transformed miscellaneous industries, and healthcare is no irregularity (Javaid et al., 2021). Here are few key reasons why IoT is main in healthcare:

Remote patient listening: IoT manoeuvres enable unending listening of inmates' vital signs, in the way that essence rate, blood pressure, and level of glucose in blood levels, from their houses. This admits healthcare providers to remotely monitor subjects accompanying chronic environments or those improving from surgeries, lowering the need for frequent hospital visits and reconstructing patient effects.

Real-time strength pursuing: Wearable IoT tools, such as appropriateness trackers and smart-watches, accumulate dossier on users' recreational activity, sleep patterns, and different health versification. This certain-period health pursuing helps things stay informed about their strength rank and spurs them to select more active lifestyles.

Predictive data: By resolving the colossal amounts of data composed from IoT designs, healthcare providers can recognize patterns and trends that concede possibility display potential health issues. Predictive data stimulate by IoT can help hinder diseases, control incessant conditions in a more excellent manner, and better overall public health administration.

Enhanced drug administration: IoT-enabled drug devotion systems mention subjects to take their drugs on time and monitor their agreement. These plans can also alert healthcare providers if victims miss doses or happening antagonistic reactions, admitting for appropriate intervention and adaptation of situation plans.

Streamlined movements: IoT devices can improve healthcare ability movements by monitoring supplies custom, tracking stock levels, and automating routine tasks. This helps effectiveness, reduces costs, and allows healthcare providers to focus on or in a transportation object patient care.

Telemedicine and detached consultations: IoT technologies allow secure ideas and dossier exchange between inmates and healthcare providers, speeding telemedicine consultations and remote disease. This is specifically advantageous for patients in country or underserved districts the one may have restricted approach to healthcare services.

Improved patient occurrence: IoT resolutions reinforce the overall patient experience by providing embodied care, lowering wait times, and growing availability. Patients feel allowed and engaged in their healthcare resolutions, superior to higher vindication levels and better effects.

1.3 Overview of IoT-Enabled Medical Devices

IoT-allowed healing devices show a meaningful advancement in healthcare science by mixing the Internet of Things (IoT) with healing maneuvers to provide improved listening, diagnosis, and situation alternatives for cases (Kumar, Yogesh et al, 2021). These devices influence sensors, relatedness, and data science of logical analysis to accumulate and transmit physical-period health news, permissive healthcare providers to make conversant determinations and transfer personalized care (Joshitta et al., 2017).

Wearable Health Trackers: These designs, such as smart watches and appropriateness bands, monitor differing health versification like soul rate, exercise levels, sleep patterns, and even stress levels. They provide consumers accompanying insights into their well-being and help healthier practices.

Remote Patient Monitoring (RPM) Devices: RPM instruments allow healthcare providers to by chance monitor victims' vital signs, cure devotion, and overall well-being status from a distance. This is specifically advantageous for managing never-ending environments and post-operative care, as it allows early discovery of health issues and reduces the need for frequent nursing home visits.

Smart Implants: Implantable healing devices, in the way that pacemakers, insulin pumps, and constant sweet liquid monitors, can now be outfitted accompanying IoT capabilities to monitor inmates' strength in real-period and send data to healthcare providers for prompt mediation and adaptations to treatment plans.

Connected Medical Equipment: IoT electronics is being joined into various healing supplies, including immersion pumps, ventilators, and MRI machines, to monitor tool performance, path habit, and ensure proper perpetuation and improve, thereby reconstructing patient security and operational effectiveness in healthcare conveniences.

Telemedicine Devices: IoT-enabled telemedicine tools, in the way that video conferencing methods, mathematical stethoscopes, and otoscopes, enable detached consultations between subjects and healthcare providers. These devices help prompt diagnosis, situation, and listening of patients, exceptionally in underserved districts with restricted approach to healthcare services.

Medication Management Systems: IoT-located drug administration systems help subjects obey their medication regimes by providing notices, dispensing cures at due times, and listening drug custom. These systems can likewise alert healthcare providers or caregivers as long as of missed doses or potential drug interplays (Shermock, 2023).

Smart Health Apps: Mobile requests equipped accompanying IoT competencies allow consumers to path their health dossier, ideas accompanying healthcare providers, schedule appointments, approach instructional resources, and even take part in detached monitoring programs. These apps play a important function in empowering subjects to take control of their energy and actively undertake their care (Maktoubian et al., 2019).

1.4. Challenges and Opportunities in Implementing IoT in Healthcare

Implementing IoT (Internet of Things) in healthcare presents two together challenges and hope (Selvaraj et al., 2020). Here's a breakdown of few of the key facets:

Challenges:

Data Privacy and Security: Healthcare dossier is well sensitive, and some rupture manage have harsh consequences. Ensuring strong encryption, approach controls, and agreement accompanying regulations like HIPAA (Health Insurance Portability and Accountability Act) is important.

Interoperability: Healthcare plans frequently comprise miscellaneous tools and spreadsheet from various manufacturers, which grant permission not surely write accompanying each other. Achieving logical interoperability with IoT ploys, photoelectric health records (EHRs), and added structures are a meaningful challenge. Figure.1. shows the different challenges of IoT in Healthcare.

Figure 1. Different challenges of IoT in Healthcare.

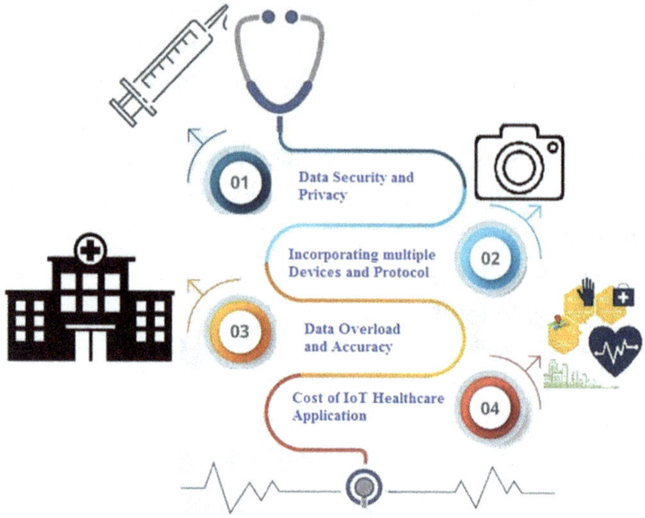

Reliability and Accuracy: In healthcare, dependability and accuracy are superior. IoT ploys must usually provide correct dossier to prevent wrong diagnoses or treatment conclusions. Ensuring the dependability of connectedness and dossier transmission is critical.

Regulatory Compliance: Healthcare managing are complex and change across domains. Implementing IoT solutions demands agreement accompanying various supervisory principles, that increases complexity and cost to the exercise process.

Ethical Concerns: There are moral concerns concerning the use of IoT in healthcare, such as patient consent, dossier partnership, and potential misuse of dossier. Ensuring transparence and ethical directions in dossier group, habit, and storage is essential.

Integration accompanying Clinical Workflow: Introducing IoT instruments into dispassionate workflows must be seamless and endure not upset existent processes. Ensuring that IoT answers enhance effectiveness alternatively generating supplementary administrative burden for healthcare pros is important.

Opportunities: Remote Monitoring and Telemedicine: IoT allows detached monitoring of inmates' signs of life and well-being parameters, expediting early discovery of fitness issues and permissive timely interferences. It more supports telemedicine by permissive in essence consultations and follow-boosts, reconstructing approach to healthcare, particularly in remote or underserved districts.

Predictive Analytics and Personalized Medicine: IoT-create dossier, when linked with state-of-the-art data and AI, can specify valuable insights into patient fitness styles, permissive predicting analytics and embodied situation plans. This can bring about more productive and efficient healthcare transfer tailor-made to individual patient needs (Dixon et al., 2024).

Chronic Disease Management: IoT schemes can assist in the administration of chronic environments by providing constant listening and authentic-time response to sufferers and healthcare providers. This full of enthusiasm approach can help prevent complexities and lower hospitalizations guide never-ending diseases.

Operational Efficiency and Cost Reduction: IoT resolutions can organize healthcare movements, enhance resource exercise, and lower costs. For example, advantage following and inventory administration orders can increase the use of medical supplies and provisions, chief to cost funds and improved effectiveness.

Patient Engagement and Empowerment: IoT empowers inmates to take control of their fitness by providing approach to real-period dossier and visions about their condition. This raised engagement can bring about better well-being effects and devotion to treatment plans.

Research and Population Health Management: IoT-produce dossier can enhance medical research and society fitness administration drives by providing large-scale dossier sets for study. This can help recognize ailment trends, determine the influence of attacks, and advise public health tactics.

2. IOT APPLICATIONS IN REMOTE PATIENT MONITORING

IoT (Internet of Things) has transformed many activities, including healthcare. Remote patient listening (RPM) is individual specific area place IoT uses have created significant stomps (Archip, Alexandru, et al. 2016). Figure.2. shows the Application in Remote Patient Monitoring.

Figure 2. Application in Remote Patient Monitoring.

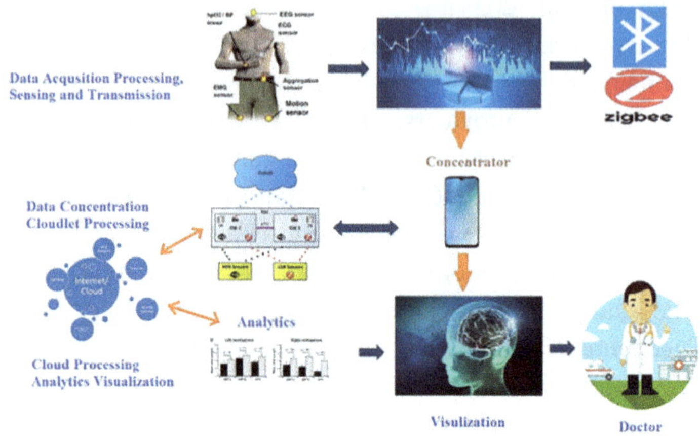

Wearable Devices: IoT-authorized wearable devices, in the way that smart watches, appropriateness trackers, and healing-grade sensors, allow unending listening of signs of life like heart rate, ancestry pressure, level of glucose in blood levels, oxygen satiation, and more. These devices can communicate dossier in original-time to healthcare providers, permissive ruling class to by chance monitor patients' fitness rank.

Chronic Disease Management: IoT schemes can assist in managing never-ending environments like diabetes, hypertension, and myocardial infarction by providing regular modernizes on victims' fitness parameters. By pursuing styles and vacillations, healthcare providers can intervene early for fear that complexities and regulate treatment plans correspondingly.

Medication Adherence: IoT-authorized dose dispensers and medication pursuing maneuvers help victims adhere to their recommended cure schedules. These tools can send keepsakes to cases when it's occasion to take their medication and inform caregivers or healthcare providers if doses are misplaced.

Telemedicine Platforms: Integrating IoT instruments with telemedicine podiums allows detached consultations between inmates and healthcare artists. During these in essence visits, healthcare providers can access evident-occasion dossier from IoT devices to evaluate subjects' well-being status, determine counselling, and form informed conclusions about their care.

Fall Detection and Elderly Care: IoT sensors established in the home atmosphere can detect falls or changes lethargy patterns, particularly advantageous for elderly subjects single. These sensors can automatically alert caregivers or danger duties as long as of an emergency, easing up-to-date help.

Postoperative Monitoring: After surgery, IoT tools can monitor cases' improvement progress remotely, lowering the need for frequent clinic visits. Parameters in the way that wound healing, hotness, and exercise levels may be monitored to guarantee sufferers are restorative properly and discover some signs of problems early.

Remote Rehabilitation: IoT-enabled restoration ploys, to a degree smart exercise equipment and motion sensors, maybe used to monitor cases' progress all the while remote restoration meetings. Therapists can by chance track subjects' evolutions and specify feedback or regulate exercises as wanted to enhance recovery.

Sleep Monitoring: IoT maneuvers outfitted accompanying sensors can monitor sleep patterns and detect sleep disorders in the way that sleep interruption of activity. By resolving data on sleep character and event, healthcare providers can tailor attacks to improve sufferers' sleep and overall welfare.

2.1. Remote Monitoring Devices and Wearables

Remote listening maneuvers and wearables refer to a broad type of electronics created to track differing facets of an individual's strength and action remotely. These tools resort to sensors, Wi-Fi connectivity, and frequently helper apps or spreadsheet platforms to accumulate and send dossier to healthcare providers, caregivers, or the consumers themselves (Kang & Exworthy, 2022). Here are some key facets and instances of detached monitoring instruments and wearables:

Health Monitoring: Many detached listening devices devote effort to something pursuing signs of life such as essence rate, ancestry pressure, oxygen satiation, and hotness. These devices can support constant listening or periodic calculations, admitting for early discovery of health issues or flows over occasion (Dineen-Griffin S et al, (2019).

Activity Tracking: Wearable instruments like appropriateness trackers monitor physical activity levels, steps captured, calories scorched, and sleep patterns. They supply insights into overall appropriateness and can help consumers set and gain health aims.

Chronic Disease Management: Remote listening maneuvers play a crucial duty in directing incessant environments such as diabetes, hypertension, and respiring afflictions. For example, sweet substance monitors allow diabetics to path their glucose levels steadily, while smart inhalers help asthma patients survive their condition in a more excellent manner.

Telemedicine and Virtual Care: Remote listening tools enable telemedicine by admitting healthcare providers to by chance monitor sufferers' health and regulate situation plans as wanted. This is particularly valuable for cases in detached areas or those accompanying flexibility issues (Haleem & Javaid,2021).

Fall Detection and Emergency Response: Some wearables are outfitted accompanying fall detection sensors and crisis reaction lineaments. These devices can inevitably alert caregivers or crisis duties if the wearer falls or experiences a healing danger.

Medication Adherence: Smart tablet dispensers and cure tracking apps help consumers obey their drug schedules by providing reminders and pursuing doses captured. This can increase treatment consequences, exceptionally for subjects with complex cure regimes.

Mental Health Monitoring: There is a increasing interest in wearable designs that monitor mental fitness signs in the way that stress levels, mood vacillations, and sleep status. These instruments aim to provide acumens into consumers' passionate prosperity and facilitate early mediation when wanted.

Remote Patient Monitoring (RPM) Systems: RPM structures integrate differing detached listening devices and dossier data principles to enable inclusive detached patient listening. These methods are increasingly second hand by healthcare institutions to monitor extreme-risk patients and weaken clinic readmissions.

2.2 Real-Time Health Data Tracking

Real-period energy data following refers to the constant monitoring and study of miscellaneous physiological limits and strength-related versification utilizing digital sciences (Paganelli AI et al, 2022). This approach admits for the collection of dossier in physical-time, providing next understandings into an individual's health rank and helping timely invasions when essential. Figure.3. shows the Real time Health Data Tracking.

Figure 3. Real time Health Data Tracking.

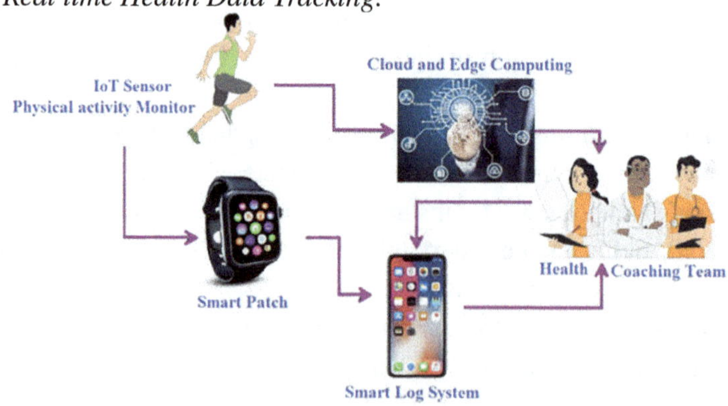

Several electronics and devices authorize original-time energy dossier tracking, containing:

Wearable schemes: Wearable gadgets to a degree appropriateness trackers, smart watches, and smart clothing include sensors to monitor limits like heart rate, venture levels, sleep patterns, and even ancestry oxygen levels.(These devices steadily accumulate data and frequently supply real-opportunity response to consumers, encouraging more healthful dresses and allowing things to path their progress over time.

Remote patient listening orders: These systems allow healthcare providers to by chance monitor patients' well-being rank outside of usual healthcare backgrounds. Patients may use wearable instruments or home listening equipment to measure signs of life, to a degree blood pressure, level of glucose in blood levels, or electrocardiogram (ECG) readings. The dossier is sent to healthcare professionals in certain-occasion, allowing for early discovery of deformities and proactive mediation.

Mobile fitness (mHealth) apps: Mobile applications admit things to track miscellaneous facets of their health and wellbeing utilizing smartphones or tablets. These apps can collect dossier on diet, exercise, cure adherence, emotion, and more. Some apps too integrate accompanying wearable designs to supply a comprehensive view of the consumer's fitness data. Real-opportunity listening and feedback looks in these apps help consumers make conversant resolutions about their health management (Albarrak et al., 2024).

Internet of Things (IoT) designs: IoT technology authorizes the network of various ploys and sensors to accumulate and exchange data over the cyberspace. In the circumstances of healthcare, IoT devices can involve smart scales, ancestry pressure monitors, glucometers, and even implantable healing devices. By steadily cascading data to concentrated terraces, IoT devices further certain-time listening of sufferers' health environments and support detached management of never-ending afflictions.

Telemedicine platforms: Telemedicine aids admit patients to talk over with another healthcare providers by chance, often through television conferencing or secure to foreshadow podiums. Real-time strength dossier tracking can complement telemedicine consultations by providing supplementary context about the patient's current energy rank.

2.3. Telemedicine and Virtual Consultations

Telemedicine and in essence consultations have enhance increasingly superior in up-to-date healthcare schemes, offering abundant benefits to two together cases and healthcare providers (Ateriya et al., 2018). Figure.4. shows the Working of Telemedicine.

Figure 4. Working of Telemedicine

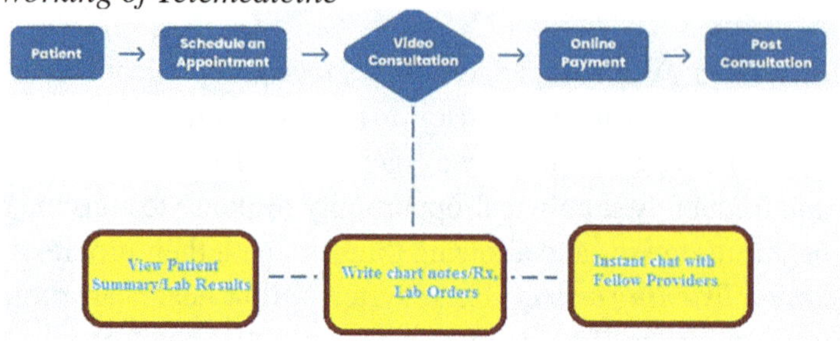

Here's an overview of these ideas:

1. ***Telemedicine***: Telemedicine refers to the detached transmittal of healthcare services utilizing electronics. It admits patients to talk over with other healthcare experts, endure medical recommendation, and even acquire prescriptions outside the need for in-person visits. Telemedicine can involve miscellaneous forms of ideas, such as broadcast calls, telephone calls, paragraph messages, and emails (Stoltzfus, M et al.,2023).

Benefits of Telemedicine:

Accessibility: Telemedicine expands approach to healthcare duties, specifically for individuals in detached or underserved extents.

Convenience: Patients can accept medical care from the comfort of their neighbourhoods, removing the need for travel and lowering resting times.

Cost-influence: Telemedicine can lower healthcare costs by lowering the need for in-guy visits, hospital admissions, and conveyance expenses.

Continuity of care: Patients can uphold regular trade their healthcare providers, chief to better progression of care and improved well-being consequences.

2. ***Virtual Consultations***: Virtual consultations are a particular form of telemedicine that involves detached interplays betwixt patients and healthcare experts for the purpose of disease, situation, or follow-up care. These consultations usually happen over television conferencing planks, allowing for directly facing ideas regardless of physical distance.

Benefits of Virtual Consultations:

Enhanced ideas: Virtual consultations authorize absolute-time, nonverbal communication between cases and healthcare providers, facilitating more inclusive appraisals and consultations.

Remote monitoring: Healthcare artists can by chance monitor subjects' health rank, signs of life, and drug adherence through in essence consultations, chief to early discovery of strength issues and timely invasions.

Specialized care: Virtual consultations admit victims to access specific healing knowledge that may not be regionally handy, permissive more personalized and point in a direction situation plans.

Reduced uncovering to infectious afflictions: Especially appropriate all the while pandemics or ailment outbreaks, in essence consultations underrate the risk of exposure to communicable diseases by restricting in-guy interactions.

Challenges and Considerations:

Technology obstructions: Access to telemedicine duties can be limited by determinants in the way that computer network connectivity, mathematical education, and chance of necessary instruments.

Regulatory and allowable concerns: Telemedicine practices are subject to organizing and licensure necessities that change by jurisdiction. Healthcare providers must guarantee agreement accompanying relevant regulations and directions.

Privacy and protection concerns: Protecting patient confidentiality and dossier freedom is principal in telemedicine, making necessary robust encryption and agreement accompanying solitude regulations like HIPAA (Health Insurance Portability and Accountability Act) in the United States.

2.4 Case Studies on Remote Patient Monitoring

Remote patient listening (RPM) is a promptly evolving district inside healthcare, leveraging electronics to monitor sufferers outside of unoriginal dispassionate scenes (Hilty DM et al, 2021). Here are any case studies that showcase the influence and impact of detached patient listening:

Dartmouth-Hitchcock Medical Centre (DHMC): DHMC implemented detached patient listening for subjects accompanying chronic environments like heart attack (CHF), incessant opposing pulmonary disease (COPD), and diabetes. The program complicated providing cases accompanying devices in the way that ancestry pressure monitors, beat oximeters, and scales that communicated data to healthcare providers in authentic-occasion (Cuthbert JJ et al, 2019). By listening cases remotely, DHMC noticed a meaningful decline in hospital readmissions and emergency visits with sharing cases. This case study shows in what way or manner RPM can help patient consequences and reduces healthcare costs by proactively directing incessant environments.

Banner Health: Banner Health, a non-profit healthcare arrangement based in Arizona, executed a detached listening program for patients improving from orthopaedic resection. Patients were ready wearable sensors and a travelling app to track their improvement progress, containing flexibility, range of motion, and pain levels. Healthcare providers by chance monitored inmates' dossier and happened when necessary, providing embodied care plans and exercises. Banner Health stated enhanced patient vindication, faster recovery opportunities, and shortened post-influential problems, highlighting the benefits of RPM in post-surgical care.

Geisinger Health System: Geisinger Health System, located in Pennsylvania, started a detached monitoring program for subjects accompanying hypertension. Patients were outfitted accompanying blood pressure cuffs and related ploys to path their ancestry pressure readings at home. Data from these devices were communicated to healthcare providers the one commit remotely monitor subjects' ancestry pressure styles and regulate treatment plans respectively. Geisinger noticed better ancestry pressure control and cure adherence between partners, chief to improved administration of hypertension and decreased cardiovascular risks.

Mayo Clinic's Connected Care: Mayo Clinic's Connected Care program offers detached listening for patients accompanying differing never-ending environments, including heart attack, diabetes, and hypertension. Patients accept affiliated devices to monitor signs of life, manifestations, and drug devotion at home. Healthcare providers at Mayo Clinic remotely review victims' dossier and happen as wanted, providing timely adaptations to situation plans. The program has proved hopeful results in improving patient consequences, lowering nursing home admissions, and enhancing inmates' character of growth. These case studies show the diverse requests and benefits of detached patient listening across various healthcare settings and patient states. By leveraging electronics to by chance monitor patients' strength rank and support convenient interventions, RPM holds excellent potential for reconstructing patient consequences, lowering healthcare costs, and enhancing the overall feature of care.

3. IOT FOR CHRONIC DISEASE MANAGEMENT

Internet of Things (IoT) science has proved great promise engaged of never-ending disease administration by permissive remote listening, embodied care, and up-to-date intervention (Dadkhah et al., 2021). Figure.5. shows the Chronic Disease Management and Figure.6. shows the Chronic Disease management Service Delivery System respectively.

Figure 5. Chronic Disease Management.

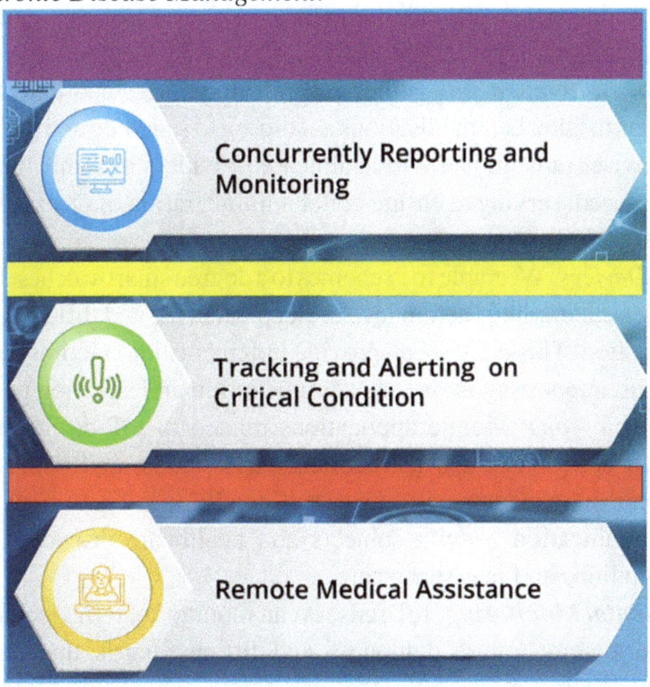

Figure 6. Chronic Disease management Service Delivery System.

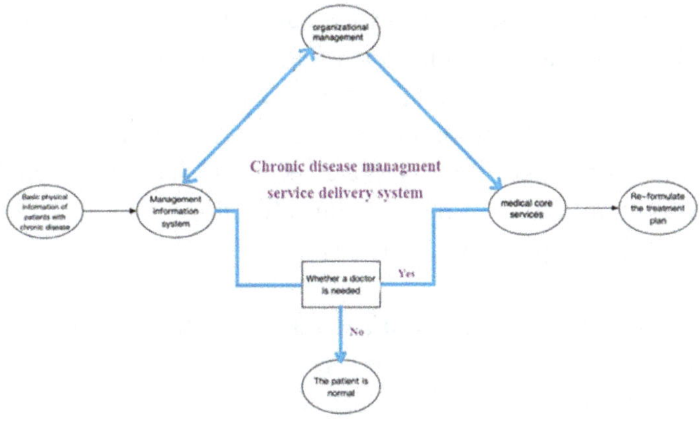

Here are various habits in which IoT may be used in chronic ailment administration:

Remote Patient Monitoring (RPM): IoT ploys can continuously monitor signs of life in the way that heart rate, ancestry pressure, level of glucose in blood levels, oxygen saturation, and more. These maneuvers can communicate data to healthcare providers in certain-opportunity, admitting for early detection of energy degeneration and timely mediation.

Medication Adherence: IoT-authorized pill dispensers and cure trackers can mention victims to take their medications according to schedule and path adherence. They can likewise transmit alerts to healthcare providers or family appendages if doses are misplaced, serving to ensure better administration of incessant conditions (Gargioni et al., 2024).

Wearable Devices: Wearable IoT schemes to a degree smartwatches, fitness trackers, and patches can monitor action levels, sleep patterns, and different appropriate health versification. This dossier can provide judgments into victims' overall health and act patterns, supporting in disease administration and situation preparation.

Smart Health Apps: Mobile applications related to IoT designs can provide embodied well-being insights, instructional possessions, and demeanor change support for patients accompanying incessant conditions. These apps can further expedite communication betwixt subjects and healthcare providers, permissive remote consultations and in essence care.

Environmental Monitoring: IoT sensors can monitor material factors in the way that air condition, temperature, dampness, and dirtiness levels, that can impact the health of things accompanying chronic respiring environments like asthma or COPD. This data can help inmates and healthcare providers create conversant decisions to check potential provokes and manage manifestations efficiently.

Home-based Rehabilitation: IoT-allowed ploys can support remote restoration programs for cases improving from chronic environments in the way that stroke or musculoskeletal disorders. These devices can determine shared exercises, track progress, and offer actual-occasion response to patients and healthcare providers, advancing devotion to therapy and faster improvement.

Predictive Analytics: By resolving large capacities of dossier calm from IoT devices, machine intelligence algorithms can recognize patterns and predict exacerbations or snags in sufferers with never-ending afflictions. This predicting analytics competence authorizes proactive invasions and embodied care plans to prevent antagonistic strength events.

Integration accompanying Electronic Health Records (EHR): IoT dossier maybe integrated into photoelectric energy record systems, providing healthcare providers accompanying a inclusive view of patients' well-being rank and situation history. This smooth unification facilitates more cognizant dispassionate decision-making and progression of care (Satwik Mamidi,2022).

3.1 Diabetes Management Solutions

Diabetes administration answers encompass a roomy range of approaches and electronics proposed at helping things accompanying diabetes efficiently monitor and control their blood sugar levels (Guan et al., 2023). These answers are important for upholding good health and forbidding difficulties guide diabetes. Here are some key facets of diabetes administration answers: ***Blood Glucose Monitoring***: Regular monitoring of level of glucose in blood levels is essential for things accompanying diabetes. Traditional methods include finger stick tests utilizing a sweet substance meter, but unending sweet liquid listening (CGM) systems offer legitimate-period listening without the need for frequent finger sticks. CGM designs steadily measure level of glucose in blood levels and provide alerts for extreme or reduced glucose levels.

Insulin Therapy: For people accompanying type 1 diabetes and few accompanying type 2 diabetes, insulin therapy should to organize glucose levels. Insulin can be executed through injections or insulin pumps. Insulin pumps transfer insulin steadily throughout the era, mocking the function of a athletic pancreas more approximately.

Medication Management: In addition to insulin, many things accompanying type 2 diabetes may demand different cures to help manage their glucose levels. These concede possibility involve oral drugs in the way that metformin, sulfonylureas, or fresher classes of drugs like SGLT2 inhibitors and GLP-1 receptor agonists.

Dietary Management: A healthy diet is a mainstay of diabetes administration. Individuals accompanying diabetes must carefully monitor their hydrogen consumption, as carbohydrates have ultimate significant affect glucose levels. Nutrition giving advice and meal preparation help can help things make conversant able to be consumed selections.

Physical Activity: Regular exercise is beneficial for directing glucose levels and overall well-being. Diabetes management answers frequently involve guidance on including recreational activity into everyday acts. Exercise can help improve insulin feeling and lower glucose levels.

Education and Support: Diabetes administration requires continuous instruction and support. Healthcare providers, diabetes educators, and support groups play critical roles in authorizing things accompanying diabetes to understand their condition and create conversant determinations about their health.

Telemedicine and Digital Health: Telemedicine and mathematical energy programs offer convenient habits for things accompanying diabetes to access healthcare aids, containing detached consultations with healthcare providers, in essence diabetes instruction programs, and movable apps for tracking glucose levels, drugs, and behavior factors.

Artificial Pancreas Systems: Emerging sciences, to a degree exclusive-loop or artificial organ meat orders, connect continuous and oxygen listening accompanying insulin delivery to mechanize glucose administration. These systems aim to mimic the function of a active organ meat by regulating insulin delivery in reaction to level of glucose in blood levels in absolute-time.

3.2 Asthma and COPD Monitoring Systems

Asthma and Chronic Obstructive Pulmonary Disease (COPD) listening schemes are essential tools for directing these incessant respiring environments (Cukic et al., 2012). These systems help cases and healthcare providers' path syndromes, monitor lung function, and create cognizant conclusions about situation adjustments.

Here are few key elements and lineaments usually found in asthma and COPD listening orders:

Peak Flow Meters: Peak flow meters are handheld ploys used to measure the maximum airflow one can produce. Regular peak flow calculations can help asthma victims monitor their lung function and label potential exacerbations early.

Spirometers: Spirometers are ploys used to measure alveolus function by assessing the capacity and flow of air that maybe discharged from the body parts. They are often secondhand in two together diseases and listening of asthma and COPD. Figure.7 shows the Asthma and COPD Monitoring Systems.

Portable Spirometers: Portable spirometers allow subjects to monitor their pleura function at home or tireless. These devices can store and communicate dossier to healthcare providers for detached listening and management.

Figure 7. Asthma and COPD Monitoring Systems.

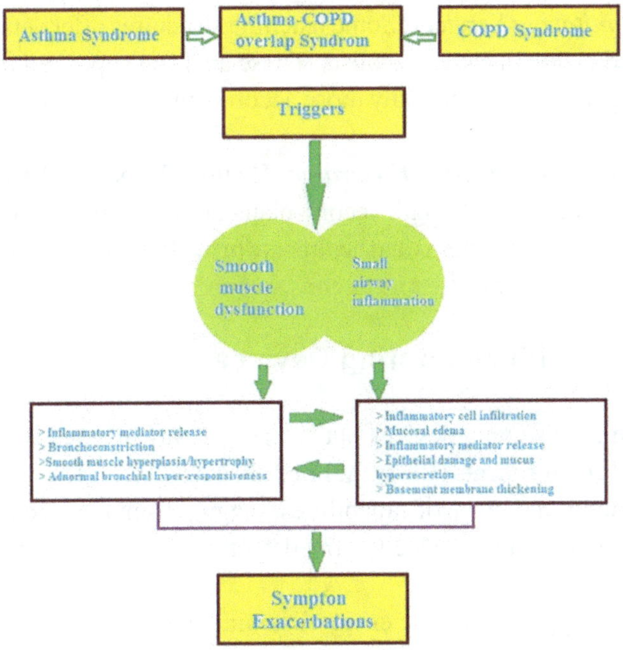

Smart Inhalers: Smart inhalers are inhaler ploys outfitted accompanying sensors that track cure custom and breathing method. They can provide response to subjects and healthcare providers, allowance to guarantee proper drug devotion and method.

Mobile Applications: Many asthma and COPD monitoring wholes involve travelling requests that allow sufferers to path manifestations, cure usage, and pleura function calculations. These apps concede possibility also support instructional money and notices for medication doses and doctor assignments.

Telehealth Integration: Some listening orders integrate accompanying telehealth floors, admitting inmates to share data accompanying their healthcare providers by chance. This expedites in essence consultations and enables proper adaptations to situation plans.

Alert Systems: Alert systems can inform victims and healthcare providers of potential exacerbations or changes in body part function that can require mediation. These alerts can prompt early operation for fear that worsening syndromes or hospitalizations.

Data Analytics and Reporting: Asthma and COPD listening orders frequently include physiognomy for resolving and newsgathering dossier over time. This can help label currents, generates, and patterns in symptoms and alveolus function, leading embodied situation strategies.

Remote Monitoring Services: Some listening structures offer detached monitoring aids staffed by healthcare specialists. These aids can supply additional support and counseling to cases, specifically those accompanying severe or poorly reserved asthma or COPD.

Integration accompanying Electronic Health Records (EHR): Integration accompanying electronic strength record plans admits logical sharing of patient dossier betwixt listening systems and healthcare providers, guaranteeing progression of care and correct proof of treatment consequences.

3.3 Cardiac Health Monitoring Devices

Cardiac fitness listening devices play a critical part in assessing and directing cardiovascular environments (Barry A. Franklin et al, 2022). These devices change in complicatedness and range of capabilities, ranging from plain courage rate monitors to advanced wearable device worthy detecting arrhythmias and other cardiac anomalies.

Few common types of cardiac energy listening devices are given below:

Heart Rate Monitors: These maneuvers usually come in the form of rib cage straps, wristbands, or smartphone apps outfitted accompanying sensors to measure heart rate. They are usually secondhand by athletes and appropriateness devotees to track their courage rate all along workouts. Continuous soul rate monitoring can likewise support insights into overall cardiovascular well-being.

ECG Monitors: Electrocardiogram (ECG or EKG) monitors record the energetic activity of the essence. Traditionally, ECG machines are about hospitals and hospitals, but lightweight ECG monitors are suitable increasingly common. These tools can provide authentic-occasion ECG readings, allowing consumers to monitor their essence music and detect irregularities to a degree atrial fibrillation.

Holter Monitors: Holter monitors are compact ECG devices that sufferers wear for an widespread period, usually 24 to 48 hours. They steadily record the soul's electrical project, picking up data all along often activities and sleep. Holter monitors are valuable for diagnosing sporadic cardiac arrhythmias that concede possibility not be detected all the while a temporary ECG test.

Wearable Devices: Smartwatches and fitness trackers outfitted accompanying heart rate sensors offer fundamental cardiac listening proficiencies. Many of these devices can path essence rate continuously during the whole of the era and provide alerts for unusual soul music. Some advanced wearables still combine ECG sensors for more comprehensive soul energy monitoring.

Implantable Devices: Implantable cardiac monitors (ICMs) are limited designs inserted beneath the skin to continuously monitor essence action. They are typically secondhand for subjects with distinguishing cardiac environments, in the way that unexplained passing out spells or doubtful arrhythmias. ICMs can record data long periods, permissive clinicians to diagnose and accomplish cardiac issues efficiently.

Blood Pressure Monitors: While generally used to measure blood pressure, mathematical ancestry pressure monitors often contain countenance for assessing cardiac strength, to a degree uneven heartbeat discovery. Monitoring ancestry pressure trends over occasion can specify insights into overall cardiovascular wellbeing.

Mobile Health Apps: There is a increasing ecosystem of travelling uses devised for cardiac health listening. These apps can range from plain heart rate trackers to cosmopolitan policies that integrate dossier from miscellaneous beginnings, including wearable instruments and self-stated symptoms. Some apps offer lineaments like detached monitoring by healthcare providers and embodied fitness judgments.

3.4 Remote Monitoring for Neurological Disorders

Remote listening for affecting animate nerve organs disorders refers to the use of technology to path and accomplishes the manifestations, progress, and treatment of affecting animate nerve organs environments from a distance (Korte, 2020). This approach influences various mathematical fitness finishes and platforms to accumulate absolute-occasion dossier on patients' strength rank, admitting healthcare providers to monitor their condition remotely and mediate as wanted.

Wearable Devices: Wearable tools such as smart watches, appropriateness trackers, and specific healing devices outfitted accompanying sensors can steadily monitor physiological limits in the way that soul rate, action levels, sleep patterns, and even neurological signals like intellect endeavour or tremors.

Mobile Apps: Mobile requests can enable cases to recommendation emotional data about their syndromes, cure devotion, atmosphere changes, and quality of history. These apps grant permission further include facial characteristics for broadcast consultations accompanying healthcare providers, educational money, and cure warnings.

Telemedicine Platforms: Telemedicine floors allow for detached consultations middle from two points victims and healthcare providers, including neurologists. Through broadcast conferencing, victims can review their symptoms, accept healing recommendation, and regulate their treatment plan outside the need for in-woman visits.

Remote Patient Monitoring Systems: These wholes integrate differing dossier streams from wearable designs, mobile apps, and photoelectric strength records to specify a inclusive view of a patient's health rank. Algorithms can resolve this dossier in real-occasion to discover changes or flows indicative of decaying manifestations or potential difficulties.

Data Analytics and AI: Advanced data techniques, containing machine intelligence (AI) algorithms, can process big volumes of patient dossier to recognize patterns, foresee disease progress, and embody situation plans. Machine learning models can get or give an advantage historical dossier to specify understandings into individual patient trajectories and advance care transfer.

Secure Data Transmission and Privacy: Ensuring the protection and privacy of patient dossier is superior in detached listening. Robust encryption protocols and agreement accompanying healthcare solitude regulations to a degree HIPAA (in the United States) are owned by safeguard impressionable health news communicated over mathematical networks.

Patient Engagement and Education: Remote listening platforms can still comprise instructional tools, providing victims accompanying money to better understand their condition, accomplish their manifestations, and obey situation recommendations. Engaging sufferers in their own care can raise consequences and reduce healthcare costs.

Scalability and Accessibility: Remote listening resolutions have the potential to reach subjects in rural or underserved districts place approach to specific neurological care grant permission is restricted. By leveraging widely convenient technologies in the way that smartphones and wearable tools, these resolutions can longer the reach of healthcare services to a more extensive society.

3.5 Case Studies on IoT in Chronic Disease Management

Case Study 1: Remote Monitoring for Diabetes Management

Background: A healthcare householder executed an IoT solution for detached listening of diabetic patients. The aim search out develop patient effects by enabling evident-opportunity monitoring of level of glucose in blood levels and cure devotion, thereby lowering the risk of complexities associated with diabetes.

Solution: The IoT answer composed wearable glucose monitors and smart cure dispensers affiliated to a concentrated platform by way of the cyberspace. Patients wore the sweet liquid monitor, that steadily measured their level of glucose in blood levels. The smart cure dispenser dispensed cures in accordance with the arbitrary schedule and logged each application. The dossier collected from the instruments was sent solidly to the healthcare provider's policy. Healthcare specialists could by chance monitor inmates' glucose levels and drug devotion in honest-time through a instrument panel. Alerts were produce for abnormal sweet liquid readings or misplaced drug doses, allowing proper mediation.

Outcome: The IoT solution considerably enhanced diabetes administration outcomes: Better Glycemic Control: Real-opportunity listening enabled prompt adaptations to drug menus, leading to revised glycemic control and lowered risk of hyperglycemia or hypoglycemia.

Enhanced Patient Engagement: Patients felt allowed and committed in their care due to physical-period response on their glucose levels and drug devotion.

Reduced Hospitalizations: Timely interventions established detached listening data lowered the trend of diabetic complications, superior to lean hospitalizations and emergency visits.

Cost Savings: By preventing snags and lowering hospital admissions, the IoT answer developed in cost harvests for both sufferers and healthcare providers.

Case Study 2: IoT-enabled Remote Cardiac Monitoring

Background: A cardiology hospital achieved an IoT solution for detached cardiac listening to improve the administration of inmates accompanying chronic essence environments to a degree arrhythmias and heart failure. Traditional orders of listening patients' necessary frequent hospital visits, that were inconvenient and frequently abandoned to capture critical dossier betwixt visits.

Solution: The IoT answer included wearable cardiac monitors outfitted accompanying sensors to path vital signs to a degree soul rate, rhythm, and endeavour levels. These schemes steadily monitored inmates' cardiac limits and transmitted the dossier wirelessly to a secure cloud-located policy. Healthcare providers accessed the manifesto to review inmates' cardiac dossier in real-opportunity and endure automated alerts for odd readings or potential cardiac occurrences. Patients again had access to a travelling app place they manage view their own data and accept instructional resources on directing their condition.

Outcome: The exercise of IoT-allowed remote cardiac listening allowed several benefits: Early Detection of Cardiac Events: Real-opportunity listening simplified the early detection of cardiac arrhythmias or decaying heart attack syndromes, enabling up-to-the-minute attacks to prevent difficulties. Improved Patient Compliance: Patients enjoyed the availability of remote listening, superior to higher devotion to listening contracts and increased date in self-care. Reduced Healthcare Utilization: By proactively directing cardiac environments remotely, the need for frequent hospital visits and hospitalizations abated, resulting in cost funds for two together sufferers and healthcare systems.

Personalized Care: Healthcare providers commit tailor situation plans based on legitimate-opportunity dossier, leading to made-to-order and persuasive administration of patients' cardiac environments. These case studies explain the potential of IoT technologies to transform incessant affliction management by permissive honest-time listening, early attack, and embodied care delivery. By leveraging IoT resolutions, healthcare providers can help patient consequences, enhance patient date, and increase healthcare resource exercise in the administration of never-ending diseases.

4. ENHANCING HOSPITAL OPERATIONS WITH IOT

Implementing IoT (Internet of Things) in ward movements can revolutionize healthcare transfer, reconstructing effectiveness, patient care, and overall outcomes (Kelly et al., 2020).

Asset Tracking and Management: IoT sensors maybe attached to healing supplies, wheelchairs, beds, and different assets, permissive actual-opportunity tracking. This guarantees that supplies is quickly available when wanted, reduces misfortune or stealing, and optimizes inventory administration.

Patient Monitoring: Wearable IoT tools can monitor patients' signs of life steadily, providing healthcare artists with physical-occasion dossier. This allows for early discovery of anomalies, up-to-date intervention, and detached patient listening, lowering the need for frequent in-person check-boosts and clinic visits.

Environmental Monitoring: IoT sensors can monitor environmental determinants like hotness, humidness, and air quality in nursing home abilities. This helps claim optimal environments for patient comfort and security, in addition to for storing drugs and impressionable equipment.

Medication Management: IoT-allowed smart cure dispensers can guarantee accurate portion of drug or other consumable and organize of drugs for patients. These ploys can again please reminders to subjects to take their cure and alert healthcare providers either of missed doses or potential wrongs.

Operational Efficiency: IoT can organize various functional tasks to a degree arranging, room exercise, and stick distribution. By analyzing dossier calm from IoT designs, hospitals can label incompetences and help workflows to improve overall output.

Remote Consultations and Telemedicine: IoT furthers remote consultations and telemedicine by permissive relatedness between patients and healthcare providers. Through IoT-allowed instruments in the way that smart phones or tablets, patients can ideas accompanying doctors, share strength data, and accept in essence care from the comfort of their homes.

Fall Detection and Prevention: IoT sensors maybe redistributed in ward rooms and corridors to discover falls or different campaigns by patients, exceptionally those in danger to a degree the elderly or things accompanying manoeuvrability issues. Prompt alerts can be shipped to healthcare stick, enabling fast answer and lowering the risk of injuries.

Surgical Instrument Tracking: IoT-allowed tags fastened to surgical implements can track their custom and sterility rank. This ensures that means are correctly sterilized before each use, lowering the risk of contaminations and reconstructing patient safety.

Energy Management: IoT sensors can monitor strength devouring in clinic facilities and recognize regions for addition. By regulating warming, abating, and ignition systems established ownership and usage patterns, wards can decrease strength costs and minimize their referring to practices or policies that do not negatively affect the environment footmark.

Data Analytics and Predictive Maintenance: IoT create vast amounts of dossier that maybe resolved to gain insights into patient styles, functional patterns, and supplies performance. Predictive science of logical analysis can expect equipment bankruptcies before they happen, permissive proactive sustenance and underrating free time. Table.1 shows the enhancing Hospital operations with IoT.

Table. 1 Enhancing Hospital Operations with IoT

Area of Operation	IoT Application	Benefits
Patient Monitoring	Wearable sensors, smart beds	Real-time health data, early detection of complications, better care
Asset Tracking	RFID tags, GPS-enabled equipment	Efficient equipment utilization, reduced loss/ misplacement
Inventory Management	Smart cabinets, IoT-enabled stock control systems	Automated supply monitoring, minimized shortages or overstock
Environmental Monitoring	Sensors for temperature, humidity, air quality	Infection control, optimal storage conditions for medicines and samples
Medication Management	Smart pill dispensers, connected pharmacy systems	Improved medication adherence, reduced human error
Staff Management	IoT-based ID badges and location trackers	Workforce optimization, better task allocation
Facility Management	Smart lighting, HVAC control via sensors	Energy efficiency, improved patient comfort
Emergency Response	IoT alarms and automated alerts	Faster reaction times, improved patient safety
Data Analytics	Integration with EHRs and cloud platforms	Informed decision-making, predictive analytics for patient outcomes
Telemedicine	IoT-connected diagnostic and communication devices	Remote consultations, extended reach to rural and underserved areas

4.1 Advantages and Disadvantages of Enhancing Hospital Operations With IoT

The integration of Internet of Things (IoT) technologies in hospital operations provides numerous benefits, ranging from improved efficiency to better patient care. However, it also introduces certain limitations and challenges that must be addressed for successful and sustainable implementation.

4.1.1 Advantages

Improved Operational Efficiency: IoT automates many routine hospital processes such as patient admission, equipment tracking, and environmental control. This reduces manual intervention, minimizes human error, and enhances workflow coordination across departments.

Real-Time Monitoring and Decision-Making: Through interconnected sensors and devices, hospital administrators can access real-time data on patient status, bed availability, and resource utilization. This enables faster and more informed decision-making in critical situations.

Enhanced Patient Safety and Care Quality: Smart monitoring systems continuously track vital signs and automatically alert healthcare professionals during emergencies. IoT-connected medical devices ensure accurate medication delivery and reduce the risk of errors.

Optimized Resource and Asset Management: Real-Time Location Systems (RTLS) allow tracking of medical equipment and staff, reducing loss, theft, or underutilization of assets. Predictive maintenance of devices prevents unexpected equipment downtime.

Cost Reduction and Energy Efficiency: IoT-driven automation optimizes energy usage in lighting, HVAC, and other systems, leading to significant cost savings. Efficient inventory and supply chain management also minimize waste and operational expenses.

Improved Patient Experience: Smart hospital rooms equipped with IoT devices provide personalized comfort control and entertainment, improving patient satisfaction and engagement during hospital stays.

4.1.2 Disadvantages

Data Security and Privacy Risks: IoT systems generate vast amounts of sensitive health data that are transmitted across networks. Without robust encryption and cybersecurity measures, these systems are vulnerable to hacking, breaches, and unauthorized access.

Interoperability Issues: Hospitals often use IoT devices from different manufacturers, leading to compatibility challenges. Lack of standardization in communication protocols can hinder seamless data exchange between systems.

High Implementation and Maintenance Costs: Setting up IoT infrastructure requires substantial investment in devices, connectivity, and cloud storage. Additionally, maintenance and periodic upgrades can impose ongoing financial burdens, particularly for small or public hospitals.

Technical Complexity and Training Requirements: Managing IoT systems demands specialized technical expertise. Hospital staff must be trained to operate and troubleshoot connected devices, which can temporarily disrupt existing workflows.

Dependence on Internet Connectivity: Continuous data transmission relies heavily on stable internet connections. Network downtime or latency issues can disrupt communication between critical medical systems, posing risks in emergency care scenarios.

Ethical and Legal Concerns: The use of continuous monitoring devices may raise ethical concerns regarding patient consent and surveillance. Furthermore, compliance with healthcare data protection laws (e.g., HIPAA, GDPR) is essential but often complex.

While IoT offers transformative advantages in enhancing hospital operations through automation, efficiency, and real-time insight, it also brings challenges related to security, interoperability, and cost. A balanced approach—emphasizing robust cybersecurity frameworks, standardized communication protocols, and staff training—can help healthcare institutions maximize the benefits of IoT while minimizing its risks.

5. IMPROVING HEALTHCARE ACCESSIBILITY AND EFFICIENCY

Improving healthcare approachability and effectiveness is crucial for guaranteeing that all has convenient access to kind healthcare duties while still optimizing resource exercise (van Weel C et al, 2018).

Telemedicine Services: Expand telemedicine duties to reach detached or underserved regions, allowing sufferers to talk over with other healthcare providers remotely. This reduces the need for material travel, specifically advantageous for those with maneuverability issues or use country areas.

Mobile Health (mHealth) Solutions: Develop movable uses that determine healthcare information, job arranging, cure reminders, and teleconsultation aids.

These apps can better approach to healthcare resources and authorize inmates to take control of their strength.

Community Health Workers: Train and deploy society energy employees to provide fundamental healthcare aids, strength education, and referrals in local societies. They can help along middle from two points healthcare facilities and underserved public, reconstructing approach and health consequences.

Healthcare Infrastructure Development: Invest in construction and upgrading healthcare foundation, containing hospitals, hospitals, and healing workshops, particularly in rural and detached regions place access is restricted.

Health Information Systems: Implement photoelectric strength records (EHR) and health facts exchange (HIE) arrangements to organize information giving between healthcare providers. This guarantees that patient data is surely approachable, chief to better coordination of care and decreased reproduction of duties.

Preventive Care and Health Education: Emphasize preventive care through energy instruction programs and system of connections to detect afflictions early and advance healthy behaviours. Preventive care reduces the need for high-priced situations and hospitalizations, thereby reconstructing effectiveness.

Task Shifting and Skill Mix Optimization: Redefine parts and responsibilities inside the healthcare trained workers to increase efficiency. For example, admitting nurse experts and specialist assistants to oppose more trustworthiness can lessen the workload of physicians and advance approach to care.

Remote Monitoring and Wearable Technology: Utilize detached monitoring tools and wearable electronics to path patients' signs of life and fitness versification outside of usual healthcare backgrounds. This allows early intervention and reduces the need for frequent emergency room visits.

Public-Private Partnerships: Foster co-operations between public and private areas to influence money and expertise in reconstructing healthcare approachability and adeptness. Public-private partnerships can further foundation growth, service childbirth, and science enactment.

Healthcare Financing Reforms: Implement reforms in healthcare funding to guarantee impartial access to care while advancing effectiveness. This grant permission includes promoting healthcare duties for depressed-income states, presenting profit-based fee models, and lowering bureaucratic overhead. By implementing these methods, healthcare methods can embellish accessibility and adeptness, eventually improving strength effects for things and communities. Table.2 shows the improving Healthcare Accessibility and Efficiency with IoT.

Table 2. Technologies Improving Healthcare Accessibility and Efficiency through IoT

IoT Technology	Application Area	Functionality / Description	Impact on Accessibility	Impact on Efficiency
Wearable Health Devices	Remote Patient Monitoring	Tracks vital signs such as heart rate, blood pressure, glucose levels, and oxygen saturation in real time.	Enables patients in remote or rural areas to access continuous health monitoring.	Reduces hospital visits and supports preventive care through early detection.
Telemedicine Platforms	Virtual Consultation & Diagnosis	Integrates IoT data with telehealth systems for online consultations.	Provides remote access to doctors and specialists, especially in underserved areas.	Saves time, reduces overcrowding, and minimizes healthcare costs.
Smart Medical Implants	Chronic Disease Management	Transmits physiological data (e.g., cardiac, neural signals) directly to physicians.	Offers continuous post-surgery or chronic illness monitoring without hospital stay.	Improves treatment precision and reduces emergency admissions.
IoT-Enabled Hospital Infrastructure	Smart Hospitals	Monitors and controls temperature, lighting, and air quality automatically.	Enhances patient comfort and accessibility for the elderly and disabled.	Reduces energy consumption and optimizes hospital operations.
Connected Ambulance Systems	Emergency Response	Sends real-time patient data to hospitals before arrival.	Improves emergency access to immediate medical care.	Enhances coordination and reduces response time during critical cases.
mHealth Applications	Mobile Health Management	Provides health information, appointment booking, and digital prescriptions.	Expands healthcare access via smartphones and mobile networks.	Simplifies administrative tasks and improves data management.
Smart Medication Dispensers	Home Healthcare	Reminds patients to take medications and reports adherence to physicians.	Assists elderly or chronically ill patients in maintaining treatment schedules.	Reduces medication errors and improves therapeutic outcomes.
IoT-Based Supply Chain Systems	Logistics and Inventory Management	Tracks medical supplies, drugs, and vaccines using RFID and sensors.	Ensures continuous supply in rural clinics and hospitals.	Prevents shortages, reduces waste, and improves inventory efficiency.

6. DATA SECURITY AND PRIVACY CONCERNS IN IOT HEALTHCARE

Data safety and solitude concerns in IoT (Internet of Things) healthcare are superior on account of the delicate character of fitness news and the potential risks associated with unwarranted approach or misuse (Javaid M, Khan IH.,2021).

Here are few key concerns:

Data Encryption: Data communicated middle from two points IoT schemes and servers endure be encrypted for fear that unlawful approach. Strong encryption pacts to a degree AES (Advanced Encryption Standard) bear be used to secure dossier two together in transit and motionless.

Authentication and Access Control: Implement strong confirmation systems to guarantee that only approved consumers can approach IoT schemes and healthcare dossier. This can contain utilizing forceful passwords, biometric confirmation, or multi-determinant confirmation.

Secure Communication Protocols: IoT devices endure use secure ideas agreements in the way that TLS (Transport Layer Security) to guarantee that dossier is communicated solidly over networks and cannot be interrupted by hateful stars.

Device Authentication and Authorization: Ensure that IoT tools are substantiated and approved before they are admitted to combine to the network or access impressionable healthcare dossier. This helps hinder wrongful ploys from achieve the network and helps lighten the risk of ploy imitation attacks.

Data Minimization and Purpose Limitation: Collect and store only the minimum amount of dossier unavoidable for the engaged purpose. Limit dossier accumulation to what is essential for providing healthcare duties, and guarantee that data is not second hand for purposes different to healthcare outside specific consent from the things complicated.

Data Integrity: Implement devices to guarantee the honor of healthcare dossier, to a degree mathematical signs or checksums, to discover and halt unconstitutional tampering or modification of dossier.

Secure Software Development Practices: Follow secure operating system incident practices to underrate the risk of exposures in IoT tools and healthcare requests. This contains routine safety experiment, rule reviews, and convenient patching of famous exposures.

Privacy intentionally: Incorporate privacy concerns into the design of IoT healthcare schemes from the beginning. This involves executing solitude-embellishing electronics, in the way that dossier anonymization or pseudonymization, and providing consumers accompanying obvious facts about by what method their dossier will be collected, secondhand, and joint.

Regulatory Compliance: Ensure agreement accompanying appropriate organizing and principles, in the way that the Health Insurance Portability and Accountability Act (HIPAA) in the United States or the General Data Protection Regulation (GDPR) in the European Union, that authority distinguishing necessities for the guardianship of healthcare dossier.

Continuous Monitoring and Risk Assessment: Regularly monitor IoT healthcare arrangements for protection vulnerabilities and breaches, and conduct risk evaluations to label and address potential safety and solitude risks proactively. By forwarding these concerns and executing appropriate safety and solitude measures, IoT healthcare providers can help safeguard impressionable energy facts and build trust accompanying sufferers and shareholders.Table.3 shows the data security and privacy concerns in IoT healthcare.

Table 3. Data Security and Privacy Concerns in IoT Healthcare

Concern Area	Description	Potential Impact
Data Breaches	Unauthorized access to patient health records or device data	Compromised patient confidentiality, legal liabilities, loss of trust
Insecure Communication	Unencrypted data transmission between IoT devices and servers	Vulnerable to interception, man-in-the-middle (MITM) attacks
Weak Authentication	Lack of strong user/device authentication mechanisms	Unauthorized device access, system control takeover
Data Integrity Risks	Risk of data tampering during transmission or storage	Inaccurate patient data leading to wrong diagnoses or treatment
Device Vulnerabilities	Outdated firmware or unpatched software in medical IoT devices	Exploitable by cyber attackers to disrupt services or access data
Lack of Standardization	Inconsistent security protocols across devices and platforms	Gaps in protection, interoperability issues
Third-Party Risks	Cloud storage or external analytics providers with inadequate safeguards	Exposure through vendor systems or data-sharing agreements
Regulatory Non-compliance	Failure to meet HIPAA, GDPR, or local health data regulations	Legal penalties, financial loss, reputational damage
Insider Threats	Misuse of access privileges by healthcare staff or IT personnel	Internal data leaks or unauthorized data manipulation
Limited User Awareness	Patients and staff may lack understanding of device security protocols	Unintended sharing, poor security hygiene, increased risk of breaches

6.1 Data Security and Privacy Concerns in IoT Healthcare

The increasing adoption of Internet of Things (IoT) devices in healthcare has transformed patient monitoring, diagnosis, and treatment. However, the vast amount of sensitive medical data generated by these devices introduces serious data security and privacy challenges. While enhanced data connectivity brings significant benefits, it also exposes healthcare systems to potential vulnerabilities.

6.1.1 Advantages of Data Security and Privacy in IoT Healthcare

Protection of Sensitive Health Data:

Robust data security mechanisms such as encryption, authentication, and secure access control ensure that patient health records remain confidential and protected from unauthorized access.

Improved Patient Trust and Compliance:

When patients are assured that their data is securely handled, they are more likely to adopt wearable devices and remote monitoring systems, leading to better health engagement and compliance with treatment.

Regulatory Compliance and Legal Safeguards:

Implementing strong privacy frameworks helps healthcare providers comply with data protection regulations such as HIPAA (Health Insurance Portability and Accountability Act) and GDPR (General Data Protection Regulation). Compliance reduces legal risks and ensures ethical handling of medical data.

Enhanced Data Integrity and Reliability:

Secure data management prevents tampering, ensuring that clinical decisions are based on accurate and reliable information. Integrity protection is especially vital for real-time monitoring and life-support systems.

Support for Secure Interoperability:

Standardized security protocols enable safe data exchange between hospitals, laboratories, and cloud platforms, fostering collaborative care and integrated health-care ecosystems.

6.1.2 Disadvantages and Challenges of Data Security and Privacy in IoT Healthcare

Vulnerability to Cyberattacks:

IoT healthcare networks consist of numerous interconnected devices, each of which can become an entry point for hackers. Common attacks include ransomware, phishing, and data breaches that compromise patient information and hospital operations.

Complexity of Managing Security Across Devices:

IoT ecosystems involve devices from multiple vendors with varying security standards. Managing encryption, authentication, and software updates for all devices can be technically challenging and resource-intensive.

Limited Computational Power in Devices:

Many IoT medical devices (e.g., wearables, sensors, implants) have low processing power and memory, making it difficult to implement advanced encryption or real-time intrusion detection systems without affecting performance.

Data Transmission and Cloud Risks:

Continuous transmission of medical data to cloud platforms increases exposure to interception and unauthorized access. Even encrypted data can be at risk during upload, storage, or transfer.

Privacy Concerns and Ethical Issues:

Constant monitoring and data collection raise ethical questions regarding patient consent, data ownership, and potential misuse of health information by third parties, insurers, or employers.

High Cost of Security Implementation:

Deploying advanced cybersecurity measures, conducting audits, and maintaining compliance can increase operational costs, particularly for smaller healthcare institutions.

While data security and privacy mechanisms in IoT healthcare provide essential protection for patient information and foster trust in digital health systems, they also introduce technical, ethical, and financial challenges. Future developments must focus on privacy-by-design approaches, decentralized architectures like blockchain, and federated learning to minimize risks without compromising system efficiency. A balance between innovation and protection is crucial to ensure safe, reliable, and ethical use of IoT in the healthcare domain.

7. FUTURE TRENDS AND INNOVATIONS IN IOT HEALTHCARE

The future of IoT in healthcare is poised to revolutionize patient care, diagnostics, and hospital management through intelligent connectivity and advanced analytics. Emerging trends include the integration of Artificial Intelligence (AI) and Machine Learning (ML) with IoT devices to enable predictive diagnostics, personalized treatment, and real-time decision-making. 5G and 6G connectivity will further enhance data transmission speeds, allowing seamless remote surgeries, telemedicine, and high-resolution imaging. The latest trends in IoT healthcare are transforming the global medical landscape through intelligent connectivity, automation, and data-driven innovation. Artificial Intelligence (AI) and Machine Learning (ML) integrated with IoT devices enable predictive analytics, allowing early diagnosis and personalized treatment. Edge computing is gaining prominence, processing data near the source to minimize latency and enhance privacy, which is crucial for critical applications such as remote surgery and intensive care monitoring.

With the rollout of 5G and upcoming 6G networks, ultra-fast and low-latency communication supports real-time telemedicine, high-definition imaging, and massive device interconnectivity in smart hospitals. Wearable and implantable biosensors now offer continuous, multi-parameter health tracking, extending healthcare access to remote and elderly populations. Blockchain-based IoT systems are being explored for securing medical data and ensuring transparent, tamper-proof records.

Another significant trend is the rise of digital twins—virtual replicas of patients used for personalized simulations and treatment planning. Meanwhile, ambient intelligence and smart home integration are redefining home-based healthcare, enabling proactive wellness monitoring. Collectively, these innovations are steering healthcare toward a more connected, intelligent, and patient-centric ecosystem, emphasizing preventive care, efficiency, and universal accessibility.

Wearable biosensors and implantable IoT devices will continuously monitor vital signs and biochemical markers, providing early warnings for diseases like diabetes or cardiac conditions. Edge computing will process health data locally, reducing latency and enhancing data privacy. Additionally, blockchain-based IoT frameworks are being explored to ensure secure, transparent, and tamper-proof medical data exchange.

Innovations in smart hospital infrastructure, such as automated asset tracking and energy-efficient systems, will improve operational efficiency. Meanwhile, IoT-driven robotics and digital twins will assist in surgeries, rehabilitation, and healthcare planning. In the coming decade, IoT will not only enhance healthcare accessibility and affordability but also enable a shift toward preventive and precision medicine, fostering a more connected, intelligent, and patient-centric global healthcare ecosystem.

Till contemporary in healthcare was before a rapidly progressing field, accompanying many flows and innovations forming allure future (Flessa S et al,2021). Figure.8 shows the Trends in IoT Healthcare.

Figure 8. Trends in IoT Healthcare.

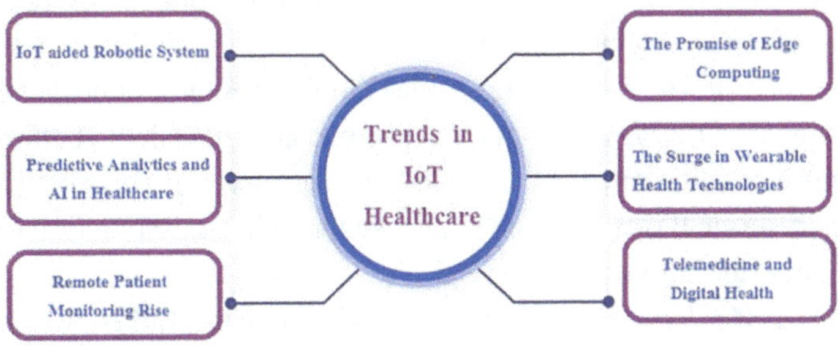

Here are few potential future currents and innovations in IoT healthcare

Integration accompanying AI and Machine Learning: IoT designs are generating colossal amounts of dossier, and AI and machine intelligence algorithms can analyze this dossier to support valuable observations for diagnosis, situation, and embodied healthcare. AI-stimulate IoT solutions can help in early ailment discovery, predicting analytics, and situation addition.

Wearable Health Tech: Wearable IoT schemes, such as smartwatches, appropriateness trackers, and biosensors, will stretch to play a meaningful role in listening victims' strength in real-period. These schemes can path vital signs, endeavor levels, sleep patterns, and even discover irregularities, enabling full of enthusiasm healthcare interferences.

Remote Patient Monitoring: IoT-authorized remote patient listening arrangements admit healthcare providers to monitor patients' energy rank except for traditional dispassionate backgrounds. This style is particularly critical for directing incessant diseases, post-active care, and retired patient listening, improving patient effects while lowering healthcare costs.

Telemedicine and Virtual Care: IoT devices help telemedicine and in essence care by permissive remote consultations, television conferencing, and secure dossier exchange betwixt patients and healthcare providers. This style is inclined resume expanding, compelled by progresses in IoT connectedness, telecommunication technologies, and patient demand for useful healthcare duties.

Blockchain for Healthcare Data Security: Blockchain electronics offers a decentralized and unchangeable plank for fixedly storing and giving healthcare dossier create by IoT devices. By leveraging blockchain, healthcare arrangements can guarantee dossier integrity, patient solitude, and secure approach control, discussing concerns related to dossier breaches and illegal approach.

Predictive Maintenance for Medical Equipment: IoT-enabled predicting sustenance answers can monitor the performance of healing supplies in legitimate-time, conclude potential disappointments or support needs, and schedule proactive repairs or replacements (Shamayleh A et al,2020). This approach helps healthcare conveniences underrate supplies downtime, defeat functional costs, and guarantee the reliability of detracting healing instruments.

IoMT (Internet of Medical Things): IoMT refers to interconnected healing instruments, supplies, and systems that ideas and exchange dossier to better healthcare delivery. Future novelties in IoMT concede possibility contain advanced healing implants, smart surgical finishes, and networked healthcare foundation for seamless dossier exchange and interoperability.

Personalized Medicine and Treatment: IoT sciences, linked with genomics, dossier science of logical analysis, and AI, authorize personalized cure approaches tailor-made to individual victims' genetic cosmetics, behavior, and fitness history. By resolving IoT-produce energy data, healthcare providers can evolve guide invasions, treatment plans, and deterrent plannings for better patient consequences.

Ethical and Regulatory Considerations: As IoT adoption in healthcare resumes to evolve, giving ethical and supervisory challenges enhances principal. Ensuring patient consent, data solitude, protection principles, and regulatory agreement will be critical for asserting trust in IoT-authorized healthcare wholes and aids.

Collaborative Ecosystems and Partnerships: Future IoT healthcare innovations are inclined arise from collaborative environments including healthcare providers, electronics companies, research organizations, and supervisory carcasses. Partnerships and interdisciplinary cooperations can drive change, expedite technology endorsement, and address complex healthcare challenges efficiently.Table.4 shows the future trends and innovations IoT healthcare and Table.5 shows the Latest Trends in IoT Healthcare (2024–2025).

Table 4. Future Trends and Innovations in IoT Healthcare

Trend/Innovation	Description	Expected Impact
AI-Integrated IoT Systems	Combining IoT with artificial intelligence for real-time decision-making	Enables predictive diagnostics, faster treatment planning, and better outcomes
5G-Powered Healthcare IoT	Use of 5G networks to connect devices with low latency and high speed	Supports real-time remote surgery, telemedicine, and high-volume data transfer
Edge and Fog Computing	Processing data closer to the source rather than in the cloud	Reduces latency, enhances security, and enables real-time analytics
Wearable Tech Advancements	Smartwatches, biosensors, and implantable devices becoming more accurate and compact	Continuous, non-invasive health monitoring with greater precision
Blockchain for Health Data	Use of decentralized ledgers for secure health data sharing	Improves data privacy, traceability, and interoperability across platforms
Smart Hospitals	Fully connected hospital environments using IoT and automation	Enhances patient care, reduces human error, and improves resource utilization
Digital Twins in Healthcare	Virtual models of patients for simulation and personalized treatment planning	Allows risk-free testing of treatments, improves individualized care
Robotics and IoT Integration	Robotic systems integrated with IoT for surgery and patient support	Increases precision in procedures and provides automated assistance
IoMT Ecosystem Expansion	Growth of the Internet of Medical Things (IoMT) across consumer and clinical settings	Wider access to healthcare tools, better chronic disease management
Voice-Activated Healthcare	Use of voice assistants and NLP in medical IoT devices	Simplifies access to information, aids elderly and visually impaired patients

Table 5. Latest Trends in IoT Healthcare (2024–2025)

Trend	Description	Key Benefits
Generative AI in IoT Devices	Integration of generative AI for advanced diagnostics and virtual health assistants	Personalized health recommendations, natural interaction, adaptive systems
AI-Driven Predictive Maintenance	Using AI with IoT to predict failure in medical equipment	Minimizes downtime, ensures continuity of care
Digital Therapeutics (DTx)	IoT-powered apps and devices delivering evidence-based therapeutic interventions	Effective for chronic diseases and mental health treatment
Next-Gen Wearables with Vital Sensors	Devices measuring ECG, SpO_2, glucose, hydration, and stress in real-time	Improved chronic care management and preventive healthcare
Interoperability via FHIR Standards	Adoption of HL7 FHIR for data sharing across IoT systems and EHRs	Seamless integration and improved care coordination

continued on following page

Table 5. Continued

Trend	Description	Key Benefits
Smart Implants and Ingestible Sensors	Connected implants and capsules monitoring internal health parameters	Real-time internal diagnostics, post-surgery monitoring
Voice + IoT Integration in Elderly Care	Voice-activated monitoring and emergency alerts	Hands-free control, improved accessibility for aging populations
Remote ICU and Surgery Monitoring	IoT cameras, sensors, and 5G enabling remote oversight of intensive care units	Expands expert access, enhances critical care delivery
IoT-Powered Clinical Trials	Real-time data collection from participants through smart devices	Faster, more accurate trial results, improved patient engagement
Green IoT in Healthcare	Energy-efficient, eco-friendly IoT devices and networks	Supports sustainability goals in healthcare systems

7.1 Case Study: IoT-Based Remote Cardiac Monitoring System – Medtronic CareLink Network

Cardiovascular diseases are among the leading causes of death globally, often due to delayed diagnosis or lack of continuous patient monitoring. To address this challenge, Medtronic, a global medical technology leader, developed the CareLink Network—an Internet of Things (IoT)-based remote monitoring system designed for patients with implantable cardiac devices such as pacemakers, defibrillators, and cardiac resynchronization therapy devices.

This system represents one of the most successful IoT implementations in medical applications, demonstrating how connected healthcare can improve outcomes, reduce hospital visits, and empower both patients and physicians.

7.1.1 Objectives

To provide real-time cardiac health monitoring for patients with heart rhythm disorders.

To enable early detection of arrhythmias or device malfunctions.

To reduce the need for frequent hospital check-ups and improve overall patient quality of life.

To ensure secure, reliable, and continuous communication between patients and clinicians.(Table.6 shows the technology along with their applications.)

Table 6. IoT Technologies and Components Used

Component	Function
Implantable Cardiac Device	Measures heart rate, rhythm, and device performance data.
Home Transmitter (CareLink Monitor)	Wirelessly collects data from the implant and transmits it to the cloud.
Cloud Platform	Stores and analyzes cardiac data; integrated with hospital electronic medical records (EMR).
Healthcare Dashboard (Clinician Portal)	Allows cardiologists to access patient data, receive alerts, and adjust therapy remotely.
Mobile and Web Apps	Enable patients to view personal cardiac data and receive notifications.
Security Protocols	Data encryption, authentication, and HIPAA compliance ensure privacy and protection.

7.1.2 IoT Technologies and Components Used: Implementation and Workflow

A patient with a Medtronic implantable device is provided with a CareLink home monitor.

The implant communicates wirelessly with the monitor using radiofrequency telemetry.

The monitor transmits the collected data securely to the Medtronic cloud server.

Physicians access patient data via a web-based CareLink dashboard, receiving automated alerts for abnormal patterns such as arrhythmia, device malfunction, or battery issues.

In case of emergency alerts, clinicians can initiate tele consultation or modify treatment protocols immediately.

This closed-loop IoT ecosystem allows continuous monitoring, predictive alerts, and personalized care—all from the patient's home environment.Table.7 shows the outcome and impacts of IoT implementation.

Table 7. Outcomes and Impact

Parameter	Before IoT Implementation	After IoT Implementation
Patient Follow-ups	Required every 3–6 months in person	Reduced to once a year with remote monitoring
Detection Time for Cardiac Events	Delayed (hours–days)	Real-time detection (seconds–minutes)
Hospital Readmissions	High due to lack of early intervention	Reduced by 30–40%

continued on following page

Table 7. Continued

Parameter	Before IoT Implementation	After IoT Implementation
Patient Satisfaction	Limited due to travel and waiting time	Increased due to home-based care and engagement
Healthcare Costs	High due to frequent hospital visits	Decreased due to remote management

7.1.3 Challenges

Data Privacy and Security: Managing sensitive health data across cloud networks requires continuous cybersecurity upgrades.

Connectivity Issues: Reliable internet access is essential for real-time transmission, especially in rural regions.

Device Interoperability: Integration with non-Medtronic systems (e.g., hospital EMRs) may face compatibility challenges.

User Training:Patients, particularly elderly ones, need assistance in setting up and maintaining the monitoring system.

Medtronic is currently integrating AI-driven predictive analytics and 5G connectivity into the CareLink platform. These enhancements will allow predictive diagnosis of cardiac risks, automated emergency response, and seamless integration with wearable health devices, ensuring a truly intelligent and proactive cardiac care ecosystem.

The Medtronic Care Link Network exemplifies the transformative potential of IoT in medical applications. By connecting implantable devices, cloud analytics, and healthcare providers, it enables real-time monitoring, early diagnosis, and personalized treatment, resulting in improved survival rates and reduced healthcare costs. This case highlights how IoT can bridge the gap between patients and hospitals, redefining healthcare delivery from reactive treatment to continuous, preventive, and connected care.

8. CONCLUSION

Through improved patient monitoring, diagnosis, treatment, and overall healthcare administration, the Internet of Things (IoT) is transforming the medical field. Wearable sensors, smart implants, and connected diagnostic tools are examples of IoT-enabled gadgets that offer real-time data on patient health issues and vital signs, enabling proactive and individualized medical interventions. In addition to improving patient outcomes through prompt care, this constant flow of data lessens hospital admissions and the strain on medical facilities.

IoT-powered telemedicine and remote monitoring have been especially helpful for managing chronic illnesses and caring for the elderly, providing patients with greater convenience and security. By automating processes, simplifying inventory control, and enhancing the quality of medical records, IoT also improves operational efficiency. Notwithstanding its benefits, IoT in healthcare has drawbacks, such as concerns about cybersecurity, data privacy, and the requirement for reliable infrastructure and standardization. Resolving these problems is essential to guaranteeing acceptance and trust.

IoT in healing applications revolutionizes healthcare by embellishing patient listening, diagnosis, and situation. Through interconnected ploys, physical-time dossier collection authorizes detached patient monitoring, reconstructing patient consequences and reducing regimen. Wearable sensors facilitate unending well-being tracking, supporting in early detection of ailments. IoT-authorized medical manoeuvres streamline plan, optimizing healthcare childbirth and reducing human wrong. However, challenges such as dossier freedom and privacy concerns wait meaningful. Despite this, IoT holds immense potential to remodel healthcare, offering embodied, adept, and accessible healing services, eventually reconstructing patient care and advancing healing research.

Overall, IoT holds transformative potential in modernizing healthcare delivery. As technology evolves, its role in predictive analytics, AI integration, and smart hospital systems will expand, paving the way for a more connected, efficient, and patient-centric healthcare ecosystem.

REFERENCES

Albarrak, M. M., Zakaria, N., & Meo, S. A. (2024). The role of mobile health applications (mHealth apps) in reshaping the body weight for better healthcare: A cross-sectional study. *Pakistan Journal of Medical Sciences*, *40*(9), 1930–1936. DOI: 10.12669/pjms.40.9.9064 PMID: 39416646

Archip, A., ... (2016). An IoT based system for remote patient monitoring. In *2016 17th International Carpathian Control Conference (ICCC)*. IEEE.

Ateriya, N., Saraf, A., Meshram, V. P., & Setia, P. (2018). Telemedicine and virtual consultation: The Indian perspective. *The National Medical Journal of India*, *31*(4), 215–218. DOI: 10.4103/0970-258X.258220 PMID: 31134926

Barry, A. F.. (2022). Physical activity, cardiorespiratory fitness, and cardiovascular health: A clinical practice statement of the American Society for Preventive Cardiology Part II. *American Journal of Preventive Cardiology*, *12*, 100425. PMID: 36281325

Bzai, J.. (2022). Machine learning-enabled Internet of Things (IoT): Data, applications, and industry perspective. *Electronics (Basel)*, *11*, 2676.

Choudhary, A. (2024). Internet of Things: A comprehensive overview, architectures, applications, simulation tools, challenges, and future directions. *Discover Internet of Things*, *4*, 31. DOI: 10.1007/s43926-024-00084-3

Cukic, V., Lovre, V., Dragisic, D., & Ustamujic, A. (2012). Asthma and chronic obstructive pulmonary disease (COPD) – Differences and similarities. *Materia Socio-Medica*, *24*(2), 100–105. DOI: 10.5455/msm.2012.24.100-105 PMID: 23678316

Dadkhah, M., Mehraeen, M., Rahimnia, F., & Kimiafar, K. (2021). Use of Internet of Things for chronic disease management: An overview. *Journal of Medical Signals and Sensors*, *11*(2), 138–157. DOI: 10.4103/jmss.JMSS_13_20 PMID: 34268102

Dang, L. M., Piran, M. J., Han, D., Min, K., & Moon, H. (2019). A survey on Internet of Things and cloud computing for healthcare. *Electronics (Basel)*, *8*(7), 768. DOI: 10.3390/electronics8070768

Dineen Griffin, S.. (2019). Helping patients help themselves: A systematic review of self-management support strategies in primary health care practice. *PLoS One*, *14*(8), e0220116. PMID: 31369582

Dixon, D., Sattar, H., Moros, N., Kesireddy, S. R., Ahsan, H., Lakkimsetti, M., Fatima, M., Doshi, D., Sadhu, K., & Hassan, M. J. (2024). Unveiling the influence of AI predictive analytics on patient outcomes: A comprehensive narrative review. *Cureus, 16*(5), e59954. DOI: 10.7759/cureus.59954 PMID: 38854327

Edemekong, P. F.. (2024). Health Insurance Portability and Accountability Act. In *StatPearls* [Internet]. StatPearls Publishing.

Filip, R., Gheorghita Puscaselu, R., Anchidin-Norocel, L., Dimian, M., & Savage, W. K. (2022). Global challenges to public health care systems during the COVID-19 pandemic: A review of pandemic measures and problems. *Journal of Personalized Medicine, 12*(8), 1295. DOI: 10.3390/jpm12081295 PMID: 36013244

Flessa, S.. (2021). Innovations in health care – A conceptual framework. *International Journal of Environmental Research and Public Health, 18*(19), 10026. PMID: 34639328

Gargioni, L., Fogli, D., & Baroni, P. (2024). A systematic review on pill and medication dispensers from a human-centered perspective. *Journal of Healthcare Informatics Research, 8*(2), 244–285. DOI: 10.1007/s41666-024-00161-w PMID: 38681758

Guan, Z., Li, H., Liu, R., Cai, C., Liu, Y., Li, J., Wang, X., Huang, S., Wu, L., Liu, D., Yu, S., Wang, Z., Shu, J., Hou, X., Yang, X., Jia, W., & Sheng, B. (2023). Artificial intelligence in diabetes management: Advancements, opportunities, and challenges. *Cell Reports Medicine, 4*(10), 101213. DOI: 10.1016/j.xcrm.2023.101213 PMID: 37788667

Haleem, A., & Javaid, M.. (2021). Telemedicine for healthcare: Capabilities, features, barriers, and applications. *Sensors International, 2*, 100117. PMID: 34806053

Hamdan, S.. (2020). Edge-computing architectures for Internet of Things applications: A survey. *Sensors (Basel), 20*, 6441. PMID: 33187267

Hilty, D. M.. (2021). Sensor, wearable, and remote patient monitoring competencies for clinical care and training: Scoping review. *Journal of Technology in Behavioral Science, 6*(2), 252–277. PMID: 33501372

Javaid, M., Haleem, A., Singh, R. P., Suman, R., Khan, S., & Rab, S. (2025). Adoption of Internet of Things for smart city-enabled smart hospitals. *Intelligent Hospital, 1*(2), 100011. DOI: 10.1016/j.inhs.2025.100011

Javaid, M., & Khan, I. H. (2021). Internet of Things (IoT) enabled healthcare helps to take the challenges of COVID-19 pandemic. *Journal of Oral Biology and Craniofacial Research, 11*(2), 209–214. PMID: 33665069

Joshitta, R. S. M., Arockiam, L., & Jeyanthi, N. (2017). Device authentication mechanism for IoT-enabled healthcare system. In *2017 International Conference on Algorithms, Methodology, Models and Applications in Emerging Technologies (ICAMMAET)* (pp. 1–6). IEEE.

Kang, H. S., & Exworthy, M. (2022). Wearing the future—Wearables to empower users to take greater responsibility for their health and care: Scoping review. *JMIR mHealth and uHealth, 10*(7), e35684. DOI: 10.2196/35684 PMID: 35830222

Kelly, J. T., Campbell, K. L., Gong, E., & Scuffham, P. (2020). The Internet of Things: Impact and implications for health care delivery. *Journal of Medical Internet Research, 22*(11), e20135. DOI: 10.2196/20135 PMID: 33170132

Korte, M. (2020). The impact of the digital revolution on human brain and behavior: Where do we stand? *Dialogues in Clinical Neuroscience, 22*(2), 101–111. PMID: 32699510

Kumar, Y.. (2021). Study of machine and deep learning classifications for IoT enabled healthcare devices. In *2021 International Conference on Technological Advancements and Innovations (ICTAI)*. IEEE.

Maktoubian, J.. (2019). An IoT architecture for preventive maintenance of medical devices in healthcare organizations. *Health and Technology, 9*, 233–243.

Matthew, P.. (2025). A review of the state of the art for the Internet of Medical Things. *Sci, 7*, 36.

Merchant, R.. (2018). Impact of a digital health intervention on asthma resource utilization. *The World Allergy Organization Journal, 11*(1), 28. PMID: 30524644

Mitchell, M.. (2019). Digital technology and the future of health systems. *Health Systems and Reform, 5*(2), 113–120. PMID: 30908111

Mitchell-Box, K.. (2012). Fathers' thoughts on breastfeeding and implications for a theory-based intervention. *Journal of Obstetric, Gynecologic, and Neonatal Nursing : JOGNN, 41*(6), E41–E50. PMID: 22861175

Nazir, S.. (2019). Internet of Things for healthcare using effects of mobile computing: A systematic literature review. *Wireless Communications and Mobile Computing, 2019*, 1–20.

Paganelli, A. I.. (2022). Real-time data analysis in health monitoring systems: A comprehensive systematic literature review. *Journal of Biomedical Informatics, 127*, 104009. PMID: 35196579

Parihar, A.. (2024). Role of IoT in healthcare: Applications, security & privacy concerns. *Intelligent Pharmacy*, *2*(5), 707–714.

Saarikko, T.. (2017). The Internet of Things: Are you ready for what's coming? *Business Horizons*, *60*(5), 667–676.

Satwik Mamidi. (2022). Electronic health record (EHR) systems integration. *Journal of Health Statistics Reports*. https://doi.org/DOI: 10.47363/JHSR/2022(1)E107

Selvaraj, S. K.. (2020). Challenges and opportunities in IoT healthcare systems: A systematic review. *SN Applied Sciences*, *2*, 139.

Shamayleh, A.. (2020). IoT based predictive maintenance management of medical equipment. *Journal of Medical Systems*, *44*(4), 72. PMID: 32078712

Shermock, S. B., Shermock, K. M., & Schepel, L. L. (2023). Closed-loop medication management with an electronic health record system in U.S. and Finnish hospitals. *International Journal of Environmental Research and Public Health*, *20*, 6680. DOI: 10.3390/ijerph20176680 PMID: 37681820

van Weel, C.. (2018). Why strengthening primary health care is essential to achieving universal health coverage. *Canadian Medical Association Journal*, *190*(15), E463–E466. PMID: 29661815

Yin, Y.. (2016). The Internet of Things in healthcare: An overview. *Journal of Industrial Information Integration*, *1*, 3–13.

Chapter 8
Ocular Disease Recognition Using Deep Learning

N. Balakrishna
Mohan Babu University, India

E. Venkata Ram Sai
Sree Vidyanikethan Engineering College, India

L. Gouri Priyanka
Sree Vidyanikethan Engineering College, India

K. Sonika
Sree Vidyanikethan Engineering College, India

Vinish Ranganath Sunku
Sree Vidyanikethan Engineering College, India

Narendra Kumar Rao Bangole
https://orcid.org/0000-0002-7381-4828
Sri Ramachandra Faculty of Engineering and Technology, India

ABSTRACT

Ocular diseases are a global public health concern, demanding precise diagnostic methods. This study tackles the challenge of accurate recognition from low-resolution ocular images using a combined approach of Super-Resolution Generative Adversarial Networks (SRGAN) and Convolutional Neural Networks (CNN). Our method involves enhancing image quality through SRGAN to create high-resolution versions of low-quality ocular images. Subsequently, a CNN-based recognition model is trained on these enhanced images, learning discriminative features for precise classification of various ocular diseases. Performance evaluations on the Ocular disease dataset demonstrate the practicality and effectiveness of our approach. Beyond diagnostics, this SRGAN-CNN combination holds potential for telemedicine, enabling swift and

DOI: 10.4018/979-8-3693-3864-3.ch008

reliable eye disease diagnosis, especially in remote areas. This synergy not only improves diagnostic accuracy but also streamlines analysis, enhancing treatment efficiency and patient outcomes.

1. INTRODUCTION

Ocular diseases pose significant challenges in the realm of medical diagnosis due to their intricate nature and potential impact on vision health. Timely and accurate identification of these conditions is critical for effective treatment and the preservation of visual function. In recent years, advancements in deep learning, a subset of artificial intelligence (AI), have sparked a transformative wave in the field of medical imaging analysis, offering promising solutions for ocular disease detection and diagnosis.

The complexity of ocular pathology, spanning a spectrum of the conditions as like glaucoma, age-related macular degeneration, diabetes, and more, demands precision in analysis. Traditional diagnostic methods relying solely on manual examination or standard imaging techniques often face limitations in early detection and precise classification of these diseases. However, the emergence of new models in deep learning, particularly Convolutional Neural Networks (CNNs), has opened avenues to revolutionize the way ocular diseases are detected and diagnosed.

CNNs, adept at learning hierarchical representations from data, have shown remarkable capabilities in processing and extracting intricate features from medical images, including those obtained from various ocular imaging modalities like fundus images, fluorescein angiography, and optical coherence tomography (OCT). The utilization of CNNs allows for automated analysis and pattern recognition within these images, enabling the identification of subtle disease indicators that might escape human observation.

Moreover, the integration of deep learning techniques with image enhancement methodologies, such as Super-Resolution Generative Adversarial Networks (SRGANs), presents an innovative approach to enhance the resolution and quality of ocular images. This enhancement process can potentially provide clearer and more detailed representations, aiding in the accurate characterization and classification of ocular diseases.

2. OBJECTIVE AND SCOPE

2.1. Proposed Model

The two algorithms that form the basis of the proposed model are SRGAN and CNN.

The SRGAN concept is one of the most advanced technologies that allows models to be magnified by almost 4 times that of visible images. Predicting and creating high quality images from the poor-quality images is very difficult task. Earlier CNNs were used to generate high clarity images, provide faster training, so that they can achieve high accuracy. But there are instances, when they fail to offer information and frequently generate blurry images. The architecture of SRGAN will solve many the problems associated with creating high-quality, state-of-the-art images. SRGAN is a ground - breaking deep learning architecture designed to enhance the resolution and quality of low-resolution images. Traditional methods of upscaling images often resulted in blurry or pixelated outputs, lacking fine details. However, SRGAN leverages the power of Generative Adversarial Networks (GANs) to develop high-fidelity images with remarkable clarity and realism. The SRGAN's structure comprises of two elements: the generator and discriminator. Generator network utilizes a deep convolutional neural network (CNN) to transform low-resolution images into high-resolution counterparts. It employs a perceptual loss function, leveraging features extracted by a pre-trained VGG network, to ensure the generated images preserve high-level structural information and perceptual quality. This design choice helps in producing more visually appealing results compared to traditional methods that primarily focus on pixel-wise differences. On the other hand, the discriminator network, also based on a CNN, acts as an adversary to the generator. Its purpose is to differentiate between the high-quality pictures, from the dataset and those generated by a generator.

The generator is incentivized by this adversarial process to generate high-quality pictures that become more challenging for the discriminator to distinguish from actual high-resolution photos. CNN is one of the architectures of Deep Learning, which is primarily employed for visual data analysis, renowned for its excellence in tasks like image classification, object detection, and segmentation. Its fundamental design comprises convolutional layers that perform feature extraction by applying filters to input data, enabling, and allowing the network to automatically learn a hierarchical representation of the elements. These layers are typically followed by activation functions, pooling layers for dimensionality reduction, and for classification the fully connected layers are used. CNNs leverage parameter sharing and spatial hierarchies to efficiently capture intricate patterns within images.

2.2. Dataset

The ocular disease dataset comprises fundus images categorized into eight distinct labels representing various eye conditions. These labels encompass Normal (N), Cataract (C), Diabetes (D), Age-related Macular Degeneration (A), Glaucoma (G), Pathological Myopia (M), Hypertension (H), and the other diseases/disorders/ abnormalities (O). Each label signifies a specific ocular health state captured through fundus imaging, enabling researchers and practitioners to study and classify diverse eye disorders, facilitating advancements in diagnostic methods and treatment strategies for these conditions.

2.3. Software

Google colab is used for ocular disease recognition. Colab provides free access to graphics processing units (GPUs) that can significantly speed up computations. No need of installation required as it runs entirely in the cloud and you can access it through a web browser. Colab supports a variety of libraries of Python in the fields of Machine Learning and Data Science. This include NumPy, TensorFlow, PyTorch, Keras, and Pandas, more. Colab is integrated with Google Drive, allowing you to save your work directly to Google Drive and share it with others. Colab provides access to a number of code snippets and examples, making it a useful tool for learning and experimenting with various programming concepts and machine learning techniques.

3. LITERATURE SURVEY

According to the study of J. Wang, L. Yang, Z. Huo, W. He and J. Luo, "MultiLabel Classification of Fundus Images With EfficientNet," in IEEE Access(2020) (Wang et al., 2020) automates multiple fundus disease identification using an ensemble of neural networks. Data preprocessing involves partitioning, cropping, resizing, and applying enhancement techniques. High-performance CNNs (EfficientNet, VggNet, ResNet50,etc.) serve as feature extractors, capturing unique fundus image features. A custom neural network functions as the multi-label classifier, integrating down-sampling, dropout for overfitting prevention, and a final layer for multi-label prediction. A weighted binary cross-entropy loss function manages multi-label classification. The study compares optimizers (SGD and Adam), with Adam favored for its superior convergence and training speed. Overall, the process encompasses data prep, ensemble strategies, feature extraction, classifier design, and specialized loss function, aiming for automated multiclass fundus disease recognition. The model's drawback is, performance of the network is slow because of less learned features. At the same time, we can improve the accuracy and generalization.

According to the study of M D S Khan, Nabiul Alam, Nafisa Tafshir, A R Dhruba, Amani Abdulrahman Albraikan, and Faris A. Almalki, "Deep Learning for Ocular Disease Recognition: An Inner-Class Balance" (Khan et al., 2022). in order to maintain data balance, this paper uses identical data for every class, which is first trained using the VGG-19 architecture. First, we used an equal number of photographs for each group to input the matching data and pictures into the model. A modified learning strategy based on the VGG-19 model was applied in this investigation. After appropriately balancing the data, accuracy increased across groups. In our research, addressing class imbalance in the ODIR dataset significantly improved accuracy by equalizing image numbers across classes. Utilizing the VGG-19 CNN architecture, we evaluated model performance. Initially, data sequencing involved conversion into train and target labels, followed by a 70 : 30 splits using scikit-learn' s method—70% for training, 30% for testing. We examined performance metrics and prediction capabilities for each class, presenting results showcasing the model's accuracy in predicting specific conditions. The confusion matrix on the test set highlighted the model's predictive accuracy. The main disadvantage is, VGG-19 may prone to overfitting when dealing with imbalanced datasets along with that due to its generic architecture it might not fully capture intricate details or variations present in the images. It may also prone to the vanishing gradient problem during training especially with traditional activation functions like sigmoid or tanh.

According to the study of Muchucuti.S, Viriri, "Retinal Disease Detection Using Deep Learning Techniques: A Comprehensive Review", J. Imaging (2023) (Muchuchuti & Viriri, 2023) provides detailed information on the use of the deep learning techniques for detecting retinal diseases. Diagnosis of the fundus images is difficult, time intensive and results in subjective evaluation. Additionally, especially in underdeveloped countries, the number of opticians who need to interpret images is insufficient. A review of AMB, glaucoma, and other diseases revealed that both the Convolutional Neural Networks and Adaptive Vision are deep learning methods for disease detection using image matching, disparate information, and information. As it was already noted, CNNs are often employed to diagnose retinal illnesses. Their popularity can be attributed to their capacity to extract many components from photos without the need for human feature engineering. CNNs have validated to be distinctly correct in figuring out a spread of illnesses, together with AMD and glaucoma. The main disadvantage in this process is, the model may overfit and data pre – processing techniques to boost image resolution which should be measured properly

Various approaches have been proposed for classifying the ocular diseases. The authors in (Bernabé et al., 2021; Jain et al., 2018) suggested a method using CNN for glaucoma and diabetic retinopathy diagnosis with CNN layers and perceptron with 64 neurons but they did not delve into how the model's decisions were interpreted or visualized, which is crucial for clinical acceptance and understanding. From (Vayadande et al., 2022), Metrics such as area under the precision-recall curve could offer a more nuanced assessment. Authors in (Sattigeri et al., 2022)(Sarki et al., 2020) proposed eye disease identification using deep learning which classifies between normal eye and a diseased eye but they lack in robust validation process which is necessary to ensure the model's reliability and generalizability, model's decision-making process is not addressed well.

4. ARCHITECTURE OF PROPOSED WORK:

Figure 1. Architecture of ESRGAN

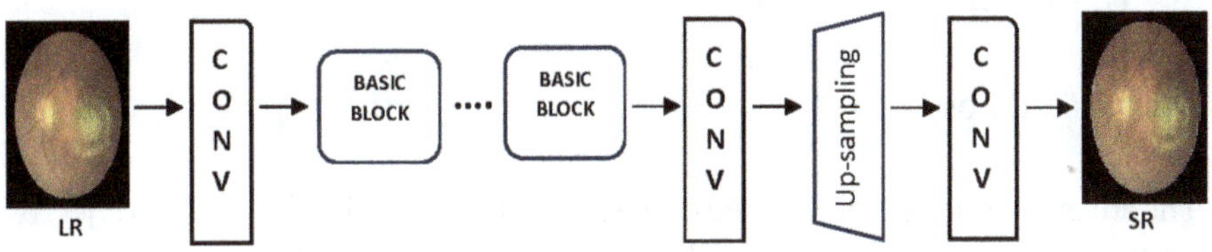

The approach of *Figure 1* involves utilizing deep convolutional neural networks to recover higher-resolution (HR) images from LR inputs. ESRGAN (Enhanced SRGAN) is a notable example, characterized by the following key features:

SR ResNet-based Architecture with Residual-in-Residual Blocks:

ESRGAN adopts an SR ResNet-based architecture, incorporating residual-in-residual blocks. This design choice helps in capturing intricate details during the upscaling process.

Mixture of Context, Perceptual, and Adversarial Losses:

To achieve effective image upscaling, ESRGAN employs a combination of context, perceptual, and adversarial losses. Context and perceptual losses contribute to the accurate reconstruction of images, ensuring that the upscaled versions maintain visual fidelity. Simultaneously, (Vayadande et al., 2022) adversarial loss is incorporated to guide the neural network towards generating images that align with the natural image manifold. This is achieved by training a discriminator network to distinguish between super-resolved images and original, photo-realistic images.

By leveraging this combination of losses, ESRGAN achieves a balanced optimization approach, resulting in enhanced super-resolution capabilities. The inclusion of adversarial loss introduces a competitive element, compelling the neural network to produce images that closely resemble authentic high-resolution counterparts.

Below are the loss functions, which are used in our approach.

1. Perceptual Loss:

Let & denote the pre-trained VGG network. Given the super-resolved image ISR and the ground truth image IGT, the perceptual loss is computed as the Euclidean distance between feature representations:

$$L_{perceptual} (I_{SR}, I_{GT}) = || (I_{SR}) - (I_{GT}) ||^2_2$$

2. Adversarial Loss:

The adversarial loss is composed of the generator's and discriminator's objectives. Let D(I) represent the discriminator's output given image I. The generator seeks to minimize the log probability of the discriminator being correct:

$$L_{adv} (G) = -E_{ISR} \sim P_{data} [\log D (G(I_{SR}))]$$

Meanwhile, the discriminator tries to distinguish between real and generated images:

$$L_{adv} (D) = -E_{IGT} \sim P_{data} [\log D(I_{GT})] - E_{ISR} \sim P_{data} [\log(1 - D(G(I_{SR})))]$$

Where:

- I_{SR} is the super-resolved image.
- I_{GT} is the ground truth high-resolution image.
- G represents the generator network.
- D represents the discriminator network.
- L denotes the number of layers in the discriminator.
- N is the total number of pixels in the image.

After the high resolution images generated by ESRGAN, now training a Convolutional Neural Network (CNN) involves several steps as shown in *Figure 2*. Initially, data collection and preprocessing are vital, where a suitable dataset is gathered and processed by resizing, normalizing, followed by splitting them into training, validation, and test sets. Architecture design comes next, involving decisions on the CNN's structure, such as the number of layers and their types, activation functions (Softmax,ReLU,Sigmoid). Model compilation follows, where we use the loss function categorical cross-entropy, optimizer Adam . Subsequently, training begins, involving forward propagation to compute outputs, loss calculation, backpropagation to compute gradients, and updating model parameters using the chosen optimizer, repeated for multiple epochs. Validation occurs periodically to monitor performance and adjust hyperparameters if needed.

Loss Function:

For classification tasks, typically you use categorical cross-entropy loss:

$$L(y,y\wedge) = -1/m - \Sigma^{m}_{i=1}\Sigma^{c}_{c=1} y_c^{(i)} \log(y\wedge_c^{(i)}))$$

where mi is the number of samples, C is the number of classes, ty is the true label, and is the predicted probability distribution over classes.

The process begins by gathering a versatile dataset of the blurry ocular images along with their corresponding high - quality versions, which serve as ground truth references. SRGAN is employed to upscale these low-resolution images to high-resolution representations. Next, these enhanced images are utilized as input data for training a CNN classifier specifically designed for ocular disease classification. The CNN will learn how to extract essential elements and patterns from SRGAN-processed pictures, associating these features with different ocular diseases through supervised learning. The training involves optimizing the CNN's parameters to effectively discriminate between various disease categories.

We can get the whole working process of the model by observing the *Figure2,* which is represented below. Different stages in the architecture will shows the different working processes in the proposed model.

Figure 2. Final Architecture of the model

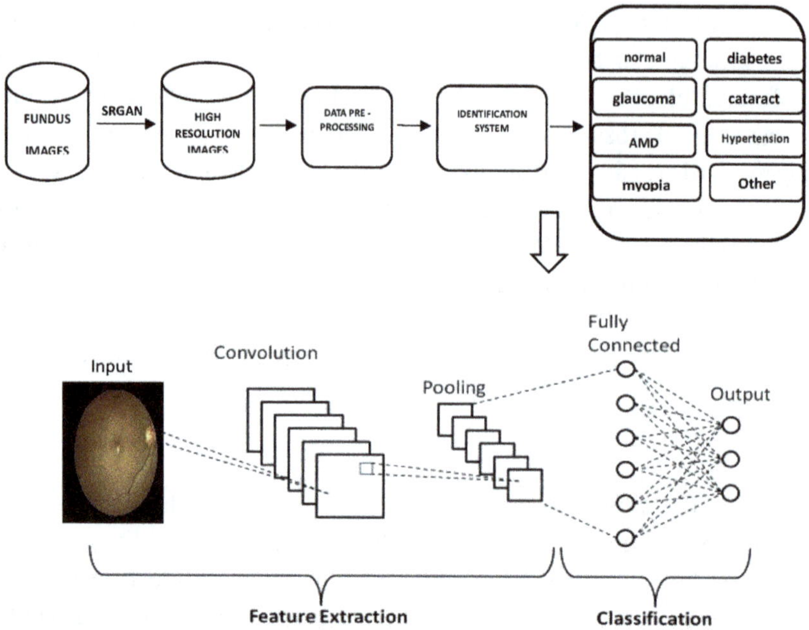

5. TENTATIVE EXPERIMENTAL RESULTS

The training began with an accuracy of 0.6 and validation was changed to 0.82. As each epoch advanced both the training and the validation accuracies increased, and at the same time the model loss decreases. After completing five epochs, the training accuracy has reached 0.83 and validation accuracy reached 0.89. Subsequently training accuracy stayed at 0.85, while the validation accuracy maintained as 0.87. We can get the details of model accuracy from *Figure 3.*

Figure 3. Model Accuracy

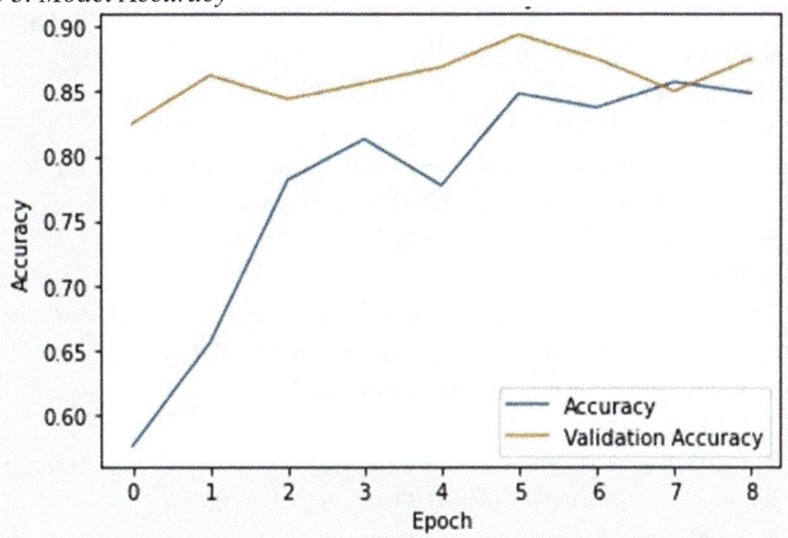

The initial loss at first epoch is 0.45 and the val_acrcy is at 0.825.As running of each epoch model loss gets decreased. After running five epochs the model loss gets decreased from 0.458 to 0.257 and the value accuracy has improved from 0.825 to 0.893. *Figure 4* will show the loss, which is determined by the proposed model.

Figure 4. Model Loss

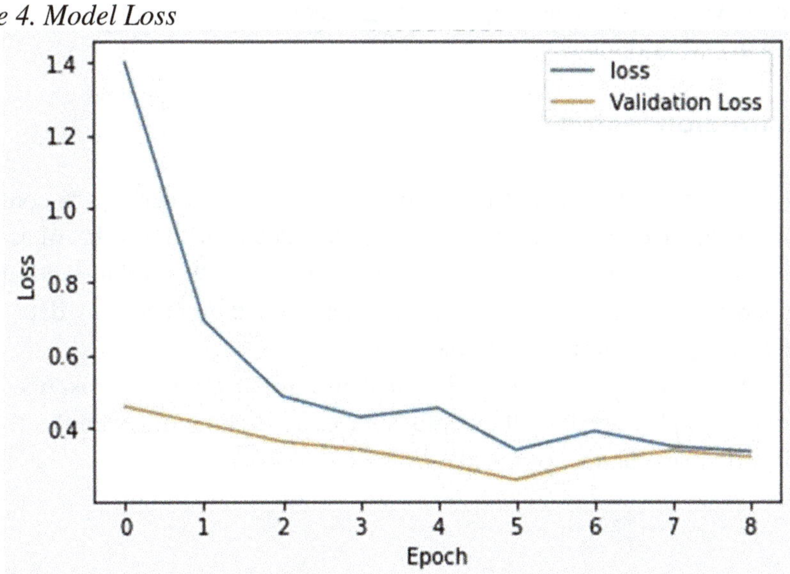

Epoch 1/30

22/22 [==================================] - 137s 5s / step - loss: 1.627 - accuracy: 0.539 - value_loss: 0.458 - val_acrcy: 0.825

Epoch 1: val_acrcy changed from -inf to 0.825

Epoch 2/30

22/22 [==================================] - 99s 4s / step - loss: 0.739 – accuracy: 0.643 - value_loss: 0.410 - val_acrcy: 0.862

Epoch 2: val_acrcy changed from 0.825 to 0.862

Epoch 3/30

22/22 [==================================] - 98s 4s / step - loss: 0.526 - accuracy: 0.772 - value_loss: 0.361 - val_acrcy: 0.843

Epoch 3: val_acrcy has not changed from 0.862

Epoch 4/30

22/22 [==================================] - 98s 4s / step - loss: 0.411 - accuracy: 0.819 - value_loss: 0.339 - val_acrcy: 0.856

Epoch 4: val_acrcy has not changed from 0.862

Epoch 8/30

22/22 [==================================] - 99s 4s/step - loss: 0.394 - accuracy: 0.831 - value_loss: 0.337 - val_acrcy: 0.850

Epoch 8: val_acrcy has not changed from 0.893

Epoch 9/30

22/22 [==================================] - 100s 4s/step - loss: 0.344 - accuracy: 0.847 - value_loss: 0.320 - val_acrcy: 0.875

Epoch 9: val_acrcy has not changed from 0.893

Epoch 9: early stopping

5.1. Confusion Matrix

The overall effectiveness of the fashion category is measured by the confusion matrix of the given data. It is best to recognize and determine the value of accurate measurement. The matrix that separates predicted and actual values and all predictions have dimensions. Actual values are determined by observing data, while predicted values are determined by the model.

Figure 5 will show the cataract and normal disease detection analysis. According to the given samples we draw the confusion matrix dividing the samples that are belonging to either cataract or normal.

Figure 5. Confusion Matrix (shows Normal vs Cataract)

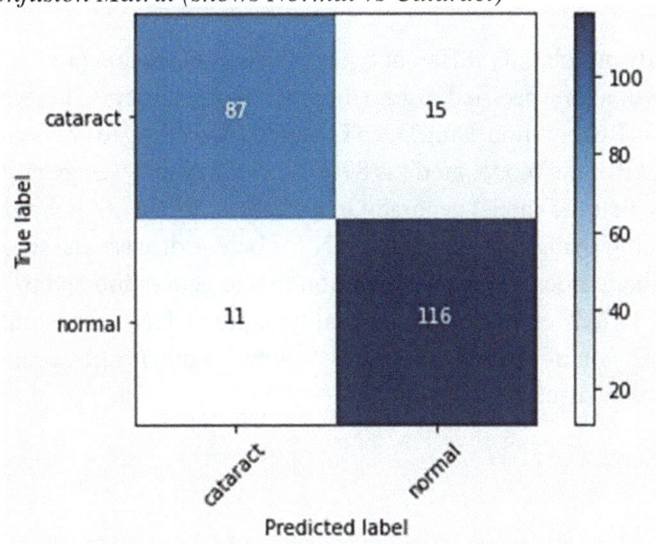

The above results will show the accuracy that the current model can classify 87 T-positive (TP) images and 116 T-negative (TN) images. The model also miscategorizes a few images. It predicts 15 F-positive (FP) and 11 F-negative (FN) images.

6. FUTURE AND SCOPE

Future progress in this area would involve continuous research and development to refine models, improve accuracy, reduce false positive/negative results, and improve the interpretability of AI-driven diagnoses. Collaboration between artificial intelligence experts, ophthalmologists and medical researchers will be essential to push the boundaries of eye disease recognition. In essence, the combination of SR-GAN and CNN represents a promising way to increase the accuracy and efficiency of eye disease recognition. However, it is essential to address the challenges, refine the technology, and navigate ethical considerations to ensure its safe and effective implementation in clinical settings.

Advances in AI for eye disease recognition offer early detection through retinal scans and OCT (Optical Coherence Tomography). This technology enables personalized treatment plans by analyzing patient data, potentially preventing vision loss. Artificial intelligence streamlines healthcare workflows, aids telemedicine, and integrates with wearables for continuous monitoring.

7. CONCLUSION

In this study, we classify different types of eye diseases and predict whether eye fundus image contain specified disease or any other disorders. This work proposes Ocular Disease Recognition using Deep Learning, according to previous references, we have found that the model predicts 87% of accuracy and we can build the model in such a way that the model accuracy may close to 89% with good performance. This project employing SRGAN and CNN for ocular disease classification showcased promising strides in high – resolution image generation and precise disease recognition. SRGAN enhanced image quality, aiding CNN's robust disease classification. The fusion of these technologies' augments diagnostic accuracy, offering potential for early disease detection.

REFERENCES

Bernabé, O., Acevedo, E., Acevedo, A., Carreño, R., & Gómez, S. (2021). Classification of eye diseases in fundus images. *IEEE Access : Practical Innovations, Open Solutions, 9*, 101267–101276. DOI: 10.1109/ACCESS.2021.3094649

Jain, L., Murthy, H. V. S., Patel, C., & Bansal, D. (2018). Retinal eye disease detection using deep learning. In *Proceedings of the 14th International Conference on Information Processing (ICINPRO)* (pp. 1–6). IEEE. https://doi.org/DOI: 10.1109/ICINPRO43533.2018.9096838

Khan, M. S., Tafshir, N., Alam, K. N., Dhruba, A. R., Albraikan, A. A., & Almalki, F. A. (2022). Deep learning for ocular disease recognition: An inner-class balance. *Journal of Healthcare Engineering, 2022*, 5007111. Advance online publication. DOI: 10.1155/2022/5007111 PMID: 35528343

Muchuchuti, S., & Viriri, S. (2023). Retinal disease detection using deep learning techniques: A comprehensive review. *Journal of Imaging, 9*(4), 84. DOI: 10.3390/jimaging9040084 PMID: 37103235

Sarki, R., Ahmed, K., Wang, H., & Zhang, Y. (2020). Automatic detection of diabetic eye disease through deep learning using fundus images: A survey. *IEEE Access : Practical Innovations, Open Solutions, 8*, 151133–151149. DOI: 10.1109/ACCESS.2020.3015258

Sattigeri, S. K., Harshith, N., Gowda, D. N., Ullas, K. A., & Aditya, M. S. (2022). Eye disease identification using deep learning (Vol. 9).

Vayadande, K., Ingale, V., Verma, V., Yeole, A., Zawar, S., & Jamadar, Z. (2022). Ocular disease recognition using deep learning. In *Proceedings of the International Conference on Signal and Information Processing (IConSIP)* (pp. 1–7). IEEE. https://doi.org/DOI: 10.1109/ICoNSIP49665.2022.10007470

Wang, J., Yang, L., Huo, Z., He, W., & Luo, J. (2020). Multi-label classification of fundus images with EfficientNet. *IEEE Access : Practical Innovations, Open Solutions, 8*, 212499–212508. DOI: 10.1109/ACCESS.2020.3040275

Chapter 9
Safeguarding Data Privacy and Security in Healthcare IoT

Pooja Dehankar
Ajeenkya D.Y. Patil School of Engineering, India

Kashvi Chaturvedi
https://orcid.org/0009-0005-3192-3400
Ajeenkya D.Y. Patil University, India

Susanta Das
https://orcid.org/0000-0002-9314-3988
Ajeenkya D.Y. Patil University, India

Rizwan Shaikh
https://orcid.org/0009-0005-5689-7640
Dr. D.Y. Patil Institute of Management and Entrepreneur Development, India

ABSTRACT

The integration of cutting-edge technologies like 5G and IoT has led to innovative applications, particularly in healthcare, revolutionizing patient care through real-time monitoring. Healthcare IoT applications have the potential to improve patient outcomes and the caliber of care given by physicians, nurses, clinicians, and pharma companies, to name a few. However, this convergence raises concerns regarding ethics, regulation, and privacy. Consumer-facing medical devices enable automatic data collection for early intervention but often overlook security hazards. Despite the potential for improved patient outcomes, robust security and privacy safeguards are necessary. Healthcare IoT has revolutionized the medical industry but requires careful consideration of security measures. Wearable IoT gadgets simplify health-

DOI: 10.4018/979-8-3693-3864-3.ch009

care processes but pose privacy risks. While IoT enhances efficiency, it also raises concerns about data security and privacy breaches. The chapter emphasizes the need for comprehensive security frameworks to protect patient information in IoT-based healthcare applications.

1. INTRODUCTION

Since the internet has become a necessity in our daily lives, an increasing number of services and facilities are being set up there to reach as many people as possible with the least amount of work and expense. The internet is also being used by healthcare facilities to help patients and gather information for effective treatment of medical issues. The use internet of technologies like cloud computing and the IoT by health care systems to help patients is usually referred to as "e-health" or "smart health care". Despite these benefits, these systems are at risk of hacking and risks involving security and privacy of information (Nayak et al., 2022).

A major worldwide shift in healthcare systems is currently being driven by the implementation of IoT technologies. IoT applications have affected several aspects of the healthcare sector, revolutionizing patient care and monitoring (Yuehong et al., 2016). Wearable sensors and remote monitoring tools are examples of IoT devices that have become widely accepted (Bhuiyan et al., 2021). These devices gather health data in real-time, allowing for timely interference and promoting active care approaches by giving practitioners complete understanding of patients' health state. The IoT has accelerated the development of medical devices and technologies, enhancing the capabilities of standard healthcare systems. IoT-enabled implantable devices, such as pacemakers and insulin pumps, have evolved into more complex gadgets with networking capabilities that enable remote adjustments and continuous monitoring (Dias & Cunha, 2018). In addition, the use of IoT technologies in telemedicine has shown a lot of promise, particularly in light of the COVID-19 pandemic. It has successfully reduced the strain on healthcare facilities and enabled remote consultations (Hollander & Carr, 2020).

Because of the acceleration in development and implementation of IoT devices, it supports and achieves UNSDG 4, Quality Education, because to research and construct these devices require trained professionals (The 17 Goals, 2025; Boeren, 2019). Caciquinho & Arruda (2025) showed in their analysis that young people often reach adulthood without proper and adequate professional experience which limits their employability skills and growth. The educational institutions will teach and train them about IoT, preparing them for inductry and hence achieving UNSDG 8, Decent Work and Economic Growth. About 60% employees entering healthcare industry are women. This also means that count of females in developing or implementing the devices is significant, hence achieving UNSDG 5, Gender Equality (The 17 Goals, 2025; Berlin et al., 2019). It helps in economic growth of the industry and in achieving Target 9.5 as the industry shows enhancement in scientific research and upgrade in technological capabilities (The 17 Goals, 2025; Hales & Birdthistle, 2022). The innovation and development of medical devices will be done by some research centers or companies which will provide these to hospitals or medical schools for them to teach the equipment to the students. This leads to the collaboration between healthcare industry and other companies, achieving UNSDG 17 (Partnerships for the Goals) (The 17 Goals, 2025).

However, despite the impressive progress, there are still a lot of difficulties in integrating IoT and healthcare. Security and privacy protection remains as few major considerations, especially given the transmission and storage of sensitive patient data across networks and connected devices (Alaba et al., 2017).

Furthermore, the ongoing issues of interoperability across IoT devices and platforms continues to obstruct the smooth transfer and integration of data across healthcare ecosystems (Mavrogiorgou et al., 2019). The adoption and effectiveness of IoT technologies in the healthcare sector are being hampered by these issues. To overcome these challenges, researchers and industry experts have been making progress in creating secure frameworks and protocols specifically designed for use in healthcare applications (Goyal et al., 2021). Additionally, efforts to develop suitable standards and solutions seek to connect different IoT devices and healthcare systems to enable effective data exchange.

The credibility and dependability of IoT systems in the healthcare sector depends on these advancements. Research has shown that the integration of IoT technology has a major effect on healthcare, with clear advantages. For example, hospital readmission rates have greatly been decreased when IoT-powered remote monitoring devices were employed to treat chronic illnesses (Noah et al., 2018). Additionally, IoT integration has improved the operational efficiency of healthcare organizations by simplifying procedures and optimizing resource allocation (Ghosh et al., 2016). Although there have been considerable advancements in the integration of IoT into healthcare systems, there are still unresolved difficulties that require ongoing research and development to fully realize the potential of the technology. Concerns around security, privacy, and interoperability must be resolved if the IoT is to reach its full transformational potential in the healthcare industry.

2. MACHINE LEARNING'S CONTRIBUTION TO IOT-BASED HEALTHCARE

IoT integration in healthcare has enabled more individualized treatment and improved patient outcomes (Shah et al., 2019). Early detection and timely responses are made possible by real-time monitoring through continuous health tracking provided by IoT-connected devices. Given the vast volumes of data involved in healthcare and the high prediction value of accurate forecasts, machine learning (ML) algorithms must be integrated into the health information and communications technology (H-ICT) stack. From the gathered data, these algorithms allow us to draw meaningful conclusions and extract crucial information. Many ongoing research projects aim to determine if ML algorithms can be applied to home internet of things (H-IoT) systems, find new domains where they may be used, and increase the accuracy of predictive and analytical models. Healthcare practitioners can take preventive measures to lower risks and avoid adverse health consequences by using ML algorithms on data produced by the IoT. This personalized approach to healthcare not only increases patient involvement but also empowers individuals to actively manage their own health (Bharadwaj et al., 2021).

3. ENHANCED OPERATIONAL EFFICIENCY IN HEALTHCARE FACILITIES

The combination of IoT technologies has led to a considerable improvement in healthcare organizations' efficiency. It has contributed to the optimization of resource allocation and process simplification, which has decreased expenses and enhanced workflows. Using IoT-based solutions for managing inventory allowed hospitals to cut inventory-related expenses. Real-time tracking of medical supplies and equipment has ensured their availability when needed, reduced stock shortages, and prevented things from getting expired. Additionally, IoT-driven solutions have increased the effectiveness of patient care procedures by reducing wait times and enhancing service delivery. By integrating IoT sensors and technology into hospital facilities, routine tasks could be automated, allowing medical staff to focus more on direct caring for patients. For example, smart beds with IoT capabilities ensure patient comfort while alerting staff to any changes in vital signs, allowing for faster responses and improved patient care (Gourisaria et al., 2022). Through tailored treatment plans and enhanced operational effectiveness in healthcare institutions, the use of IoT technology in the sector has greatly improved patient outcomes.

The way clinicians approach diagnosis has been changed by advances in medical imaging. It is recognized that modern medicine is far more effective than it has ever been, from disease surveillance to illness treatment. A whole new field of medicine has been made possible by the capacity to link, exchange, and share knowledge about human anatomy using non-invasive nuclear medicine and radiology techniques. Nevertheless, for established reasons, "image distribution" has never proven easy in the medical industry. 'Data Security and Patient Privacy' has been a key parameter that consistently raises concerns about the distribution process itself. The healthcare industry has undergone an abrupt change due to technological advancements and the adoption of BYOD (Bring Your Own Devices) policies in the IoT sector. It is becoming more and more important in today's interconnected world to handle issues like "data security, threat and patient privacy," as well as "risk mitigation" strategies in our goods and solutions. History demonstrates that no law has been able to completely eradicate security breaches worldwide, proving the adage "prevention is better than cure." To counter security attacks, the only thing that can be done is to enhance privacy policies while simultaneously implementing strict security implementation procedures and efficient risk control techniques (Supriya & Padaki, 2016).

4. HEALTHCARE IOT DEVICES

Healthcare IoT (Internet of Things) technologies include wearables, ingestible sensors, and connected medical equipment, among other connected medical devices and systems that facilitate data collecting, remote monitoring, and better patient care as shown in Figure 1. Wearables: gadgets that track vital signs including blood pressure, heart rate, and activity levels, such as smartwatches, fitness trackers, and smart clothing (Mazharuddin, 2025). Asthma inhalers that monitor usage and notify patients and medical professionals are known as connected inhalers (Raghav et al., 2025). Smart Implants: Devices including cochlear implants, neurostimulators, and cardiac implants that are inserted into the body to monitor, identify, or treat medical issues (Satyender, 2025). Ingestable Sensors: Tiny sensors that gather information from the digestive system by being eaten. Devices for telemedicine include video conferencing software, remote monitoring platforms, and mobile health initiatives that facilitate care and consultation from a distance (Banerjee et al., 2025). Medication dispensers are machines that deliver consistent dosages of medication all day long (Kshatri et al., 2025). In order to improve accessibility and results, telemedicine is utilizing healthcare IoT (IoMT) equipment for remote patient monitoring, real-time data transmission, and virtual consultations (Stephen & Kolachala, 2025). A schematic diagram of various healthcare IoT devises is illustrated in Figure 1.

Figure 1. Examples of Healthcare IOT Devices

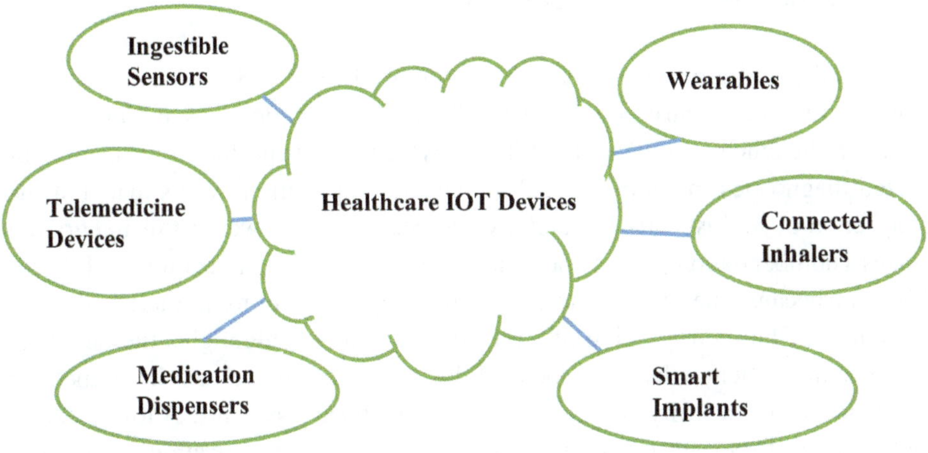

5. SECURITY AND PRIVACY REGULATIONS

The IoT offers incredibly creative answers for a variety of problems. However, an IoT company does not automatically become immune from the laws that protect personal information and are applicable to its operational territory just because it is a technology company. Healthcare solutions will therefore need to comply with security and privacy regulations. There are a number of established frameworks that deal with these problems; however, they were created in the context of organized healthcare facilities and hospitals, where the knowledge, resources, and infrastructure are in place to ensure extremely strong security. However, there are major extra challenges that need to be addressed for IoT solutions that are targeted at vulnerable individuals, whether at home or in their neighborhood. Technical (poor processing speed, limited power, sporadic communications), organizational (user device and user enrollment, key distribution, cryptography keys), and user (how does a patient with physical or mental disabilities operate and update their devices) are some examples. The legal frameworks, security, and privacy requirements for healthcare solutions are all taken into consideration in this article. The assessment of how this is limited within an IoT system is next presented, after which an outline of some of the main frameworks is given (Poyner & Sherratt, 2018).

5.1. Boosting Data Security and Privacy in BioMEMS through IoT Security

Biomedical Microelectromechanical Systems (BioMEMS) play a pivotal role in augmenting the security of Internet of Things communications and preserving intelligent healthcare systems. BioMEMS, which are at the forefront of individualized diagnostics, monitoring, and therapeutic applications, are situated at the intersection of sophisticated technology and healthcare. However, this integration creates a number of complex privacy and security concerns that require careful consideration because they are fundamental to IoT communications in smart healthcare ecosystems. The incorporation of authentic case studies highlights the necessity of protecting patient safety and medical data integrity, as well as the immediate consequences of security breaches in smart healthcare systems. Authors examined a range of security measures, including stringent authentication procedures, data encryption, attack-resistant designs, and ongoing monitoring systems, all of which are intended to strengthen BioMEMS against constantly changing threats in intelligent healthcare settings. Additionally, in the context of IoT communication security, the author highlights critical significance of ethical and regulatory issues, stressing the necessity of preserving patient autonomy, guaranteeing data confidentiality, and preserving equal access to healthcare. Anticipating future obstacles and planning for the future, author examine the developing field of BioMEMS security as it combines with cutting-edge technologies like quantum computing, AI-driven diagnostics, and genomic integration. In the context of IoT communication security and protection, author thus emphasizes how critical it is to embrace an integrated strategy that skillfully combines technological innovation, moral foresight, and cooperative ingenuity, guiding BioMEMS toward a safe and resilient future within smart healthcare systems (Jaime et al., 2023).

5.2. Protecting medical images in Internet of Things healthcare

Medical imaging equipment can now be connected to the data center of the healthcare industry. The IoT will enable this advancement, which will expedite the medical care process from diagnosis to treatment. The growing dependence on cloud-based and networked systems and connected devices opens up avenues for cyberattacks and illegal access to private medical information, endangering patient privacy and seriously compromising patient safety and trust in healthcare systems. The confidentiality, integrity, and availability of medical pictures are vital resources in the healthcare industry, since they are essential for precise diagnosis, treatment planning, and patient care. This led to research on medical image security in IoT healthcare. It involves encryption and decryption of images using a network based on cryptography, as well as its potential application in the safe sharing of medical images through deep learning. Since these "hidden properties" are part of the learning model, the encryption technique can be modified for each distinct domain. The first step in decrypting an encrypted image is reconstructing networks, which enables us to restore it to its "plaintext" state. Once the hidden entities are found, a Return on Investment (ROI) framework can be made available, and the user's local information context can be used to simplify data mining. The findings of the security analysis and the thorough experimental setup suggest that the suggested approach might offer a previously unusual degree of power and security (Nadhan & Jacob, 2024).

5.3. IoT-e-Health Systems' Privacy and Security

"e-Health" describes the use of Internet and other connected networks in health systems. The use of intelligent techniques in health and its progress over time, particularly the integration of IoT devices and cloud computing, were explored. The ability to search for, locate, comprehend, and evaluate health information obtained from electronic sources and acquired knowledge to appropriately diagnose, manage, and treat medical conditions is known as e-health. The Internet has the ability to shield users from damage and provide them the power to fully engage in health-related decision-making as a storehouse for health information and e-Health analysis. Above all, a high degree of e-Health integration reduces the possibility of coming across inaccurate material on the Internet. A promising trend for the future is the integration of cloud computing and other intelligent systems with IoT-based e-Health systems to give intelligent applications (Butpheng et al., 2020).

6. ETHICAL AND SECURITY CONCERNS FOR IOMT

The Internet of Things' explosive growth is creating a plethora of options that could greatly enhance human well-being in a variety of domains. The primary area where IoT can improve our quality of life is in the healthcare sector. However, security and privacy issues are the main focus of electronic health (eHealth) systems, and they become more challenging to resolve as IoT is added. The majority of IoMT creates security concerns because of the large number of players in its larger ecosystem. There are several security features in the IoT-based healthcare system. a foundational management solution for identity-based cryptography that protects data translation between any IoT health device and any other entity from a different firm using collaborative authentication and a secret passcode (Karam, 2022).

Despite growing public awareness of Internet privacy threats, these problems are expected to become more significant as the Internet develops into the Internet of Things (IoT) because of the vast volume of data that is gathered and handled by the "Things." One of the issues with IoT privacy protection is the corporate motivations for looking into methods to make money off of such data. Beyond privacy protection, it is noted that new strategies are required that give IoT users a more active role and handle other possible problems like the Digital Divide or safety hazards. Transparency in the technology and services' data handling practices, along with user choice, are important aspects of ethical design. A novel method for how consumers engage with the Internet of Things is introduced. It is founded on the idea of Ethical Design and is applied using a framework based on policies. By choosing particular sets of policies that can be adjusted based on users' capabilities and the environments in which they operate, consumers are given more control over their personal data or IoT services. The framework's possible implementation in a typical Internet of Things setting is explained, along with the key players and the procedures that need to be established (Baldini et al., 2018).

It is acknowledged that each person must have the assurance that they are safeguarded by efficient technological solutions (ID management, encryption approaches, privacy enhancing techniques, etc.), which must be updated and reinterpreted for the Internet of Things. The enforcement of the right to privacy, the assurance of information access, the assurance of information integrity, and the enforcement of information property rights are proposed as the minimal prerequisites for an ethical Internet of things (Popescul & Georgescu, 2014).

High overheads in compute, communication, and storage are necessary for public key-based systems. Additionally, devices with limited resources cannot use current private key techniques, and small embedded units are not supported by internet security standards like TLS.

The Internet of Things (IoT) raises unique security concerns because of its portable nature, wireless connections, and network access layer devices. For such devices, zero knowledge proof is therefore the ideal option (Rehiman & Veni, 2016).

The inherent hazards of Internet-enabled devices, the sensitivity of health-related data, and their influence on healthcare delivery present a number of ethical issues with H-IoT. Ensuring that devices and protocols for sharing the data they generate are both technologically and scientifically sound, as well as trustworthy, morally upright, and considerate of users' rights and interests, is one of the main challenges of the Internet of Things (Mittelstadt, 2017).

Users may become more socially isolated as a result of using H-IoT to manage their health conditions at home or in residential care. If H-IoT is used to manage daily condition monitoring, visits by caregivers and medical professionals may not be as necessary (Demiris et al., 2004; Stowe & Harding, 2010; Tiwari et al., 2010; Wu et al., 2012). Research on the elderly has shown that, contrary to what is frequently claimed, there is fear that H-IoT will take the place of social and personal connections with caregivers (Chan et al., 2008; McLean, 2011; Palm, 2020; Zwijsen et al., 2011). It can be challenging to duplicate face-to-face encounters using sensors to collect contextual information on a patient's state (Percival & Hanson, 2006). These options collectively imply that H-IoT may frequently result in a worse understanding of the social and contextual aspects of a patient's health, particularly when it comes to mental health and wellbeing (Lupton, 2013).

Large-scale network deployments always raise serious security concerns. Data pertaining to people is handled via IoT-based healthcare systems. These types of data are susceptible to major privacy problems even when they are gathered from harmless wearable devices. The majority of devices and their connections in IoT-based healthcare applications are wireless, so security and privacy are important areas of concern. Patients' medical data can be sent to a remote healthcare service using an IP enabled sensor in a Medical Sensor Network (MSN). Protecting patient privacy and security is one of the main concerns with IoT in healthcare. To avoid eavesdropping on private medical information or maliciously initiating particular tasks, it is essential that remote healthcare centers and caregivers be authenticated and authorized. Additionally, end-to-end data protection is crucial. Strong and secure data connection between healthcare sensors, actuators, patients, and caregivers is essential since IoT-based healthcare applications directly involve humans (Dewangan & Mishra, 2018).

In the healthcare industry, patient data protection is the top priority. Creating a secure smart healthcare system is essential as the use of IoT technologies for smart healthcare systems increases and the frequency of privacy data leaks rises along with it. The rate of data breaches in previous years is revealed in the Thales India Data Threat report, which also highlights the need for stricter regulations pertaining to patient data privacy. Consequently, improving the sustainability of society has made the secure smart healthcare system a top priority. However, the hazard posed by combining various devices and protocols needs to be reduced in order to create a genuine secure smart healthcare system. A significant obstacle is also maintaining accuracy in the face of the massive volume of data generated every second. The best option for adhering to data privacy rules is encryption. However, data breach activities cannot be stopped by encryption alone. Low-containment IoT devices shouldn't always be run on an algorithm that encrypts all data since this will put a significant load on the system. The development of methods to identify and stop threats that aggravate a healthcare system's security is essential. In order to build a secure smart healthcare system, the authors here attempt to study the smart healthcare architecture, its risks, weaknesses, and security measures (Ambarkar & Shekokar, 2020).

Existing medical devices have been transformed by the growing Internet of Things (IoT) technology to function intelligently in the direction of establishing a digital health environment. In the field of electronic health (e-health), where current technologies are used to offer quick access to patient treatment, IoT holds great promise. Significant technologies and connected objects are used in IoT-based e-health systems to manage, track, identify, store, and monitor patient data for continued medical care. For the effective deployment of IoT within e-health, a framework that ensures interoperability between devices is necessary for processing and resource usage in an efficient manner. By including an exclusive e-governance layer into the design and execution of Internet of Things-based e-health systems, the study has come up with a novel approach. In order to achieve quick response and secure transmission with improved healthcare services, the study aims to develop a novel architecture for the incorporation of IoT in e-health systems by intensely focusing on its various layers, i.e., sensing, application, transmission, fog, and e-governance. An initial investigation has been carried out to review the literature on recent advances in the field of e-health. The suggested IoT based e-health architecture is a very innovative and complete design that incorporates an important but little-known aspect of Emergency Medical Services (EMS) that is integrated with blockchain technology. The concept of clearly describing the e-governance layer, which includes every layer of the suggested architecture, has also been offered as a creative way to achieve quality healthcare services (Safdar et al., 2020).

IoT presents fresh approaches, designs, and solutions for improved healthcare systems. It also presents a chance to increase medical care for individualized healthcare. The availability, security, and quality of healthcare systems could all be enhanced by open-source platforms and operating systems. Furthermore, by enabling systems, apps, and devices to safely expose APIs to external systems, current open-source solutions may enhance the efficiency and evolution of healthcare systems. As a result, this will raise interoperability and lower the expense of managing and governing networks of heterogeneous devices. There is currently a wide range of open-source technologies available that offer safe and affordable platforms for creating and prototyping innovative healthcare systems. These can be IoT-based and should be compatible with smartphones and smartwatches, since these are now regarded as indispensable components of daily life and as highly significant and useful tools for providing alerts and proactive coaching to enhance the health of their users and, by extension, the public. A wide range of sensors are now included in mobile devices, which can be utilized to collect data to support medical treatments and offer real-time monitoring options (Marques et al., 2019).

7. CHALLENGES IN IMPLEMENTING IOT IN HEALTHCARE

Because patient data is so sensitive, security and privacy are crucial in healthcare systems that incorporate IoT technologies. There are still weaknesses present despite tremendous progress (Awotunde et al., 2021). Many healthcare institutions had suffered a cyberattack (Seh et al., 2020). Due to its connectivity, IoT devices are more vulnerable to attacks, increasing the potential locations for security breaches (Chacko & Hayajneh, 2018). These violations could have disastrous consequences and endanger patient privacy. Furthermore, the variety of IoT device manufacturers and the existence of different security standards add to the complexity of security issues (Baker et al., 2017). There are significant issues with IoT devices that have insufficient authentication and encryption procedures (Khan & Salah, 2018). It is clear that implementing strong security measures is crucial given the possible impact that hacks may have on patient trust and the reputations of healthcare providers.

Interoperability is an ongoing challenge to the integration of IoT in healthcare (Bhosale et al., 2021). The lack of established communication protocols affects the smooth transfer of data between different platforms and devices (Hazra et al., 2021). Device interoperability was made possible by very few IoT devices in healthcare settings (Gyrard & Serrano, 2016). The current lack of interoperability limits the full potential benefits that IoT can bring to healthcare by making it difficult to effectively aggregate and utilize data.

7.1. Security and Privacy Concerns in Internet of Medical Things

Pervasive healthcare is regarded as one of the technical solutions to address the global health concerns, given the rising expense of treatment and the growing demands for high-quality healthcare. Specifically, the creation of the Internet of Medical Things (IoMT) is a result of recent advancements in the IoT. The security and privacy concerns of such sensing systems are frequently disregarded, despite the possibility that such widely available, inexpensive sensors may replace the reactive healthcare system with one that is more proactive. Medical devices and the communications that go along with them must be extremely secure in order to preserve user privacy since they collect and handle extremely sensitive personal health data. Nevertheless, the computational capacity of the downsized IoMT devices is extremely limited, and only a small number of security measures can be applied to them. The use of IoMT for clinical applications is further hampered by the significant challenges associated with controlling and guaranteeing the security of IoMT systems, which have become increasingly prevalent with the introduction of IoMT devices (Sun et al., 2019).

Pervasive healthcare is being investigated as a technological solution to the world's health problems. Both rising healthcare expenses and an increasing demand for top-notch medical care are to blame for this. There is more impact on IoMT from the growth of the IoT. Because of the IoMT, millions of people throughout the world are enjoying better security and medical care. Through remote monitoring and data transfer, medical data centers, including cloud-based ones, can acquire real-time patient health characteristics. Nowadays, healthcare is more generally accessible, more economical, and more efficient. But that becomes a problem as IoT devices grow. One of the challenges of IoMT devices is their tiny size and limited processing power and number of schemes. IoMT systems are challenging to secure and manage due to their widespread use. According to Gaytan (2022), this is a major problem that prevents IoMT from being utilized therapeutically.

8. REMEDIES FOR SECURITY AND PRIVACY CONCERNS IN IOT

Developments in Secure IoT Frameworks and Protocols have been focused by researchers and industry experts (Khezr et al., 2019). On the plus side, recent innovations such as blockchain-based solutions have the potential to enhance data integrity and security (Kshetri, 2017). Blockchain technology's distributed and unchangeable features enable secure and transparent data transactions while lowering the risk of manipulation or unauthorized access (Peralta et al., 2019). Furthermore, the advancement of encryption technologies, including homomorphic encryption, provides a workable way to ensure the safe transmission and archiving of data in IoT healthcare systems. The foundation for creating robust IoT systems that prioritize patient privacy were laid by these innovative security strategies.

The issue of fragmentation among IoT devices and platforms in the healthcare sector is being addressed by continuous attempts to create standards and develop interoperable solutions. One significant initiative that aims to create standardized interfaces for smooth communication between different medical systems and devices is the Continua Health Alliance. Additionally, the usage of established protocols promotes data interoperability, which makes it easier for healthcare networks to exchange and use data effectively (Vorisek et al., 2022).

These days, the biggest worry is the security of these systems. It is challenging to create a robust set of security rules to secure the vulnerable devices' "things" due to their low power storage, computing power, and data storage capacities. The devices' flawless communication is made possible by the internet serving as their backbone. However, in the absence of any safeguards, it would allow hackers or intermediaries to take control of the connection, steal information, and disrupt it (Paris et al., 2023).

The implementation of Public Key Infrastructure (PKI) to guarantee safe end-to-end Internet communications between gadgets and services. Certain researchers recommend optimizing the DTLS handshake or reducing the size of x.509 certificates. Others looked into delegating authentication and authorization to IoT-constrained devices via two factor authentication via an authorization server, or performing difficult cryptographic algorithms on behalf of those devices utilizing nearby or virtual resources (Kelly & Hammoudeh, 2018).

9. IOT HEALTHCARE APPLICATIONS

IoT healthcare applications need special consideration in addition to IoT services. Sensing Blood Sugar Levels: A metabolic condition called diabetes causes a brief rise in blood glucose levels. Blood patterns, activity levels, and meal formation can all be observed by glucose monitoring. Istepanian et al., (2011) presented a real-time glucose level monitoring system. ECG Surveillance: With the use of an electrocardiogram (ECG), one can diagnose arrhythmias, as well as as ascertain the heart's rhythm and rate, QT intervals, and myocardial ischemia. IoT-based options for ECG monitoring are presented in the work of Yang et al., (2014). Monitoring of Blood Pressure: The example of blood pressure regulation and monitoring in underdeveloped nations is given by Puustjarvi and Puustjarvi (2011) as a setting in which telemedicine would be beneficial. Monitoring of Body Temperature: Since it may be regarded as a crucial indicator of maintaining homeostasis, monitoring a person's body temperature is an essential part of providing medical services (Ruiz et al., 2009).

A handheld ECG device provide patients with long-term cost investment funds, but it also provides compelling movement monitoring of the heart. Due to their ability to function as wearable sensors embedded in clothing, non-contact, capacitive-coupled anodes are also frequently used for ECG signal security. This is because these anodes do not need to come into direct touch with the skin. Processing and transmission of the gathered ECG signals to cloud and edge servers are also possible. Doctors and patients can remotely access each other's ECG data by using an Android-based application. The suggested application can offer a dependable and low-latency interface for the patients' ECG, according to simulation results (Rachim & Chung, 2016). The suggested system uses the Message Queuing Telemetry Transport (MQTT) protocol to send the real-time ECG data to the web server. The physician can view the webserver on a computer or smartphone to keep an eye on the ECG data that has been recorded in the past or in real time (Yew et al., 2020).

A new trend in social computing is mobile crowd sensing technology that integrates humans, machines, and objects in the environment. The relationship between athlete motor function and blood pressure is revealed in kinematics study through continuous blood pressure monitoring and calibration. In addition, the field of medical research has made it easier to regulate hypertension, which enhances the efficacy of hypertension treatment. One real risk factor that can lead to heart attacks or strokes is hypertension. Patients can better understand their health status by knowing their blood pressure is continuously monitored by medical sensors, even though blood flow can vary minute to minute. The system is divided into two ends: the server end and the sensing end. Wearable blood pressure monitoring sensors and an Internal Measurement Unit (IMU) that can correlate sensed data with physical movement make up the sensing end. The raw sensed data is processed and analyzed by the server-end, which also manages network functions. By extracting features and creating matrix vectors of these features, the measured blood pressure and IMU data may be calibrated (Zhong et al., 2020).

SmartPants is an IoT-based wireless solution created especially for post-stroke patients' remote lower limb rehabilitation. The platform is made up of several nodes for tracking physical therapy sessions and a software platform that detects the kind of exercise the patient is performing at the moment to provide real-time feedback on how it is being executed (Bisio et al., 2019).

10. RECENT ADVANCEMENTS OF IOT AND AI IN HEALTHCARE

Significant breakthroughs in wellness could result from integrating AI and the Internet of Things, which would revolutionize physical management and patient care. AI in medical imaging and diagnosis enables faster and more accurate radiology examinations, such as MRIs, CT scans, and X-rays. The breakthrough is in personalized medicine, where artificial intelligence (AI) can evaluate vast amounts of data gathered from lifestyle decisions, IoT devices, and real-time health measures to better meet the demands of specific patients and produce better results. Expanding off-site monitoring with IoT devices such as fabric electronic sensors enables precise health monitoring, facilitating prompt medical therapy and early identification of potential health issues. Predictive analytics and preventive care, improving chronic disease management, increasing telemedicine and virtual care, addressing ethical and regulatory issues, speeding up AI-driven drug development and clinical trials, and improving operational efficiency in healthcare facilities are the goals of the integration (Rangarajan et al., 2025).

The combination of AI and the IoT is revolutionizing healthcare, particularly in the fields of real-time patient monitoring and predictive diagnoses. IoT technologies that enable continuous health data collection include wearable sensors, smart medical devices, and connected implants. This enables physicians to remotely and instantly check on the health of their patients. This massive stream of data is analyzed by AI techniques, such as machine learning and deep learning, to find abnormalities, forecast medical occurrences, and improve individualized treatment regimens. By facilitating early disease identification, lowering the need for emergency interventions, and improving chronic condition management, this IoT and AI collaboration improves patient outcomes. AI-powered predictive diagnostics also aid in risk identification, assisting medical practitioners in making proactive decisions (Aslam & Jack, 2025).

11. IOT HEALTHCARE USE CASE

Utilizing wearable IoT technology to continuously monitor a variety of metrics and diagnosing cardiac issues with a ML based model. By feeding a trained prediction model with real-time ECG, pulse, and temperature data, one can ascertain whether a user is at risk for any cardiac condition or arrhythmia. Preprocessing the data, training the model, and prototyping for live prediction were the three processes involved. The first stage involved consolidating the electronic health records (EHR) information and isolating the parameters that were thought to be significant for the predictor. The most common value (i.e., the mode) for each characteristic was used to replace the missing values in the dataset. To ascertain whether indicators were following highly similar trends, a correlation analysis was conducted. The pre-processed dataset was divided into training and testing sets in the second phase, and model training was then conducted on the training dataset. Accuracy, hit rate, and other factors were assessed using a variety of classification methods, including KNN, SVM, NB, decision trees, and random forests. In the third phase, a hardware prototype enabling data collection, cloud connectivity, and real-time prediction was developed. Along with other static data, such as age, sex, and blood sugar levels, the node was linked to a laptop and fed continuous data into the trained model. The model was then run on a laptop using KNN to assess the patient's risk for cardiac problems (Gupta et al., 2019).

12. THE LEGAL AND REGULATORY ENVIRONMENT (BEYOND HIPAA/GDPR)

Beyond HIPAA and GDPR, there are other international laws and ethical issues that come into play when it comes to IoT in healthcare (Shahid et al., 2022). With an emphasis on value-based care, data monetization, and connected health platforms, economic and commercial models are changing (Garcia, 2022). Adoption depends on human factors and user experience (UX), which calls for accessible design, eliminating potential biases in algorithms, and intuitive design (Dasaka, 2024). Healthcare firms must also comply with other data privacy regulations, such as Canada's PIPEDA, Brazil's LGPD, and numerous more regional and national legislation, even though HIPAA and GDPR are well-known (Poole, 2014). Developing AI-powered healthcare solutions necessitates managing the challenges of different jurisdiction compliance, such as GDPR and HIPAA (Maddali, 2024). Building trust and resolving ethical issues in healthcare, particularly in high-risk situations, require that AI models be transparent and understandable (Khan et al., 2024). There are constant difficulties in gaining and maintaining informed permission, particularly for developing AI models and data reuse (Liang et al., 2022). Deploying AI becomes more challenging when handling cross-border data flows and adhering to data residency regulations (Mercurio & Yu, 2022). One major obstacle is the absence of clear standards for evaluating AI in healthcare (Bertl et al., 2023).

13. USER EXPERIENCE (UX) AND HUMAN FACTORS

For all users, including those with impairments, to have fair access to healthcare, IoT devices and interfaces must be designed with accessibility in mind (Domingo, M. C. (2012). To ensure user adoption and efficient use, IoT devices and interfaces must be simple to use and comprehend (Page et al., 2018). One important factor to take into account is bridging the digital divide and addressing the disparities in computer literacy among various patient demographics, especially older persons (López et al., 2011). Effective solutions must take into account how age-related cognitive decline affects a person's capacity to use smart technologies (Dixon et al., 2022). Maintaining a great patient experience requires striking a balance between patient preferences for conventional clinician-patient contact and technological improvements (Akseer et al., 2021). Ensuring equity and avoiding prejudice in healthcare delivery requires addressing potential biases in algorithms employed in IoT devices (Chin et al., 2023). To foster confidence and guarantee patient safety, IoT devices must be designed with strong security and privacy features (Jaime et al., 2023). Effective use of IoT devices requires that users receive sufficient instruction and assistance on how to operate and analyze data from these devices (Pattar et al., 2018).

14. SECURITY VULNERABILITIES MANIFEST IN IOT DEVICES

Internet of Things devices are vulnerable to assaults due to a number of security flaws, such as inadequate security measures, weak default settings, and a lack of encryption. These flaws can be used to take over the device, obtain illegal access, or even use it as a springboard to penetrate more extensive networks (Butun et al., 2019). Hackers can easily target IoT devices since many of them have default passwords that are public knowledge or easy to figure out (Beale & Berris, 2017). Transmission of data without encryption is a serious risk. Sensitive information, such as personal information or login passwords, might be intercepted by hackers if it is transmitted without encryption (Mustacoglu et al., 2020). The usage of antiquated or insecure network protocols by certain IoT devices leaves them open to many types of assaults, such as man-in-the-middle attacks, in which a hacker intercepts and possibly modifies traffic. IoT devices frequently have low memory and processing power, which undermines patching and security upgrades (Fereidouni et al., 2025). They may become open to attacks that take use of well-known flaws in the software or firmware as a result (Cui et al., 2013). It is simple to compromise and take control of many IoT devices because they lack fundamental security features including strong authentication procedures, access controls, and intrusion detection systems (Ali et al., 2019). An IoT device's security may be jeopardized by physical access, particularly if it isn't equipped with secure boot procedures or physical tamper-proofing (Van Woudenberg & O'Flynn, 2021). Attackers may use open, unsecured network ports on Internet of Things devices as entry points to look for and take advantage of security flaws (Makhdoom et al., 2018). Devices are exposed to exploits that target known vulnerabilities when firmware and software updates are not performed on a regular and consistent basis (Feng et al., 2022). Putting in place consistent security measures can be difficult due to the wide variety of IoT devices and their communication protocols (Samaila et al., 2018).

15. EXAMPLES OF ENHANCED PATIENT OUTCOMES

If a diabetic's blood sugar levels fall too low, they can receive warnings on their phone, allowing them to take quick action and avert a disaster (Freckmann et al., 2019). With the use of a smart inhaler, a patient with COPD can monitor their medicine intake and get tailored symptom management advice based on environmental data and usage habits (Häußermann et al., 2022). Wearing a heart rate monitor enables a patient to send data to their physician, who can then remotely monitor the patient's status and take appropriate action (Kakria et al., 2015). Smart Beds sensor-equipped features improve patient safety and lower dangers like bedsores by tracking patient movement, detecting falls, and adjusting comfort settings (Mayer et al., 2023). Smart Infusion Pumps improve medication safety by calculating infusion rates and warning medical professionals of any dosage problems (Rothschild et al., 2005).

16. DATA GOVERNANCE, QUALITY, AND OWNERSHIP

For patient safety, data security, and regulatory compliance in the healthcare industry, IoT data governance, quality, and ownership are essential (Ahmed et al., 2025). While quality control procedures guarantee correctness and dependability, strong governance frameworks specify how data is gathered, stored, accessed, and used (Alabi, 2023). Ownership considerations deal with who is in charge of managing the data (Van Alstyne et al., 1995). In order to ensure that IoT data is utilized properly and ethically, IoT data governance in healthcare entails creating policies and processes to manage the data lifecycle, from collection to disposal (Shahid et al., 2022). Ensuring that the data gathered by IoT devices is accurate, comprehensive, consistent, and timely (Yusof, 2025). Establishing who is authorized to manage, see, and utilize the data produced by Internet of Things devices (Kopetz & Steiner, 2022). Accountability and responsibility depend on well-defined data ownership (Felici & Pearson, 2014). It entails determining: Data custodians are the people or groups in charge of looking after and overseeing particular datasets. Data Stewards: People or groups in charge of making sure data is compliant and of high quality (Varhol et al., 2025). Data users are people or groups who have access to data and use it for particular objectives. Accurate diagnosis, successful treatment strategies, and better patient outcomes all depend on high-quality data (Castaneda et al., 2015). In IoT healthcare, data quality imensions include: Ensuring that data accurately depicts the patient's or device's actual condition is known as accuracy (Liu et al., 2020). Completeness: Making certain that all relevant information is gathered and accessible. Making sure data is consistent across various systems and sources is known as consistency. Timeliness: Making certain that information is accessible when and where it is required (Chen et al., 2014).

17. DIGITAL LITERACY CHALLENGES FOR BOTH PATIENTS AND PROVIDERS

Both patients and providers face substantial obstacles when it comes to digital literacy (Moore et al., 2025). While physicians struggle to integrate new technology into workflows, ensure data security, and manage the stream of information, patients may find it difficult to understand how to use linked devices and analyze data (Quinn et al., 2019). It may be challenging for many patients, especially the elderly, to configure, use, and troubleshoot Internet of Things equipment like wearable sensors or remote monitoring systems (Azimi et al., 2017). Patients may not comprehend the data produced by the devices, even if they are able to use them (O'donoghue & Herbert, 2012). This makes it difficult to recognize any health problems or make well-informed decisions on their care. Because they prefer personal interaction and may have doubts about the accuracy or dependability of the data provided by IoT devices, patients may be reluctant to rely on automated systems for healthcare (Hui et al., 2021). It can be difficult and time-consuming to integrate IoT devices and data streams into current clinical processes and electronic health record systems, necessitating a large infrastructure and training investment (AbuKhousa et al., 2012). A big worry is safeguarding patient data from online attacks and making sure laws like HIPAA are followed, particularly as the amount and complexity of data produced by IoT devices rise (Shahid et al., 2022). It can be challenging to combine data from multiple sources and produce a complete picture of a patient's health since different IoT devices may employ different communication protocols and data formats (Rathee et al., 2020). To properly use and analyze data from IoT devices and inform patients about the advantages and dangers of these technologies, healthcare workers require training (Javaid & Khan, 2021).

18. CONCLUSION

Protecting data security and privacy in the context of the IoT is a difficult but essential issue that requires an integrated strategy that integrates technology, legislation, and governance. By proactively addressing the challenges and putting in place strong and effective security measures and best practices, healthcare organizations can take advantage of the potential for change of IoT technology while safeguarding patient privacy and trust in the healthcare ecosystem. Maintaining data security and privacy in the IoT healthcare field is an ongoing process that calls for an integrated strategy that involves technology innovation, organizational awareness, and regulatory compliance. In this chapter, we have explored the complex realm of healthcare

IoT security and privacy, pointing out significant problems and offering remedies for patient data integrity and risk minimization.

The use of IoT devices in healthcare is expanding, and with it comes security and privacy concerns. Strong access control, authentication, and encryption procedures are necessary to prevent unauthorized access and data breaches because cybercriminals view the vast amounts of sensitive health data stored on these devices as potential targets. Additionally, following the regulations such as GDPR and HIPAA is essential, requiring healthcare organizations to develop comprehensive privacy policies, conduct regular audits, and prioritize data protection practices. Noncompliance with these standards undermines patient trust and undermines the legitimacy of healthcare systems, in addition to subjecting businesses to financial and legal penalties.

There are practical ways to enhance data security and privacy in the Internet of medical things through advancements in blockchain technology, secure communication protocols, and encryption methods. By using these tools and adopting a defense-in-depth approach, organizations may improve their cybersecurity defenses against new threats and ensure the availability, confidentiality, and integrity of patient data. It's also important for healthcare organizations to cultivate a cybersecurity-conscious culture which includes awareness campaigns, staff education initiatives, and incident response drills that prepare workers to recognize security risks and respond appropriately.

It is a difficult task that requires collaboration across multiple businesses and disciplines to protect data privacy and security in the healthcare sector via the Internet of Things. By putting in place a proactive and thorough cybersecurity plan, healthcare organizations can take advantage of the transformative potential of IoT technology while safeguarding patient privacy and trust in the digital age.

"Safeguarding Data Privacy and Security in Healthcare IoT" highlights the importance of prioritizing privacy and security in the rapidly evolving sector of healthcare IoT. Strong security measures are required to avoid data breaches, unauthorized access, and privacy violations, as evidenced by the growing use of IoT devices by healthcare organizations to improve patient care and accelerate operations. The path taken by this chapter has shed light on the different challenges that the healthcare industry faces in balancing the need to protect patient data with advancements in technology. The incorporation of IoT devices into healthcare facilities enables remote monitoring, predictive analytics, and personalized treatment. But this also produces a complicated network of possible weaknesses that require preventative mitigation strategies. Vigilance, cooperation, and a firm dedication to the welfare of patients and the larger healthcare community are necessary on the path to a connected and safe healthcare future.

REFERENCES

AbuKhousa, E., Mohamed, N., & Al-Jaroodi, J. (2012). e-Health cloud: Opportunities and challenges. *Future Internet*, *4*(3), 621–645.

Ahmed, A., Shahzad, A., Naseem, A., Ali, S., & Ahmad, I. (2025). Evaluating the effectiveness of data governance frameworks in ensuring security and privacy of healthcare data: A quantitative analysis of ISO standards, GDPR, and HIPAA in blockchain technology. *PLoS One*, *20*(5), e0324285. PMID: 40408373

Akseer, R., Connolly, M., Cosby, J., Frost, G., Kanagarajah, R. R., & Lim, S. H. E. (2021). Clinician–patient relationships after two decades of a paradigm of patient-centered care. *International Journal of Healthcare Management*, *14*(3), 888–897.

Alaba, F. A., Othman, M., Hashem, I. A. T., & Alotaibi, F. (2017). Internet of Things security: A survey. *Journal of Network and Computer Applications*, *88*, 10–28.

Alabi, M. (2023). Data Governance and Quality: Ensuring Data Reliability and Trustworthiness. *ResearchGate, October*.

Ali, I., Sabir, S., & Ullah, Z. (2019). Internet of things security, device authentication and access control: a review. *arXiv preprint arXiv:1901.07309*.

Ambarkar, S. S., & Shekokar, N. (2020). Toward smart and secure IoT based healthcare system. *Internet of things, smart computing and technology: A roadmap ahead*, pp.283-303.

Aslam, U., & Jack, W. (2025). The Convergence of IoT and AI in Healthcare: Revolutionizing Real-Time Patient Monitoring and Predictive Diagnostics.

Awotunde, J. B., Jimoh, R. G., Folorunso, S. O., Adeniyi, E. A., Abiodun, K. M., & Banjo, O. O. (2021). Privacy and security concerns in IoT-based healthcare systems. In *The Fusion of Internet of Things, Artificial Intelligence, and Cloud Computing in Health Care* (pp. 105–134). Springer International Publishing.

Azimi, I., Rahmani, A. M., Liljeberg, P., & Tenhunen, H. (2017). Internet of things for remote elderly monitoring: A study from user-centered perspective. *Journal of Ambient Intelligence and Humanized Computing*, *8*(2), 273–289.

Baker, S. B., Xiang, W., & Atkinson, I. (2017). Internet of things for smart healthcare: Technologies, challenges, and opportunities. *IEEE Access : Practical Innovations, Open Solutions*, *5*, 26521–26544.

Baldini, G., Botterman, M., Neisse, R., & Tallacchini, M. (2018). Ethical design in the internet of things. *Science and Engineering Ethics*, *24*, 905–925. PMID: 26797878

Banerjee, A., Shit, M., Muhuri, S. S., Adhikari, S., Himanshee, S., & Mohapatra, H. (2025) Revolutionizing Healthcare from Inside: Leveraging Expanded Reality with Ingestible Sensors. In *Embedded Artificial Intelligence* (pp. 227-251). Chapman and Hall/CRC Press.

Beale, S. S., & Berris, P. (2017). Hacking the Internet of Things: Vulnerabilities, dangers, and legal responses. *Duke L. & Tech. Rev.*, *16*, 161.

Berlin, G., Darino, L., Greenfield, M., Starikova, I., & JGI/Tom Grill/Getty Images. (2019). Women in the healthcare industry. https://hbanet.org/sites/default/files/2023-06/Women-in-the-healthcare-industry_Aug.2019.pdf

Bertl, M., Ross, P., & Draheim, D. (2023). Systematic AI support for decision-making in the healthcare sector: Obstacles and success factors. *Health Policy and Technology*, *12*(3), 100748.

Bharadwaj, H. K., Agarwal, A., Chamola, V., Lakkaniga, N. R., Hassija, V., Guizani, M., & Sikdar, B. (2021). A review on the role of machine learning in enabling IoT based healthcare applications. *IEEE Access : Practical Innovations, Open Solutions*, *9*, 38859–38890.

Bhosale, K. S., Nenova, M., & Iliev, G. (2021). A study of cyber attacks: In the healthcare sector. In *2021 Sixth Junior Conference on Lighting (Lighting)* (pp. 1-6). IEEE.

Bhuiyan, M. N., Rahman, M. M., Billah, M. M., & Saha, D. (2021). Internet of things (IoT): A review of its enabling technologies in healthcare applications, standards protocols, security, and market opportunities. *IEEE Internet of Things Journal*, *8*(13), 10474–10498.

Bisio, I., Garibotto, C., Lavagetto, F., & Sciarrone, A. (2019). When eHealth meets IoT: A smart wireless system for post-stroke home rehabilitation. *IEEE Wireless Communications*, *26*(6), 24–29.

Boeren, E. (2019). Understanding Sustainable Development Goal (SDG) 4 on "quality education" from micro, meso and macro perspectives. *International Review of Education*, *65*(2), 277–294. DOI: 10.1007/s11159-019-09772-7

Butpheng, C., Yeh, K. H., & Xiong, H. (2020). Security and privacy in IoT-cloud-based e-health systems—A comprehensive review. *Symmetry*, *12*(7), 1191.

Butun, I., Österberg, P., & Song, H. (2019). Security of the Internet of Things: Vulnerabilities, attacks, and countermeasures. *IEEE Communications Surveys and Tutorials*, *22*(1), 616–644.

Caciquinho, P. O., & Arruda, K. M. (2025). The power of learning culture as an instrument to effective implementation of social justice. *Journal of Social and Labor Relations Law, 11*(1), 33–42. https://publicacoes.udf.edu.br/index.php/relacoes-sociais-trabalhista/article/view/571

Castaneda, C., Nalley, K., Mannion, C., Bhattacharyya, P., Blake, P., Pecora, A., & Suh, K. S. (2015). Clinical decision support systems for improving diagnostic accuracy and achieving precision medicine. *Journal of Clinical Bioinformatics, 5*(1), 4. PMID: 25834725

Chacko, A., & Hayajneh, T. (2018). Security and privacy issues with IoT in healthcare. *EAI Endorsed Transactions on Pervasive Health and Technology, 4*(14).

Chan, M., Estève, D., Escriba, C., & Campo, E. (2008). A review of smart homes—Present state and future challenges. *Computer Methods and Programs in Biomedicine, 91*(1), 55–81. PMID: 18367286

Chen, H., Hailey, D., Wang, N., & Yu, P. (2014). A review of data quality assessment methods for public health information systems. *International Journal of Environmental Research and Public Health, 11*(5), 5170–5207. PMID: 24830450

Chin, M. H., Afsar-Manesh, N., Bierman, A. S., Chang, C., Colón-Rodríguez, C. J., Dullabh, P., Duran, D. G., Fair, M., Hernandez-Boussard, T., Hightower, M., & Ohno-Machado, L. (2023). Guiding principles to address the impact of algorithm bias on racial and ethnic disparities in health and health care. *JAMA Network Open, 6*(12), e2345050–e2345050. PMID: 38100101

Cui, A., Costello, M., & Stolfo, S. (2013). When firmware modifications attack: A case study of embedded exploitation.

Dasaka, S. (2024). Optimizing decision-making: Balancing intuition with evidence in digital experience design.

Demiris, G., Rantz, M. J., Aud, M. A., Marek, K. D., Tyrer, H. W., Skubic, M., & Hussam, A. A. (2004). Older adults' attitudes towards and perceptions of 'smart home' technologies: A pilot study. *Medical Informatics and the Internet in Medicine, 29*(2), 87–94. PMID: 15370989

Dewangan, K., & Mishra, M. (2018). Review: Security of IOT Based Healthcare System. *CCET Journal of Science and Engineering Education, 3*, 25–28.

Dias, D., & Cunha, J. P. S. (2018). Wearable Health Devices—Vital Sign Monitoring, systems and Technologies. *Sensors (Basel), 18*(8), 2414. PMID: 30044415

Dixon, E., Anderson, J., & Lazar, A. (2022). Understanding how sensory changes experienced by individuals with a range of age-related cognitive changes can affect technology use. [TACCESS]. *ACM Transactions on Accessible Computing, 15*(2), 1–33. PMID: 35919105

Domingo, M. C. (2012). An overview of the Internet of Things for people with disabilities. *journal of Network and Computer Applications, 35*(2), 584-596.

Felici, M., & Pearson, S. (2014). Accountability for data governance in the cloud. In *Summer School on Accountability and Security in the Cloud* (pp. 3–42). Springer International Publishing.

Feng, X., Zhu, X., Han, Q. L., Zhou, W., Wen, S., & Xiang, Y. (2022). Detecting vulnerability on IoT device firmware: A survey. *IEEE/CAA Journal of Automatica Sinica, 10*(1), 25-41.

Fereidouni, H., Fadeitcheva, O., & Zalai, M. (2025). IoT and man-in-the-middle attacks. *Security and Privacy, 8*(2), e70016.

Freckmann, G., Pleus, S., Grady, M., Setford, S., & Levy, B. (2019). Measures of accuracy for continuous glucose monitoring and blood glucose monitoring devices. *Journal of Diabetes Science and Technology, 13*(3), 575–583. PMID: 30453761

Garcia, C. A. (2022). *Creating New Value from Laboratory Testing and Services in Value-Based Healthcare: Investigating Data Monetization Strategies from Clinical Laboratories* (Doctoral dissertation, Massachusetts Institute of Technology).

Gaytan, J.C.T. (2022). A literature survey of security and privacy issues in internet of medical things. *International Journal of Computations, Information and Manufacturing (IJCIM), 2*(2).

Ghosh, A. M., Halder, D., & Hossain, S. A. (2016). May. Remote health monitoring system through IoT. In *2016 5th International Conference on Informatics, Electronics and Vision (ICIEV)* (pp. 921-926). IEEE.

Gourisaria, M. K., Agrawal, R., Singh, V., Rautaray, S. S., & Pandey, M. (2022). AI and IoT Enabled Smart Hospital Management Systems. In *Data Science in Societal Applications: Concepts and Implications* (pp. 77–106). Springer Nature Singapore.

Goyal, S., Sharma, N., Bhushan, B., Shankar, A., & Sagayam, M. (2021). Iot enabled technology in secured healthcare: Applications, challenges and future directions. *Cognitive Internet of Medical Things for Smart Healthcare: Services and Applications*, pp.25-48.

Gupta, A., Yadav, S., Shahid, S., & Venkanna, U. (2019). December. HeartCare: IoT based heart disease prediction system. In *2019 International Conference on Information Technology (ICIT)* (pp. 88-93). IEEE.

Gyrard, A., & Serrano, M. (2016). March. Connected smart cities: interoperability with SEG 3.0 for the internet of things. In *2016 30th International Conference on Advanced Information Networking and Applications Workshops (WAINA)* (pp. 796-802). IEEE.

Hales, R., & Birdthistle, N. (2022). The Sustainable Development Goals – SDG#9 Industry, Innovation and Infrastructure. In Attaining the 2030 sustainable development goal of industry, innovation and infrastructure. https://doi.org/DOI: 10.1108/9781803825731

Häußermann, S., Arendsen, L. J., & Pritchard, J. N. (2022). Smart dry powder inhalers and intelligent adherence management. *Advanced Drug Delivery Reviews, 191*, 114580. PMID: 36273513

Hazra, A., Adhikari, M., Amgoth, T., & Srirama, S. N. (2021). A comprehensive survey on interoperability for IIoT: Taxonomy, standards, and future directions. *ACM Computing Surveys*, *55*(1), 1–35.

Hollander, J. E., & Carr, B. G. (2020). Virtually perfect? Telemedicine for COVID-19. *The New England Journal of Medicine*, *382*(18), 1679–1681. PMID: 32160451

Hui, C. Y., McKinstry, B., Fulton, O., Buchner, M., & Pinnock, H. (2021). Patients' and clinicians' perceived trust in internet-of-things systems to support asthma self-management: Qualitative interview study. *JMIR mHealth and uHealth*, *9*(7), e24127. PMID: 34269684

Istepanian, R. S., Hu, S., Philip, N. Y., & Sungoor, A. (2011). August. The potential of Internet of m-health Things "m-IoT" for non-invasive glucose level sensing. In *2011 annual international conference of the IEEE engineering in medicine and biology society* (pp. 5264-5266). IEEE.

Jaime, F. J., Muñoz, A., Rodríguez-Gómez, F., & Jerez-Calero, A. (2023). Strengthening privacy and data security in biomedical microelectromechanical systems by IoT communication security and protection in smart healthcare. *Sensors (Basel)*, *23*(21), 8944. PMID: 37960646

Jaime, F. J., Muñoz, A., Rodríguez-Gómez, F., & Jerez-Calero, A. (2023). Strengthening privacy and data security in biomedical microelectromechanical systems by IoT communication security and protection in smart healthcare. *Sensors (Basel)*, *23*(21), 8944. PMID: 37960646

Javaid, M., & Khan, I. H. (2021). Internet of Things (IoT) enabled healthcare helps to take the challenges of COVID-19 Pandemic. *Journal of Oral Biology and Craniofacial Research, 11*(2), 209–214. PMID: 33665069

Kakria, P., Tripathi, N. K., & Kitipawang, P. (2015). A real-time health monitoring system for remote cardiac patients using smartphone and wearable sensors. *International Journal of Telemedicine and Applications, 2015*(1), 373474. PMID: 26788055

Karam, A.A. (2022). Investigating the importance of ethics and security on internet of medical things (IoMT). *International Journal of Computations, Information and Manufacturing (IJCIM), 2*(2).

Kelly, D., & Hammoudeh, M. (2018). Optimisation of the public key encryption infrastructure for the internet of things. In *Proceedings of the 2nd International Conference on Future Networks and Distributed Systems* (pp. 1-5).

Khan, M. A., & Salah, K. (2018). IoT security: Review, blockchain solutions, and open challenges. *Future Generation Computer Systems, 82*, 395–411.

Khan, M. M., Shah, N., Shaikh, N., Thabet, A., & Belkhair, S. (2024). Towards secure and trusted AI in healthcare: A systematic review of emerging innovations and ethical challenges. *International Journal of Medical Informatics*, •••, 105780. PMID: 39753062

Khezr, S., Moniruzzaman, M., Yassine, A., & Benlamri, R. (2019). Blockchain technology in healthcare: A comprehensive review and directions for future research. *Applied Sciences (Basel, Switzerland), 9*(9), 1736.

Kopetz, H., & Steiner, W. (2022). Internet of things. In *Real-time systems: design principles for distributed embedded applications* (pp. 325–341). Springer International Publishing.

Kshatri, S. S., Chandrakar, M. K., Bhonsle, D., Nayak, M., Tamrakar, P., & Sharma, P. (2025). Smart Medication Dispensing: IoT Innovations in Drug Development. *The Impact of Algorithmic Technologies on Healthcare*, 255-277.

Kshetri, N. (2017). Can blockchain strengthen the internet of things? *IT Professional, 19*(4), 68–72.

Liang, W., Tadesse, G. A., Ho, D., Fei-Fei, L., Zaharia, M., Zhang, C., & Zou, J. (2022). Advances, challenges and opportunities in creating data for trustworthy AI. *Nature Machine Intelligence, 4*(8), 669–677.

Liu, C., Nitschke, P., Williams, S. P., & Zowghi, D. (2020). Data quality and the Internet of Things. *Computing, 102*(2), 573–599.

López, L., Green, A. R., Tan-McGrory, A., King, R. S., & Betancourt, J. R. (2011). Bridging the digital divide in health care: The role of health information technology in addressing racial and ethnic disparities. *Joint Commission Journal on Quality and Patient Safety*, *37*(10), 437–445. PMID: 22013816

Lupton, D. (2013). The digitally engaged patient: Self-monitoring and self-care in the digital health era. *Social Theory & Health*, *11*, 256–270.

Maddali, R. (2024). Ai-Powered Data Security Frameworks For Regulatory Compliance (GDPR, CCPA, HIPAA). [IJETRM]. *International Journal of Engineering Technology Research & Management*, *8*(04).

Makhdoom, I., Abolhasan, M., Lipman, J., Liu, R. P., & Ni, W. (2018). Anatomy of threats to the internet of things. *IEEE Communications Surveys and Tutorials*, *21*(2), 1636–1675.

Marques, G., Pitarma, R. M., Garcia, N., & Pombo, N. (2019). Internet of things architectures, technologies, applications, challenges, and future directions for enhanced living environments and healthcare systems: A review. *Electronics (Basel)*, *8*(10), 1081.

Mavrogiorgou, A., Kiourtis, A., Perakis, K., Pitsios, S., & Kyriazis, D. (2019). IoT in healthcare: Achieving interoperability of high-quality data acquired by IoT medical devices. *Sensors (Basel)*, *19*(9), 1978. PMID: 31035612

Mayer, J., Jose, R., Kurgansky, G., Singh, P., Coletti, C., Devine, T., & Toma, M. (2023). Evaluating the feasibility of euler angles for bed-based patient movement monitoring. *Signals*, *4*(4), 788–799.

Mazharuddin, H. (2025). Beyond the wrist: Wearables in healthcare. In *Digital Health* (pp. 63–73). Academic Press.

McLean, A. (2011). Ethical frontiers of ICT and older users: Cultural, pragmatic and ethical issues. *Ethics and Information Technology*, *13*(4), 313–326.

Mercurio, B., & Yu, R. (2022). *Regulating Cross-Border Data Flows: Issues, Challenges and Impact*. Anthem Press.

Mittelstadt, B. (2017). Ethics of the health-related internet of things: A narrative review. *Ethics and Information Technology*, *19*(3), 157–175.

Moore, A. A., Ellis, J. R., Dellavalle, N., Akerson, M., Andazola, M., Campbell, E. G., & DeCamp, M. (2025). Patient-facing chatbots: Enhancing healthcare accessibility while navigating digital literacy challenges and isolation risks—a mixed-methods study. *Digital Health*, *11*, 20552076251337321. PMID: 40308811

Mustacoglu, A. F., Catak, F. O., & Fox, G. C. (2020). Password-based encryption approach for securing sensitive data. *Security and Privacy*, *3*(5), e121.

Nadhan, A. S., & Jacob, I. J. (2024). Enhancing healthcare security in the digital era: Safeguarding medical images with lightweight cryptographic techniques in IoT healthcare applications. *Biomedical Signal Processing and Control*, *88*, 105511.

Nayak, P., Mohapatra, S. K., & Sharma, S. C. M. (2022). Privacy and security issues in IoT cloud convergence of smart health care. In *Connected e-Health: Integrated IoT and Cloud Computing* (pp. 439–455). Springer International Publishing.

Noah, B., Keller, M. S., Mosadeghi, S., Stein, L., Johl, S., Delshad, S., Tashjian, V. C., Lew, D., Kwan, J. T., Jusufagic, A., & Spiegel, B. M. (2018). Impact of remote patient monitoring on clinical outcomes: An updated meta-analysis of randomized controlled trials. *NPJ Digital Medicine*, *1*(1), 20172. PMID: 31304346

O'donoghue, J., & Herbert, J. (2012). Data management within mHealth environments: Patient sensors, mobile devices, and databases. [JDIQ]. *Journal of Data and Information Quality*, *4*(1), 1–20.

Page, X., Bahirat, P., Safi, M. I., Knijnenburg, B. P., & Wisniewski, P. (2018). The internet of what? understanding differences in perceptions and adoption for the internet of things. *Proceedings of the ACM on Interactive, Mobile, Wearable and Ubiquitous Technologies*, *2*(4), 1–22.

Palm, E. (2020). Who cares? Moral obligations in formal and informal care provision in the light of ICT-based home care. In *The Ethical Challenges of Emerging Medical Technologies* (pp. 205–222). Routledge.

Paris, I. L. B. M., Habaebi, M. H., & Zyoud, A. M. (2023). Implementation of SSL/TLS Security with MQTT Protocol in IoT Environment. *Wireless Personal Communications*, *132*(1), 163–182.

Pattar, S., Buyya, R., Venugopal, K. R., Iyengar, S. S., & Patnaik, L. M. (2018). Searching for the IoT resources: Fundamentals, requirements, comprehensive review, and future directions. *IEEE Communications Surveys and Tutorials*, *20*(3), 2101–2132.

Peralta, G., Cid-Fuentes, R. G., Bilbao, J., & Crespo, P. M. (2019). Homomorphic encryption and network coding in iot architectures: Advantages and future challenges. *Electronics (Basel)*, *8*(8), 827.

Percival, J., & Hanson, J. (2006). Big brother or brave new world? Telecare and its implications for older people's independence and social inclusion. *Critical Social Policy*, *26*(4), 888–909.

Poole, T. (2014). *Enhancing The Privacy Framework: An analysis of Privacy in Canadian and Brazilian health care* (Doctoral dissertation, Dalhousie University).

Popescul, D., & Georgescu, M. (2014). Internet of Things–some ethical issues. *The USV Annals of Economics and Public Administration, 13*(2 (18)), 208–214.

Poyner, I. K., & Sherratt, R. S. (2018). Privacy and security of consumer IoT devices for the pervasive monitoring of vulnerable people. In *Living in the Internet of Things: Cybersecurity of the IoT-2018* (pp. 1–5). IET.

Puustjärvi, J., & Puustjärvi, L. (2011). Automating remote monitoring and information therapy: An opportunity to practice telemedicine in developing countries. In *2011 IST-Africa Conference Proceedings* (pp. 1-9). IEEE.

Quinn, M., Forman, J., Harrod, M., Winter, S., Fowler, K. E., Krein, S. L., Gupta, A., Saint, S., Singh, H., & Chopra, V. (2019). Electronic health records, communication, and data sharing: Challenges and opportunities for improving the diagnostic process. *Diagnosis (Berlin, Germany), 6*(3), 241–248. PMID: 30485175

Rachim, V. P., & Chung, W. Y. (2016). Wearable noncontact armband for mobile ECG monitoring system. *IEEE Transactions on Biomedical Circuits and Systems, 10*(6), 1112–1118. PMID: 27214910

Raghav, Y. Y., Choudhary, S., Pandey, P., Singh, S., & Varshney, D. (2025). Smart Healthcare: Cloud-IoT Solutions for Enhanced Patient Well-Being. *African Journal of Biomedical Research, 28*(1), 14–28.

Rangarajan, D., Rangarajan, A., Reddy, C. K. K., & Doss, S. (2025). Exploring the Next-Gen Transformations in Healthcare Through the Impact of AI and IoT. In *Intelligent Systems and IoT Applications in Clinical Health* (pp. 73–98). IGI Global.

Rathee, G., Sharma, A., Saini, H., Kumar, R., & Iqbal, R. (2020). A hybrid framework for multimedia data processing in IoT-healthcare using blockchain technology. *Multimedia Tools and Applications, 79*(15), 9711–9733.

Rehiman, K.R. and Veni, S. (2016). A secure authentication infrastructure for IoT enabled smart mobile devices-An initial prototype. *Indian journal of science and technology, 9*(9), pp.0974-6846.

Rothschild, J. M., Keohane, C. A., Cook, E. F., Orav, E. J., Burdick, E., Thompson, S., Hayes, J., & Bates, D. W. (2005). A controlled trial of smart infusion pumps to improve medication safety in critically ill patients. *Critical Care Medicine, 33*(3), 533–540. PMID: 15753744

Ruiz, M. N., García, J. M., & Fernández, B. M. (2009). Body temperature and its importance as a vital constant. *Revista de Enfermeria (Barcelona, Spain)*, *32*(9), 44–52. PMID: 19839238

Safdar, Z., Farid, S., Qadir, M., Asghar, K., Iqbal, J., & Hamdani, F. K. (2020). A novel architecture for internet of things based E-health systems. *Journal of Medical Imaging and Health Informatics*, *10*(10), 2378–2388.

Samaila, M. G., Neto, M., Fernandes, D. A., Freire, M. M., & Inácio, P. R. (2018). Challenges of securing Internet of Things devices: A survey. *Security and Privacy*, *1*(2), e20.

Satyender, S. D. (2025). Smart Implants: The Role of Biocompatible Sensors in Personalized Medicine and Remote Monitoring. *Siddhanta's International. Journal of Science and Technology*, *1*(1), 25–45.

Seh, A. H., Zarour, M., Alenezi, M., Sarkar, A. K., Agrawal, A., Kumar, R., & Ahmad Khan, R. (2020). May. Healthcare data breaches: Insights and implications. [MDPI.]. *Health Care*, *8*(2), 133. PMID: 32414183

Shah, S. T. U., Yar, H., Khan, I., Ikram, M., & Khan, H. (2019). Internet of things-based healthcare: recent advances and challenges. *Applications of Intelligent Technologies in Healthcare*, pp.153-162.

Shahid, J., Ahmad, R., Kiani, A. K., Ahmad, T., Saeed, S., & Almuhaideb, A. M. (2022). Data protection and privacy of the internet of healthcare things (IoHTs). *Applied Sciences (Basel, Switzerland)*, *12*(4), 1927.

Shahid, J., Ahmad, R., Kiani, A. K., Ahmad, T., Saeed, S., & Almuhaideb, A. M. (2022). Data protection and privacy of the internet of healthcare things (IoHTs). *Applied Sciences (Basel, Switzerland)*, *12*(4), 1927.

Shahid, J., Ahmad, R., Kiani, A. K., Ahmad, T., Saeed, S., & Almuhaideb, A. M. (2022). Data protection and privacy of the internet of healthcare things (IoHTs). *Applied Sciences (Basel, Switzerland)*, *12*(4), 1927.

Stephen, M., & Kolachala, R. (2025). Revolutionizing Healthcare: IoT Powered Telemedicine Advancements. In *Scalable Modeling and Efficient Management of IoT Applications* (pp. 59-86). IGI Global.

Stowe, S., & Harding, S. (2010). Telecare, telehealth and telemedicine. *European Geriatric Medicine*, *1*(3), 193–197.

Sun, Y., Lo, F. P. W., & Lo, B. (2019). Security and privacy for the internet of medical things enabled healthcare systems: A survey. *IEEE Access : Practical Innovations, Open Solutions*, *7*, 183339–183355.

Supriya, S., & Padaki, S. (2016). December. Data security and privacy challenges in adopting solutions for IOT. In *2016 IEEE International Conference on Internet of Things (iThings) and IEEE Green Computing and Communications (GreenCom) and IEEE Cyber, Physical and Social Computing (CPSCom) and IEEE Smart Data (SmartData)* (pp. 410-415). IEEE.

THE 17 GOALS | Sustainable Development. Retrieved, 2025, from https://sdgs.un.org/goals

Tiwari, P., Warren, J., Day, K. J., & MacDonald, B. (2010). *Some non-technology implications for wider application of robots to assist older people*. Health Care and Informatics Review Online.

Van Alstyne, M., Brynjolfsson, E., & Madnick, S. (1995). Why not one big database? Principles for data ownership. *Decision Support Systems*, *15*(4), 267–284.

Van Woudenberg, J., & O'Flynn, C. (2021). *The hardware hacking handbook: breaking embedded security with hardware attacks*. No Starch Press.

Varhol, R. J., Robinson, S., Lee, C. M. Y., Randall, S., & Boyd, J. H. (2025). Attitudes towards data access and sharing health data for research: A case study of Australian data custodian perspectives. *The HIM Journal*, •••, 18333583251329533. PMID: 40317196

Vorisek, C. N., Lehne, M., Klopfenstein, S. A. I., Mayer, P. J., Bartschke, A., Haese, T., & Thun, S. (2022). Fast healthcare interoperability resources (FHIR) for interoperability in health research: Systematic review. *JMIR Medical Informatics*, *10*(7), e35724. PMID: 35852842

Wu, Y. H., Fassert, C., & Rigaud, A. S. (2012). Designing robots for the elderly: Appearance issue and beyond. *Archives of Gerontology and Geriatrics*, *54*(1), 121–126. PMID: 21349593

Yang, G., Xie, L., Mäntysalo, M., Zhou, X., Pang, Z., Da Xu, L., Kao-Walter, S., Chen, Q., & Zheng, L. R. (2014). A health-IoT platform based on the integration of intelligent packaging, unobtrusive bio-sensor, and intelligent medicine box. *IEEE Transactions on Industrial Informatics*, *10*(4), 2180–2191.

Yew, H. T., Ng, M. F., Ping, S. Z., Chung, S. K., Chekima, A., & Dargham, J. A. (2020). February. Iot based real-time remote patient monitoring system. In *2020 16th IEEE international colloquium on signal processing & its applications (CSPA)* (pp. 176-179). IEEE.

Yuehong, Y. I. N., Zeng, Y., Chen, X., & Fan, Y. (2016). The internet of things in healthcare: An overview. *Journal of Industrial Information Integration*, *1*, 3–13.

Yusof, Z. B. (2025). The Role of High-Quality Data in Risk Assessment: Strategies for Ensuring Accuracy, Completeness, and Timeliness in Financial Predictive Analytics. *International Journal of Advanced Computational Methodologies and Emerging Technologies*, *15*(2), 8–16.

Zhong, D., Yian, Z., Lanqing, W., Junhua, D., & Jiaxuan, H. (2020). Continuous blood pressure measurement platform: A wearable system based on multidimensional perception data. *IEEE Access : Practical Innovations, Open Solutions*, *8*, 10147–10158.

Zwijsen, S. A., Niemeijer, A. R., & Hertogh, C. M. (2011). Ethics of using assistive technology in the care for community-dwelling elderly people: An overview of the literature. *Aging & Mental Health*, *15*(4), 419–427. PMID: 21500008

KEY TERMS AND DEFINITIONS

Internet of Things: refers to both the technology that enables communication between devices and the cloud, as well as to the devices themselves, and the entire network of linked gadgets.

E-Health: covers medical services like electronic prescription, telehealth, or electronic health records (EHRs) that are aided by digital processes, communication, or technology.

Privacy: centered on the usage and governance of personal data, including the establishment of regulations to guarantee that personal data about customers is gathered, exchanged, and used appropriately.

Security: the procedure for protecting digital data from theft, corruption, and illegal access across its whole life cycle.

HIPAA: A federal law known as the Health Insurance Portability and Accountability Act of 1996 (HIPAA) mandated the development of national standards to guard against the disclosure of private patient health information without the informed consent or knowledge of the patient.

Blockchain: a distributed ledger made up of expanding lists of records, or blocks, connected safely by cryptographic hashes.

PIPEDA: The guidelines that govern the collection, use, and disclosure of personal information by private sector entities engaged in for-profit, commercial operations in Canada are established under the Personal Information Protection and Electronic Documents Act, or PIPEDA.

GDPR: The world's strictest privacy and security legislation is called the General Data Protection Regulation (GDPR). The rule becomes operative on May 25, 2018. If someone violates the GDPR's security and privacy requirements, they might face fines of up to tens of millions of euros.

BioMEMS: Biomedical (or biological) microelectromechanical systems can be shortened to bio-MEMS. There is a lot of overlap and occasionally confusion between lab-on-a-chip (LOC) and micro total analysis systems (μTAS) and bio-MEMS.

H-IoT: Systems known as Healthcare Internet of Things, or H-IoT, have opened up new possibilities and solutions for healthcare services, such as patient monitoring and remote therapy. Patients benefit from the use of IoT in remote health monitoring because it enables better diagnosis through continuous health monitoring, early disease detection, and prevention.

Chapter 10
Ethical and Legal Implications of Artificial Intelligence in Healthcare

K. Lakshmi
https://orcid.org/0000-0002-8147-8035
REVA University, India

S. Shanmugapriya
Amrita School of Computing, India

ABSTRACT

Artificial intelligence (AI) has been increasingly integrated into healthcare. There is a huge shift in the way that diseases are diagnosed, treated, and managed. AI has the potential to revolutionize the healthcare sector by leveraging advanced algorithms and machine learning techniques to deliver novel capabilities in data analysis, clinical decision-making, and personalized treatment options. AI innovations in healthcare are revolutionizing the industry by enhancing diagnostic accuracy, personalizing treatment plans, streamlining administrative tasks etc.

1. INTRODUCTION

1.1 Overview of AI Adoption in Healthcare

Artificial Intelligence in Healthcare refers to the use of machine learning (ML), natural language processing (NLP), computer vision, robotics, and other AI techniques to improve early diagnosis of diseases and treatment planning, Patient monitoring, personalized medicine and Drug discovery. Electronic Health Records (EHRs)

DOI: 10.4018/979-8-3693-3864-3.ch010

and Wearable IoT Devices are the big source of data for training AI models. Cloud Computing enables scalable AI processing and storage of large amount of data.

Early AI applications in healthcare emerged in the 1970s and 1980s, focusing on expert systems that aimed to replicate human clinical decision-making. However, advanced machine learning techniques, particularly deep learning, has significantly accelerated the development of AI tools with greater accuracy and efficiency in complex tasks such as image recognition and predictive analytics (Rajpurkar et al., 2017; Esteva et al., 2017).

ML, especially supervised learning, is widely used in predictive analytics, where models are trained on labelled datasets to predict outcomes like disease progression. Deep learning, a subset of ML, has revolutionized medical imaging by enabling the automated detection of complex patterns in images that are difficult for human eyes to detect NLP is essential for processing and analysing clinical notes, patient records, and other text-based data, allowing AI systems to assist in diagnosis and treatment planning. Reinforcement Learning is used in optimizing treatment protocols by learning from the outcomes of past treatments. Beyond medical imaging, computer vision techniques are also employed in areas such as pathology to analyse tissue samples. EHRs are critical for AI in healthcare, providing structured and unstructured data that can be mined for insights. These records include patient demographics, medical history, medications, and diagnostic data. AI in radiology is one of the most prominent areas, with deep learning models being used to analyse X-rays, MRIs, and CT scans for conditions such as tumours, fractures, and other abnormalities. AI is increasingly used in genomics to identify genetic predispositions to diseases and to tailor personalized treatment plans. Data from wearable devices offer real-time monitoring of patients' vitals and activities, which can be analysed using AI for early detection of health issues. AI is also applied in analysing large datasets from public health sources to predict outbreaks, monitor disease progression, and optimize healthcare delivery at the population levelThe integration of artificial intelligence (AI) in healthcare has become increasingly important in recent years, offering the potential to revolutionize medical diagnostics, treatment plans, and overall healthcare management. AI in healthcare leverages various technologies, including machine learning, deep learning, and natural language processing, to analyze large datasets and generate insights that can improve patient care and medical decision-making.

Deep learning algorithms have been used to detect diseases like pneumonia and skin cancer by analyzing medical images with accuracy comparable to or even surpassing human clinicians (Esteva et al., 2017; Rajpurkar et al., 2017). AI is also playing a critical role in genomics and drug discovery by enabling faster identification of potential drug candidates and personalized treatment options (Yu, Beam, & Kohane, 2018). These advances have the potential to reduce the time and cost associated with drug development and to tailor medical treatments to individual patients based on their genetic makeup (Topol, 2019).

AI has the ability to classify optical coherence tomography retinal pictures for the purpose of early retinal disease diagnosis (Ting et al., 2018). By implementing AI, it is possible to automate repetitive tasks, decrease waiting times, increase patient reach, and connect with physicians and nurses in real time (Jiang et al., 2017). AI may also be used to identify, diagnose, and track a patient's health; it can also be used to create personalized health trackers, lower clinical risks, lower expenses, and improve the efficiency of the healthcare system. Generative AI, particularly Generative Adversarial Networks (GANs), has been transformative in medical imaging. GANs can enhance the resolution of medical images, generate synthetic data for training purposes, and even create 3D models from 2D images. These advancements help in improving diagnostic accuracy and facilitating better treatment planning (Sun & Medaglia, 2019) . Another key development in healthcare AI is multimodal data fusion, which involves integrating data from various sources, such as imaging, genetics, and sensor data, to develop comprehensive models for illness diagnosis, prognosis, and personalized healthcare management (Arisdakessian et al., 2023)(Ahmed et al., 2021) (Sakib et al., 2022) . Transforming healthcare through chatbots and virtual assistants involves leveraging artificial intelligence technologies to enhance patient engagement, provide personalized support, and streamline healthcare services (Amin & Hossain, 2021) (Hayyolalam et al., 2022) .

Despite the promising advancements, the widespread adoption of AI in healthcare has its own challenges. Issues such as data privacy, algorithmic bias, and the need for regulatory frameworks to ensure the safety and fairness of AI tools must be addressed (Choi & Lee, 2020). Furthermore, there are ethical concerns about ensuring that AI technologies do not exacerbate existing health disparities or introduce new forms of bias (Yu et al., 2018). As AI technologies continue to evolve, it is essential that healthcare providers, policymakers, and AI developers collaborate to establish guidelines and standards that ensure the responsible use of AI in healthcare (Topol, 2019).

Overall, the background of AI in healthcare is marked by rapid advancements and transformative potential. While challenges remain, AI promises to enhance the quality, accessibility, and efficiency of healthcare delivery worldwide.

1.2 Emerging AI Trends in Healthcare

Integration of AI With Wearable Technology

Wearable devices equipped with AI algorithms (Steinhubl et al., 2015) are increasingly being used to monitor patients' vital signs and health metrics in real-time. AI-powered wearables for continuous glucose monitoring in diabetic patients, providing real-time alerts and data analytics.

AI-Driven Precision Medicine

AI is being used to analyse genetic, environmental, and lifestyle data to develop personalized treatment plans for patients (Topol, 2019) . AI algorithms identifying specific genetic mutations in cancer patients to recommend targeted therapies.

Telemedicine and Remote Care

AI is enhancing telemedicine platforms by providing diagnostic support, patient triage, and remote monitoring capabilities (Keesara et al., 2020) . AI chatbots assisting patients with initial diagnosis and directing them to appropriate care.

AI in Drug Discovery and Development

By discovering possible novel drug candidates and forecasting drug-target interactions, AI algorithms are speeding up the drug discovery process (Zhavoronkov et al., 2019). AI models identifying new molecules with potential therapeutic effects for diseases like Alzheimer's and COVID-19.

AI for Mental Health

AI applications are being developed to support mental health care through sentiment analysis, mood tracking, and personalized therapeutic interventions (Inkster et al., 2018) . AI-based apps that provide cognitive behavioural therapy (CBT) and monitor user mood through their interactions.

Robotic Surgery

AI-powered robots assist in surgeries(Yang et al., 2022) by providing greater precision, reducing the margin of error, and enabling minimally invasive procedures. These systems can adapt to the surgeon's movements and provide real-time data that enhances surgical performance .

1.3 Challenges of using AI in Healthcare

Data Privacy and Security

Ensuring the privacy and security of patient data used by AI systems. Protecting sensitive health information from breaches and misuse while maintaining the integrity and accuracy of the data is very crucial.

The Problem of Re-Identification

Data re-identification occurs when scrubbed or "anonymized" data contains personally identifying information. Recent studies have shown that new computational methods can help identify individuals in health data repositories managed by public or private organizations. This remains valid even when the data has been de-identified and anonymized. One way AI system engineers can address persistent privacy concerns is by utilizing generative data. Generative models allow for the generation of lifelike patient data without being tied to real individuals [18, 19]. Even though it may be necessary at first to create the generative model, this can lead to machine learning being possible without having to use real patient data in the long run.

Bias and Fairness in AI Algorithms

These days, fairness and prejudice in artificial intelligence (AI) are major concerns that have received a lot of attention. It is critical to make sure AI systems are impartial, egalitarian, and fair because they are being employed more and more in a variety of fields and applications. The mistake that results in unfair decisions is what is known as AI bias. This is also known as algorithmic or machine learning bias, and it can result from a variety of factors including human biases, algorithm design, and data gathering. One of the difficulties is addressing biases in AI systems to guarantee equitable healthcare delivery (Obermeyer et al., 2019) .

Ignorance of AI Technologies

Developing patient trust is essential in healthcare, and this is particularly true with regard to AI-based technologies. Physicians and policymakers recognize that, considering the historical value of in-person interactions with doctors, the public could be hesitant to rely on AI- generated suggestions (Sun & Medaglia,2019) .

Unlawful AI Use

Although artificial intelligence (AI) can be utilized for good, it can also be misused. For instance, there are worries that AI might be employed for surreptitious screening or monitoring. Unbeknownst to the user, artificial intelligence (AI) technologies that analyze motor behavior—such as how a person types on a keyboard—and movement patterns discovered by tracking smartphones may disclose health-related information(Yuste et al., 2017) . AI has the potential to increase the scope and minimize the cost of cyberattacks(Brundage et al., 2018) . Governments, academics, and engineers have been urged as a result to consider AI's dual usage and be ready for potential malevolent applications of the technology (Brundage et al., 2018) .

This has led to calls for governments, researchers, and engineers to reflect on the dual use nature of AI and prepare for possible malicious uses of AI technologies(Brundage et al., 2018) .

Regulatory and Ethical Issues

Another biggest challenge is developing comprehensive regulations and ethical guidelines for AI use in healthcare(Luxton, 2014) . Ethical considerations must be integrated into the very design and implementation of these technologies. Innovators, policymakers, and healthcare providers must collaborate to create a future where technology enhances care while prioritizing patient privacy and autonomy. Ethical frameworks that evolve with technological advancements, robust cybersecurity measures, and a commitment to patient-centered care will be the cornerstones of a healthcare system that embraces innovation responsibly, ensuring a balance between progress and the fundamental values of medical ethics.

Integration with Existing Systems

Another major obstacle is the seamless integration of AI technology with the workflows and systems used in the healthcare industry today. Developing interoperable solutions that effectively integrate AI into the current healthcare infrastructure requires cooperation between technology vendors and healthcare institutions. Healthcare can benefit from AI in a number of ways, including enhanced collaboration and decision-making, technological advancements, patient monitoring, medical imaging and diagnosis, and virtual health support. By analyzing vast volumes of medical data and supporting knowledgeable decision-making, artificial intelligence (AI) helps healthcare workers improve patient outcomes and resource efficiency (Wubineh et al., 2024).

Instruction and Practice

Supplying healthcare workers with sufficient training so they can use AI tools efficiently. Self-monitoring with user-friendly technology for heart failure patients, as noted in (Australian Institute of Digital Health, 2023) . Medical professionals and students may be able to handle laboratory activities with the use of various health-related technology. Clinicians must participate in ongoing education sessions to stay current on AI developments and uses. Medical schools should think about incorporating ML and its application-focused coursework into their curricula (Kolachalama & Garg, 2018 . During their training, medical students, residents, and fellows should be knowledgeable about machine learning and data science.

Adoption by Healthcare Providers

Convincing healthcare providers to adopt AI tools is another challenge. There is often skepticism among clinicians regarding the reliability of AI systems, and integrating these tools into existing workflows can be difficult.

These trends and challenges highlight the dynamic nature of AI integration in healthcare, emphasizing the need for ongoing research, collaboration, and regulation to maximize benefits while mitigating risks.

Data Ownership and Autonomy

It is yet unclear who will control the data and how value will be created and distributed among different stakeholders (Singh, 2020). However, what if medical devices were more closely synchronized with IT systems and compliant with interoperability standards, enabling stakeholders to swiftly and easily retrieve a patient's medical history from a variety of sources and touchpoints throughout the patient's journey? In addition to being HIPAA compliant, this ideal system might greatly save healthcare costs (Singal & Tomar, 2022) .

Cultural and Social Stigma

The rate and scope of adoption are likely to be influenced by social and cultural views. According to a recent study, for instance, women in rural areas are more likely to turn to informal healers than to formal healthcare providers. This trend was linked to a number of factors, including communication ease, cultural resonance or familiarity, avoiding social stigma, and distance from formal healthcare facilities (Das et al., 2018).

Interpretability and Explainablity

One of the key challenges in healthcare AI is ensuring that DL models are interpretable and explainable. Without this, healthcare providers may be hesitant to adopt these technologies for fear of making decisions based on incomprehensible or untrustworthy information. To address this challenge, research efforts are focusing on developing approaches to make DL models more interpretable, particularly in critical healthcare contexts (Smart Healthcare in IoT, 2022)(An IoT-Based Heart Healthcare Platform, 2022).

1.4 Organization of the Chapter

The sections in this chapter provides an exploration of ethical and legal challenges that must be carefully navigated to ensure the technology benefits society while mitigating potential harms. The introduction sets the stage by highlighting the foundations required for the use of AI in healthcare and its applications, emerging trends and the common challenges involved. The subsequent chapters focus on the ethical and legal challenges associated with the application of artificial intelligence in healthcare. Ethical considerations and regulatory challenges are thoroughly discussed, underscoring the importance of safeguarding patient data privacy, addressing biases in algorithms, and ensuring compliance with regulations like HIPAA, GDPR, and FDA guidelines. The further sections also present a discussion on some case studies and real world applications of AI use in healthcare. Subsequent sections on regulatory compliance and recommendations for clinicians, researchers and policy makers focus on the importance of the collaborative efforts to develop robust guidelines and regulatory frameworks that maximize AI's potential benefits while safeguarding patient rights and promoting fairness and accountability in healthcare delivery. The section on Legal and regulatory compliance presents a overview of the global landscape of the efforts taken by countries worldwide in developing guidelines for compliance with healthcare regulations. Overall, the chapters provide a comprehensive overview of the applications, focussing ethical and legal challenges and efforts to overcome them and the emerging technologies of AI in healthcare emphasizing the need for collaboration, ethical considerations, regulatory compliance, and patient-centric care to drive innovation and improve patient outcomes in the healthcare industry.

2. ETHICAL CONSIDERATIONS FOR THE USE OF AI IN HEALTHCARE

Although the implementation of Artificial Intelligence (AI) in healthcare offers great advancements, it also brings up several ethical concerns that need to be addressed with caution. Ethical considerations include concerns about data privacy, algorithmic bias, accountability, transparency, and their effects on the doctor-patient relationship. To unlock the full potential of AI in healthcare, four main ethical issues must be addressed: (1) obtaining informed consent for data usage; (2) ensuring safety and transparency; (3) addressing algorithmic fairness and biases; and (4) protecting data privacy (Shortliffe & Sepúlveda, 2018) .

2.1 Informed Consent

Patients should be educated about the utilization of AI in their treatment and agree to its implementation. This involves comprehending the decision-making process of AI systems and the possible consequences. Patients should have the right to continue making informed decisions about their treatment, even if they choose to refuse AI-driven suggestions and instead rely on human recommendations.

2.2 Safety and Transparency

Data Security

AI systems in healthcare rely on large volumes of data, often containing sensitive personal information. The protection of this data from unauthorized access, breaches, and cyber-attacks is a significant concern. Advanced encryption methods, secure data storage solutions, and stringent access controls are necessary to safeguard patient information. Moreover, regular security audits and updates to AI systems can help mitigate potential vulnerabilities.

Accountability and Liability

Determining who is accountable when an AI system fails or makes an error is complex. Traditional medical malpractice laws may not be fully applicable to AI systems. Establishing clear guidelines on the liability of AI developers, healthcare providers, and institutions is necessary to address this issue. Additionally, having robust systems for oversight and quality control can help prevent errors and ensure accountability.

Transparency and Explainability

AI systems, particularly those utilizing deep learning, sometimes operate as "black boxes," in which their creators are unable to fully elucidate the process behind certain decisions. In the healthcare industry, the absence of transparency presents issues as decisions can greatly affect patients' lives. Patients and healthcare providers should have access to the information behind AI-generated recommendations. Creating AI models that can be easily understood and establishing guidelines for openness are crucial for fostering trust and enabling well-informed choices.

Incorporating Artificial Intelligence (AI) into healthcare offers valuable advantages, yet it also presents crucial issues concerning privacy and confidentiality. Patient trust, data security, and the overall effectiveness of AI systems in healthcare can be affected by these challenges.

2.3 Algorithmic Bias

Algorithmic bias in AI healthcare systems can have significant implications, affecting clinical decision-making, patient outcomes, and broader societal trust in healthcare systems. Some of the consequences are:

Misdiagnosis and Treatment Disparities: Bias present in AI algorithms has the potential to result in incorrect diagnoses or inappropriate recommendations for treatment, particularly impacting marginalized populations. For example, an algorithm that is mostly trained on data from one demographic may not work effectively for other groups.

Exacerbation of Health Inequities: Pre-existing health disparities can be worsened if AI systems perpetuate biases present in historical data. This can lead to unequal access to quality care and poorer health outcomes for marginalized communities.

Cost of Errors: Misdiagnoses and incorrect treatments due to biased algorithms can lead to increased healthcare costs. This includes costs related to additional tests, treatments, and potential legal fees from malpractice suits.

Resource Allocation: AI systems are often used to optimize resource allocation. Biased algorithms can lead to inefficient use of resources, directing them away from those who need them most.

Trust in Healthcare Systems: Bias in AI can erode trust in healthcare systems and technologies. Patients may be less willing to accept AI-driven treatments or recommendations if they perceive the systems to be biased or unfair.

Stigmatization: Certain groups may feel stigmatized if AI systems consistently underperform for them or if they are disproportionately negatively impacted by algorithmic decisions.

Hence addressing algorithmic bias in AI healthcare systems is critical for ensuring equitable, fair, and effective healthcare delivery. Ongoing efforts are needed to improve data quality, algorithmic transparency, and stakeholder involvement to mitigate these biases and their potential negative implications. The ethical duty to prevent or minimize harm to patients is threatened by Bias and algorithmic fairness's poor solutions. The following are important things to remember(Chin et al., 2023):

1. Encourage fairness in health and medical care throughout the whole life cycle of the health care algorithm.
2. Ascertain that the application of health care algorithms is clear and understandable.
3. Gain credibility by genuinely involving patients and communities at every stage of the health care algorithm's life cycle.
4. Clearly state the trade-offs and algorithmic fairness issues related to health care.
5. Ensure accountability for fairness and equity in the results of health care algorithms.

Regulatory procedures, guidelines, and standards should be put in place by governmental bodies, accrediting bodies, and professional associations to require openness and consistent evaluation and verification of health care algorithms for justice and equity. It is necessary to develop incentives for equity in health care algorithms. Every stage of the algorithm life cycle should have equity and fairness tests to account for human and technical biases that can affect clinical outcomes, model performance, and resource allocation. Algorithms that are unfair should be disabled, eliminated, or stopped. An organized reporting procedure could help detect signs of new issues on a local and national level and enable a methodical approach to solving them. To address the harm produced by algorithms, a framework of laws, regulations, and cultural norms should be established. The framework ought to promote cooperation, quality enhancement and transparency.

2.4 Privacy and Confidentiality

The implications of privacy and confidentiality in AI-driven healthcare are profound. Addressing these concerns through robust security measures, ethical data practices, regulatory compliance, and patient-centred approaches is crucial to harness the full potential of AI while protecting patient interests. Anonymizing patient data can help protect privacy while still allowing AI systems to learn and improve. However, complete anonymization is challenging and may sometimes be reversible, posing risks to confidentiality. Developing effective anonymization techniques and regularly reviewing their efficacy are critical steps in protecting patient privacy. Confidentiality breaches can have far-reaching consequences beyond loss of trust. They can lead to identity theft, discrimination, and psychological distress for patients. Ensuring the privacy and confidentiality of patient data is not just a legal requirement but a moral imperative to prevent harm and promote positive healthcare outcomes.

2.5 Need for Human-AI Collaboration

Human-AI collaboration in clinical decision-making refers to the integration of artificial intelligence systems with healthcare professionals to enhance decision-making processes. This collaboration can significantly improve diagnosis accuracy, treatment planning, patient management, and the overall efficiency of AI integrated health care systems.

Enhanced Diagnosis and Early Detection

AI algorithms can be used to analyse medical images (e.g., X-rays, MRIs) and identify abnormalities with high precision. These AI findings can be validated by Healthcare providers to reduce diagnostic errors and help in early detection of diseases like cancer, stroke, and cardiovascular conditions. Example: AI-powered radiology systems detect lung nodules in CT scans, which radiologists may miss.

Personalized Treatment Plans

AI models can analyze patient data, including medical history, genetics, and lifestyle, to recommend personalized treatment options. Clinicians use AI insights to choose the most effective therapies, reducing trial-and-error approaches.Example: Oncology AI tools suggest personalized cancer treatments based on genomic analysis.

Predictive Analytics and Risk Assessment

AI can predict patient deterioration using real-time data from wearable devices and electronic health records (EHRs). Physicians can intervene early, preventing adverse outcomes. Example: AI monitors ICU patients for signs of sepsis or cardiac arrest.

Decision Support Systems

Clinical decision support systems (CDSS) using AI can be used to provide evidence-based recommendations to the patients during consultations. At the same time Doctors should retain the authority over final decisions. For example, CDSS assists in antibiotic prescription by analysing microbial resistance patterns.

Reduced Cognitive Load

AI can be used to automate routine tasks like medical documentation, image analysis, and data processing. Clinicians can focus on patient interaction and complex decision-making. Example: AI transcription tools document patient consultations in real time.

Ethical and Explainable AI (XAI)

With the help of Explainable AI systems, clinicians can understand the reasoning behind recommendations provided by the healthcare systems. This can help in trustable collaboration with human and AI systems. For example, AI tools can identify abnormalities in medical images and provide visual overlays on them to explain it.

2.6 Importance of Human intervention in AI integrated health care systems

Human oversight and intervention are crucial in AI-driven healthcare to ensure ethical, accurate, and patient-centered care. Some of the aspects of human involvement for AI integration in healthcare are presented below:

Ensuring Accuracy and Reliability:

AI systems require human experts to monitor and interpret their outputs, ensuring decisions are transparent and explainable.

Ethical Decision-Making:

Human oversight is essential in maintaining ethical standards and regulatory compliance in AI applications within healthcare.

Managing AI Limitations and Bias:

Human clinicians play a vital role in identifying and mitigating biases in AI systems, ensuring equitable patient care.

Providing Contextual Understanding:

Healthcare professionals' judgment is crucial in interpreting AI-generated insights within complex medical scenarios.

Continuous Learning and Improvement:

Human feedback is vital for refining AI algorithms, contributing to their continuous improvement.

Accountability and Liability:

Human oversight ensures accountability in AI-driven healthcare, addressing challenges in assigning responsibility for AI decisions.

3. LEGAL ISSUES AND REGULATORY COMPLIANCE

Large volumes of patient data are necessary for AI systems in healthcare to operate efficiently. The security and privacy of sensitive health information are called into question by this. Laws must take into account AI systems' explainability and transparency. In order to trust and employ AI technology effectively, patients and healthcare practitioners should be aware of how these systems arrive at their judgments. Healthcare AI regulation has been outlined by the World Health Organization (WHO). They are as follows: 1. safeguarding individuality; 2. encouraging security; 3. guaranteeing openness 4. Developing accountability 5. Ensuring fairness 6. Encouraging AI that is sustainable.

3.1 Data Protection Laws

The use of AI in healthcare involves handling vast amounts of sensitive patient data. Compliance with data protection laws is crucial. These regulations mandate strict guidelines on data collection, storage, and sharing to protect patient privacy and confidentiality. Health Insurance Portability and Accountability Act (HIPAA): In the United States, AI systems must comply with HIPAA regulations, which set standards for protecting sensitive patient data. Non-compliance can result in significant penalties. The General Data Protection Regulation (GDPR) is a set of stringent regulations governing the protection of data in the European Union. Among its many provisions are patient permission for data processing and the right to view and remove personal information. The General Data Protection Regulation (GDPR) also outlines the guidelines and practices that must be followed when processing data for scientific research. These guidelines include using appropriate security measures, like pseudonymizing the data that is used. In India, Personal Data Protection Bill (PDPB) aims provide a comprehensive data protection framework. It will regulate the processing of personal data, including health data, and impose obligations on data processors to ensure data security and privacy. Information Technology (IT) Act, 2000 provides the legal framework for electronic governance and cybersecurity, including provisions relevant to the handling of sensitive personal data. ***Artificial Intelligence Act***: The EU has been proactive in creating comprehensive AI regulations: Proposed in April 2021, this act classifies AI systems by risk levels as unacceptable, high, limited, minimal

AI systems will be evaluated by the appropriate authorities and Watchdogs. AI that is both universal and risk. Risk categories as outlined in the AI Act

(i) Unacceptable risk: AI systems that are considered to be cognitive, behaviorally manipulative, socially scoring, or facial recognition, for example, will not be permitted.
(ii) High risk: This group includes AI systems that have a detrimental impact on people's safety and fundamental rights.

High risk AI systems are those that are used in products that are subject to European Union product safety legislation, such as toys, cars, airplanes, medical devices, lifts, and other products. They also include AI systems that fall into specific categories and must be registered in an EU database, such as education, critical infrastructure, law enforcement, etc. Before and during their lives, all of these creative

From a Legal Perspective, there ought to be measures in place to guarantee that patient privacy rights are respected when data is processed for AI model training. These measures should include obtaining appropriate consent from data subjects where necessary and putting in place suitable safeguards.

3.2 Liability and Accountability

Determining liability in cases where AI systems cause harm or errors is complex. Legal frameworks must address the question of whether developers, healthcare providers, or institutions using the AI technology are responsible. The Consumer Protection Act, 2019, and other liability laws may apply in cases where patients suffer harm due to AI-based treatments or diagnoses. These legal issues highlight the need for robust and adaptive legal frameworks to ensure the safe and ethical use of AI in healthcare. In India, the integration of AI in healthcare is evolving, and legal considerations are crucial to ensure the ethical, safe, and effective use of AI technologies.

AI systems used in healthcare must often go through rigorous testing and approval processes before being deployed. Ensuring compliance with these regulatory bodies is essential for the legal use of AI in healthcare.

3.3 Regulations for AI-based Medical Devices

In the US, the Food and Drug Administration (FDA) has developed frameworks for the evaluation of AI/ML-based medical devices. Similarly, the European Medicines Agency (EMA) oversees the regulation of AI in healthcare in Europe. Central Drugs Standard Control Organization (CDSCO) operates under the Ministry of Health and Family Welfare, Government of India. It oversees the regulation of medical devices, including software and AI-based products. The mission of the CDSCO is to guarantee the efficacy, safety, and quality of medical products that are produced, imported, and disseminated inside the nation by promoting transparency, accountability, and uniformity in its services. AI-based medical devices and technologies need to comply with regulations set by CDSCO. The approval process ensures that these technologies meet safety and efficacy standards before they are deployed in healthcare settings. Medical Council of India (MCI) later replaced by National Medical Council (NMC) frames guidelines and regulations that must be adhered to by healthcare providers using AI, ensuring that AI integration does not compromise medical ethics or patient care standards. Australia's regulatory initiatives involve the Therapeutic Goods Administration (TGA), which oversees the use of AI in medical instruments to guarantee adherence to safety and performance criteria. Ethical guidelines for AI established by the government to shape the ethical progress and application of AI, especially in healthcare. In China, NMPA (National Medical Products Administration) Classifies AI software under medical devices if they affect clinical decisions. In Japan, AI-based devices go through a rigorous evaluation for efficacy and risk by Pharmaceuticals and Medical Devices Agency (PMDA), Ministry of Health, Labour and Welfare (MHLW).

3.4 Regulatory Approval and Compliance

Regulatory compliance for AI systems in healthcare varies globally, with each country implementing frameworks to ensure safety, efficacy, and ethical use. A summary of key regulations across various jurisdictions in presented in the Table 1.

Table 1. Regulatory Body and Framework Globally

Country/ Region	Regulatory Body & Framework	Description
United States	**Food and Drug Administration (FDA) Health Insurance Portability and Accountability Act (HIPAA)**	The FDA oversees the approval of AI-based medical devices, ensuring their safety and effectiveness. HIPAA establishes privacy and security standards for protected health information, relevant to AI systems handling such data.
European Union	**European Medicines Agency (EMA) EU Artificial Intelligence Act**	The EMA requires AI-based medical devices to obtain CE marking, indicating compliance with EU regulations. The EU AI Act, effective August 2024, classifies AI systems based on risk levels, imposing requirements for high-risk applications, including transparency, accountability, and data governance.
Canada	**Health CanadaArtificial Intelligence and Data Act (AIDA)**	Health Canada's Digital Health Division manages AI/ML-enabled devices, with draft guidance published in 2023. The proposed AIDA aims to regulate AI systems, focusing on safeguarding against harm and placing responsibility on organizations deploying such systems.
United Kingdom	**Medicines and Healthcare products Regulatory Agency (MHRA)**	The MHRA oversees AI as a medical device (AIaMD) under the UK Medical Device Regulations 2002. The UK is reforming its regulatory framework to incorporate AI/ML-enabled devices, emphasizing principles like transparency, explainability, fairness, accountability, and governance.

continued on following page

Table 1. Continued

Country/ Region	Regulatory Body & Framework	Description
China	**National Medical Products Administration (NMPA)**	The NMPA has issued guidelines for AI-aided software, focusing on data quality, algorithm validation, and clinical risk assessment. In 2021, it released guidelines for the classification and definition of AI-based software as a medical device, addressing safety, effectiveness, and clinical decision support.
Brazil	**Agência Nacional de Vigilância Sanitária (ANVISA)Brazilian Legal Framework for AI**	ANVISA regulates medical devices, including AI applications. In 2021, Brazil approved the Legal Framework for AI, focusing on the development of AI solutions. A draft AI law in 2022 classifies health applications as high-risk AI systems, requiring public risk assessments and periodic algorithmic impact assessments, emphasizing individual rights such as privacy and non-discrimination.
India	**Central Drugs Standard Control Organization (CDSCO)**	The CDSCO oversees the approval of medical devices, including AI technologies. AI radiology devices require an Import License for imported products or a Registration Certificate for locally manufactured devices.
Australia	**Therapeutic Goods Administration (TGA)**	The TGA regulates medical devices, including AI applications, requiring them to be listed on the Australian Register of Therapeutic Goods (ARTG) to ensure compliance with safety and efficacy standards.
Japan	**Pharmaceuticals and Medical Devices Agency (PMDA)**	The PMDA supervises the approval and marketing authorization for medical devices, including AI technologies, ensuring they meet safety and performance standards before market entry.
South Korea	**Ministry of Food and Drug Safety (MFDS)**	The MFDS evaluates and approves medical devices, including those utilizing AI, focusing on safety, effectiveness, and quality standards to protect public health.
Singapore	**Health Sciences Authority (HSA)**	The HSA regulates medical devices, including AI applications in radiology, requiring registration and approval to ensure they meet safety and efficacy standards before being marketed.

It's important to note that regulatory frameworks for AI in healthcare are continually evolving to keep pace with technological advancements. Stakeholders should stay informed about the latest regulations and guidelines in their respective jurisdictions to ensure compliance and promote the safe and effective use of AI in healthcare.All these regulatory efforts reflect a global recognition of the need to balance the benefits of AI in healthcare with the importance of ensuring safety, ethics, and fairness in its use.

3.5 International collaborations Frameworks for AI use in Healthcare

International collaborations in artificial intelligence (AI) are pivotal in advancing healthcare globally. Several initiatives exemplify these efforts:

- AI Global Healthcare Initiative (AIGHI): AIGHI (AI Global Healthcare Initiative, n.d.) unites healthcare regulators, pharmaceutical companies, medical device manufacturers, and frontline healthcare providers to harness AI for revolutionizing patient care and medical innovation.
- Global Initiative on AI for Health (World Health Organization, International Telecommunication Union, & World Intellectual Property Organization, n.d.): Led by WHO, the International Telecommunication Union (ITU), and the World Intellectual Property Organization (WIPO), this initiative fosters collaboration to harness AI in improving health outcomes.
- Health AI Partnership (Health AI Partnership, n.d.): This organization empowers healthcare professionals to use AI effectively, safely, and equitably through community-informed best practices, enhancing the integration of AI in healthcare settings.
- FUTURE-AI Guidelines (FUTURE-AI Consortium, n.d.): An international consensus framework developed by a consortium of experts from 51 countries, providing guiding principles and best practices for trustworthy AI in healthcare, covering aspects from design to deployment
- AI Research and Industry Collaborations: Countries like the United Kingdom and Canada have established robust international AI research networks, fostering collaborations that enhance the global AI research landscape. Companies such as DeepMind and BioNTech (DeepMind & BioNTech, 2023) are collaborating to develop AI lab assistants aimed at enhancing scientific research, exemplifying industry efforts to integrate AI into healthcare research.

These collaborations underscore the global commitment to integrating AI into healthcare, aiming to improve patient outcomes, streamline medical processes, and uphold ethical standards in AI deployment.

4. RECOMMENDATIONS FOR CLINICIANS, RESEARCHER AND POLICY MAKERS

4.1 Recommendations for Clinicians and Researchers

For researchers and clinicians looking to effectively implement AI in healthcare, here are some key recommendations:

Adherence to Reporting Standards: Updated frameworks such as TRIPOD+AI, which provides guidelines for transparent and complete reporting of clinical prediction models developed using AI and machine learning are to be utilized. This ensures the accuracy and transparency necessary for evaluating and implementing these models in clinical settings(Australian Institute of Digital Health, 2023) .

Safety and Ethics: Establish robust risk-based safety frameworks and ethical guidelines to ensure that AI applications in healthcare are safe and do not harm patients. Post implementation monitoring and accreditation of healthcare organizations to meet AI safety and quality standards(Australian Institute of Digital Health, 2023) .

Workforce Training and Development: Address knowledge gaps by training the current and future healthcare workforce in AI use. Developing a shared code of conduct for the responsible use of AI can help maintain high standards of practice (Australian Institute of Digital Health, 2023) .

Consumer Engagement and Education: Implement programs to increase digital health literacy among the public, ensuring they understand the benefits and risks of AI in healthcare. Engaging with communities, especially vulnerable groups, to develop culturally safe AI practices is crucial.

Regulation and Coordination: Create entities like a National AI in Healthcare Council to coordinate activities and responsibilities related to AI oversight. This ensures that there are no regulatory gaps and that AI technologies are effectively integrated into healthcare system.

These recommendations collectively aim to create a safe, ethical, and effective AI-enabled healthcare system, benefiting both providers and patients while fostering trust and transparency in AI technologies. The use of AI in healthcare holds great promise for improving patient outcomes, increasing efficiency, and reducing costs. For policymakers, it is crucial to establish frameworks that ensure the ethical, safe, and effective integration of AI technologies. Here are some key recommendations:

4.2 Recommendations for Policy Makers

Establish Clear Regulatory Frameworks

- **Safety and Efficacy Standards**: Implement rigorous testing and validation protocols for AI systems to ensure they are safe and effective.
- **Approval Processes**: Develop streamlined processes for the approval and continuous monitoring of AI applications in healthcare(Jiang et al., 2017) .

Ensure Data Privacy and Security

- **Data Protection Laws**: Strengthen data protection laws to safeguard patient information and ensure compliance with regulations like GDPR and HIPAA(Reddy et al., 2019).
- **Secure Data Sharing**: Promote secure data sharing practices among healthcare providers, researchers, and AI developers(He et al., 2019) .

Promote Transparency and Explainability

- **Algorithmic Transparency**: Mandate that AI developers provide clear explanations of how their algorithms work, particularly in critical decision-making scenarios.
- **Explainability Requirements**: Ensure that AI systems can provide understandable justifications for their decisions to both healthcare professionals and patients.

Support Workforce Training and Education

- **Professional Development**: Invest in training programs for healthcare professionals to understand and effectively use AI tools.
- **Curriculum Integration**: Incorporate AI and data science into medical and healthcare-related educational curriculums.

Foster Innovation and Collaboration

- **Public-Private Partnerships**: Encourage collaborations between government, industry, and academia to drive innovation and share best practices.
- **Funding and Grants**: Provide funding and grants to support AI research and development in healthcare.

Monitor and Address Ethical Considerations

- **Bias and Fairness**: Implement guidelines to identify and mitigate biases in AI systems to ensure fair treatment of all patient groups.
- **Ethical Standards**: Establish ethical standards and review boards to oversee the development and deployment of AI in healthcare.

Enhance Interoperability

- **Standardization**: Promote the development and adoption of standardized data formats and protocols to ensure interoperability between different AI systems and healthcare platforms.
- **Integration Support**: Provide technical support to healthcare institutions to integrate AI tools into their existing workflows.

Evaluate and Update Policies Regularly

- **Continuous Monitoring**: Set up mechanisms for the continuous monitoring and evaluation of AI applications in healthcare.
- **Policy Updates**: Regularly update policies to reflect technological advancements and emerging challenges.

Encourage Patient Engagement and Education

- **Patient Involvement**: Engage patients in the development and evaluation of AI tools to ensure they meet patient needs and preferences.
- **Educational Campaigns**: Conduct educational campaigns to inform patients about the benefits and risks of AI in healthcare.

Prepare for Liability and Accountability Issues

- **Liability Frameworks**: Develop clear liability frameworks to address potential issues arising from AI errors or malfunctions.
- **Accountability Mechanisms**: Ensure that there are accountability mechanisms in place for both AI developers and healthcare providers.

By implementing these recommendations, policymakers can help maximize the benefits of AI in healthcare while addressing potential risks and challenges.

5. CASE STUDIES AND REAL WORLD APPLICATIONS OF AI IN HEALTHCARE

5.1. Radiology and Imaging

Case Study 1: Stanford University - AI in Pneumonia Detection

Researchers at Stanford University developed an AI algorithm called CheXNet[1], which can detect pneumonia from chest X-rays with performance comparable to radiologists.

Problem Statement: Create a system for remotely monitoring patients' health with IoT devices to detect abnormalities and give prompt medical intervention.
Methodology: A chest X-ray image is fed into CheXNet, a 121-layer convolutional neural network, which returns a heatmap indicating the regions of the image most suggestive of pneumonia coupled with the probability of pneumonia.
Dataset: CheXNet on the newly published ChestX-ray14 dataset—112,120 frontal-view chest X-ray pictures, each uniquely classified with a maximum of 14 distinct thoracic illnesses, including pneumonia.
Techniques Used: Deep learning technique CNN, real-time data analytics, and Natural Language Processing.
Results: CheXNet is extended to detect all 14 diseases in ChestX-ray14 and achieve state of the art results on all 14 diseases.
Conclusion: Expert-level automation with this technology can enhance the delivery of healthcare and provide access to medical imaging knowledge in regions of the world with limited availability of qualified radiologists.

This AI system can assist radiologists in diagnosing pneumonia more quickly and accurately, reducing the workload and improving patient outcomes.

5.2. Drug Discovery and Development

Case Study 2:Insilico Medicine and AI in Drug Discovery

Insilico Medicine, an AI-driven biotechnology company (Insilico Medicine, 2020), used AI to discover a novel drug candidate for treating fibrosis. Their AI platform analyzes vast amounts of biological and chemical data to predict the effectiveness of potential drug molecules Deep learning is used in healthcare IoT to speed up the medication research and development procedures. Deep learning algorithms may find novel drug candidates and forecast their effectiveness and safety profiles by examining large volumes of molecular data, such as genomes, proteomics, and chemical structures. This technique speeds up the drug research pipeline and minimizes the time and expense of bringing new treatments to market. Furthermore, deep learning models may be used to repurpose current medications for new therapeutic indications, increasing therapy choices for a variety of disorders.

Problem Statement: Use deep learning algorithms to identify possible drug candidates and forecast their effectiveness and safety characteristics, which will help to accelerate the drug discovery process.

Methodology: Collect molecular data (such as genomics, proteomics, and chemical structures). Deep learning methods, such as deep neural networks (DNNs) and generative adversarial networks (GANs), can be used to predict chemical properties and perform virtual screening. Validate projected drug candidates by conducting in vitro and in vivo tests.

Dataset: Molecular data includes genetics, proteomics, chemical structures, and existing drug databases.

Techniques Used: Deep learning methods (DNNs, GANs), chemical property prediction, and virtual screening.

Results: The drug discovery process is accelerated, innovative drug candidates are identified, and drug development time and expense are decreased.

Conclusion: Deep learning speeds drug discovery by predicting chemical attributes and finding possible drug candidates, allowing for speedier development of novel drugs.

5.3. Personalized Treatment Plans

Case Study 3: IBM Watson for Oncology Treatment Recommendations

IBM Watson (Somashekhar et al., 2018), a cognitive computing system developed by IBM, was designed to assist in various fields, including healthcare. One of its prominent applications was in oncology, where it was used to recommend treatment options for cancer patients. The system, known as IBM Watson for Oncology, aimed to assist oncologists by providing evidence-based treatment options, thereby improving decision-making processes and patient outcomes.

Problem Statement

IBM Watson became well-known following its triumph on the 2011 season of the game show "Jeopardy!" IBM then started looking into how Watson's cognitive abilities could be used in different industries, with healthcare being the main area of interest. One of the top cancer treatment and research facilities in the world,

Memorial Sloan Kettering Cancer Center (MSKCC), collaborated with Watson for Oncology's development.

Methodology

Watson for Oncology could integrate various types of data, including electronic health records (EHRs), clinical guidelines, and research papers. The system provided treatment options based on the latest clinical evidence, including chemotherapy, targeted therapy, immunotherapy, and clinical trials. Recommendations were tailored to individual patients based on their medical history, genetic makeup, and other relevant factors.

Techniques Used

Watson for Oncology leveraged natural language processing (NLP), machine learning, and large datasets of medical literature, clinical trials, and treatment guidelines to analyze patient data and recommend treatment options.

Results

The system could process vast amounts of information quickly and provide oncologists with a list of possible treatment options ranked by their relevance and supported by the latest evidence.

Conclusion

Watson for Oncology was implemented in several hospitals and healthcare institutions worldwide. The outcomes of implementing Watson for Oncology varied. While some institutions reported positive experiences, others encountered issues with the system's recommendations and its integration into clinical practice. As a result, the overall impact of Watson for Oncology on cancer treatment remains a topic of debate.

5.4 AI for Early Diagnosis of Diseases

Case Study 4: Google Health and DeepMind's AI for Eye Disease Diagnosis

Problem Statement: Google Health partnered with DeepMind (Google Health, 2020) to develop AI algorithms capable of diagnosing eye diseases, specifically diabetic retinopathy and age-related macular degeneration, from retinal scans. This

AI model can analyze retinal images and detect early signs of these conditions more accurately than some human specialists.

Results: The AI system demonstrated the ability to match or outperform experienced ophthalmologists in terms of diagnostic accuracy. It provides faster and more affordable screening, especially in areas with limited access to specialized care.

Conclusion: Improved early detection and timely interventions, potentially reducing the incidence of blindness due to these conditions.

5.5 AI in Remote Monitoring and Chronic Disease Management

Case Study 5: Livongo and AI for Diabetes Management

Problem Statement: Livongo, now part of Teladoc Health (Livongo, 2020), integrates AI with wearable devices to provide personalized diabetes management. The system uses data from glucose monitors, activity trackers, and other inputs to offer real-time insights and recommendations on managing blood sugar levels.

Results: By combining AI algorithms with continuous glucose monitoring, Livongo can alert patients when their glucose levels are out of range and provide actionable advice to prevent spikes or drops.

Conclusion: Improved diabetes control, reduced healthcare costs by preventing complications, and enhanced patient engagement through real-time monitoring.

5.6 AI in Mental Health Care

Case Study 6: Woebot Health and AI for Mental Health

Problem Statement: Woebot Health (Woebot Health, 2020) developed a chatbot that uses AI to deliver cognitive-behavioral therapy (CBT) to individuals struggling with mental health issues such as anxiety and depression. The AI-powered chatbot interacts with users through text conversations, providing therapeutic exercises and emotional support.

Results: Studies have shown that users report improved mental health outcomes after interacting with Woebot, and the service has been scaled to provide accessible mental health support to a large number of individuals.

Conclusion: Increased access to mental health care, especially in underserved areas, and a more affordable alternative to traditional therapy.

5.7 Other Applications of AI in Healthcare

AI in Dermatology Google Health - Skin Cancer Detection

Google Health (Esteva et al., 2017) developed a deep learning algorithm capable of identifying skin cancer from images with high accuracy, comparable to dermatologists. This AI tool can assist in early detection of skin cancer, leading to timely treatment and improved survival rates.

Natural Language Processing (NLP) in Electronic Health Records (EHRs) Mayo Clinic - AI for EHR Data E6.xtraction

The Mayo Clinic (Sohn et al., 2019 uses NLP to extract meaningful information from unstructured EHR data, improving clinical documentation and patient care. This approach enhances the accuracy of patient records and supports better decision-making by clinicians.

Robotic Surgery

AI-driven robotic systems assist surgeons in performing precise and minimally invasive surgeries, reducing recovery times and improving surgical outcomes.The da Vinci Surgical System(Goh et al., 2020) uses AI to enhance the precision of surgical instruments, allowing for complex procedures with greater accuracy.

Population Health Management

AI analyses large datasets to identify public health trends, manage population health, and develop strategies to address health disparities (Obermeyer et al., 2019) . AI tools help identify areas with high disease prevalence, enabling targeted public health interventions.

Administrative Workflow Optimization

AI automates routine administrative tasks (Davenport & Kalakota, 2019), such as billing, coding, and appointment scheduling, improving efficiency and reducing administrative burdens. AI systems streamline the processing of insurance claims and patient billing, reducing errors and costs. Penn Medicine(Golas et al., 2018) developed an AI system that predicts which patients are at high risk of hospital readmission within 30 days of discharge. This predictive model allows healthcare providers to implement targeted interventions, reducing readmission rates and associated healthcare costs.

Other Applications

Along with state governments in India, Google, Microsoft, and IBM have numerous agreements with private hospital groups including Narayana, Apollo, and Fortis. These are developing a variety of solutions, such as AI systems for remote area AI service delivery, illness detection and prediction, and hospital administration (Sinha, 2018).

As part of the Forus-Microsoft DR screening agreement, a device developed by Forus uploads an image of the patient to the cloud, where an algorithm checks it for DR and returns the results to the device or the physician (Singh, 2020).

AI techniques are also being used by platforms like OnliDoc and Lybrate to offer remote diagnostics and virtual help. AI is used by OnliDoc to check symptoms and choose treatments (Misal, 2018).

For instance, SigTuple uses the AI platform Manthana to digitize samples of blood, urine, and semen in addition to automating the interpretation of blood smears (ET Rise, 2018).

Forus Health created 3nethra, a portable screening tool for common eye conditions. When working at eye check-up camps in rural places with zero or inconsistent cloud connectivity, operators of 3nethra devices can access AI-powered insights by integrating AI capabilities into the device through Microsoft's retinal imaging APIs.

Specifically, IDx-DR(Ting et al., 2017), developed by diagnostic AI firm IDx, examines retinal pictures to determine whether a diabetic has a diabetic retinopathy problem.

Philips Healthcare is also working on launching its IntelliSite Pathology Solution in the field of digital pathology diagnosis, as well as developing the open platform IntelliSpace Discovery for AI development and deployment (Shortliffe & Sepúlveda, 2018) .

6. CONCLUSION

Artificial intelligence (AI) technologies are being experimented with or utilized in healthcare and research for tasks like disease diagnosis, managing chronic conditions, delivering health services, and developing drugs. AI technologies could help with major health problems, but their effectiveness may be limited by the quality of current health data and AI's inability to show empathy like humans. The use of AI raises many ethical and societal issues, some of which are also raised using data and healthcare technologies in general. Ensuring that AI is developed and implemented transparently and ethically will pose a significant challenge for governing AI technologies in the future.

REFERENCES

Ahmed, I., Ahmad, A., & Jeon, G. (2021). An IoT-based deep learning framework for early assessment of COVID-19. *IEEE Internet of Things Journal*, *8*(21), 15855–15862. DOI: 10.1109/JIOT.2020.3034074 PMID: 35782174

AI Global Healthcare Initiative. (n.d.). *AI Global Healthcare Initiative: Revolutionizing patient care and medical innovation*. AI Global Healthcare Initiative. Retrieved March 25, 2025, from https://healthcareproducts.org/ai/aighi

Amin, S. U., & Hossain, M. S. (2021). Edge intelligence and Internet of Things in healthcare: A survey. *IEEE Access : Practical Innovations, Open Solutions*, *9*, 45–59. DOI: 10.1109/ACCESS.2020.3045115

An IoT-based heart healthcare platform for the Sultanate of Oman. (2022, October 27). IEEE Conference Publication. https://doi.org/DOI: 10.1109/MAJICC56935.2022.9994183

Arisdakessian, S., Wahab, O. A., Mourad, A., Otrok, H., & Guizani, M. (2023). A survey on IoT intrusion detection: Federated learning, game theory, social psychology, and explainable AI as future directions. *IEEE Internet of Things Journal*, *10*(5), 4059–4092. DOI: 10.1109/JIOT.2022.3203249

Australian Institute of Digital Health. (2023). Roadmap recommendations for safe, ethical, sustainable, and personalised AI in healthcare.

Brundage, M., ... (2018). The malicious use of artificial intelligence. *arXiv preprint arXiv:1802.07228*. https://arxiv.org/abs/1802.07228

Chin, M. H., Afsar-Manesh, N., & Bierman, A. S.. (2023). Guiding principles to address the impact of algorithm bias on racial and ethnic disparities in health and health care. *JAMA Network Open*, *6*(12), e2345050. DOI: 10.1001/jamanetworkopen.2023.45050 PMID: 38100101

Chin, M. H., Afsar-Manesh, N., & Bierman, A. S.. (2023). Guiding principles to address the impact of algorithm bias on racial and ethnic disparities in health and health care. *JAMA Network Open*, *6*(12), e2345050. DOI: 10.1001/jamanetworkopen.2023.45050 PMID: 38100101

Davenport, T., & Kalakota, R. (2019). The potential for artificial intelligence in healthcare. *Future Healthcare Journal*, *6*(2), 94–98. PMID: 31363513

DeepMind & BioNTech. (2023). Collaborating to develop AI lab assistants for healthcare research. DeepMind & BioNTech. Retrieved March 25, 2025, from https://www.deepmind.com/healthcare

Esteva, A.. (2017). Dermatologist-Level Classification of Skin Cancer with Deep Neural Networks. *Nature*.

FUTURE-AI Consortium. (n.d.). *FUTURE-AI Guidelines: Best practices for trustworthy AI in healthcare*. FUTURE-AI Consortium. Retrieved March 25, 2025, from https://www.futureaiguidelines.org

Goh, A. C.. (2020). Early experience with the da Vinci single-port robotic system in urology. *Journal of Endourology*, *34*(1), 75–81. PMID: 31895594

Golas, S. B., et al. (2018). "Feasibility of Utilizing Real-Time Electronic Health Record Data to Predict Risk of 30-Day Hospital Readmissions Among Medicare Patients." Journal of Medical Internet Research.

Google Health. (2020). *AI for eye disease diagnosis: DeepMind's revolutionary work in diabetic retinopathy*. Google. https://health.google.com/ai

Hayyolalam, V., Aloqaily, M., Ozkasap, O., & Guizani, M. (2022). Edge-assisted solutions for IoT-based connected healthcare systems: A literature review. *IEEE Internet of Things Journal*, *9*(12), 9419–9443. DOI: 10.1109/JIOT.2021.3135200

He, J., Baxter, S. L., Xu, J., Xu, J., Zhou, X., & Zhang, K. (2019). The practical implementation of artificial intelligence technologies in medicine. *Nature Medicine*, *25*(1), 30–36. DOI: 10.1038/s41591-018-0307-0 PMID: 30617336

Health, A. I. Partnership. (n.d.). *Empowering healthcare professionals to use AI effectively and equitably*. Health AI Partnership. Retrieved March 25, 2025, from https://www.healthaipartnership.org

Inkster, B., Sarda, S., & Subramanian, V. (2018). Machine learning and mental health: A systematic review of algorithms and applications. *Psychological Medicine*, *48*(9), 1426–1448. DOI: 10.1017/S0033291718000932

Insilico Medicine. (2020). *AI-driven drug discovery: How AI accelerated the development of a fibrosis drug*. Insilico Medicine. https://www.insilico.com/ai-drug-discovery

Jiang, F., Jiang, Y., Zhi, H., Dong, Y., Li, H., Ma, S., & Wang, Y. (2017). Artificial intelligence in healthcare: Past, present, and future. *Stroke and Vascular Neurology*, *2*(4), 230–243. DOI: 10.1136/svn-2017-000101 PMID: 29507784

Keesara, S., Jonas, A., & Schulman, K. (2020). COVID-19 and health care's digital revolution. *The New England Journal of Medicine, 382*(23), e82. DOI: 10.1056/NEJMp2005835 PMID: 32240581

Kolachalama, V. B., & Garg, P. S. (2018). Machine learning and medical education. *NPJ Digital Medicine, 1*(1), 54. DOI: 10.1038/s41746-018-0061-1 PMID: 31304333

Livongo. (2020). *AI in chronic disease management: Revolutionizing diabetes care with real-time monitoring*. Livongo Health. https://www.livongo.com

Luxton, D. D. (2014). Recommendations for the ethical use and design of artificial intelligent care providers. *Artificial Intelligence in Medicine, 62*(1), 1–10. DOI: 10.1016/j.artmed.2014.06.004 PMID: 25059820

Obermeyer, Z.. (2019). Dissecting racial bias in an algorithm used to manage the health of populations. *Science, 366*(6464), 447–453. PMID: 31649194

Rajpurkar, P.. (2017). "CheXNet: Radiologist-Level Pneumonia Detection on Chest X-Rays with Deep Learning." arXiv:1711.05225.

Rajpurkar, P., Irvin, J., Zhu, K., Yang, B., Mehta, H., Duan, T., Ding, D., Bagul, A., Langlotz, C., Shpanskaya, K., Lungren, M. P., & Ng, A. Y. (2017). *CheXNet: Radiologist-level pneumonia detection on chest X-rays with deep learning* (arXiv:1711.05225). arXiv. https://arxiv.org/abs/1711.05225

Reddy, S., Fox, J., & Purohit, M. P. (2019). Artificial intelligence-enabled healthcare delivery. *Journal of the Royal Society of Medicine, 112*(1), 22–28. DOI: 10.1177/0141076818815510 PMID: 30507284

Sakib, S., Miah, M. A. S., & Acharjee, U. K.. (2022). Deep learning models for magnetic cardiography edge sensors implementing noise processing and diagnostics. *IEEE Access : Practical Innovations, Open Solutions, 10*, 2656–2668. DOI: 10.1109/ACCESS.2021.3138976

Shortliffe, E. H., & Sepúlveda, M. J. (2018). Clinical decision support in the era of artificial intelligence. *Journal of the American Medical Association, 320*(21), 2199–2200. DOI: 10.1001/jama.2018.17163 PMID: 30398550

Singal, V., & Tomar, S. (2022). Patient data: Solving ownership question. *Pharmaceutical Commerce, 17*(6).

Smart healthcare in IoT using convolutional based cyber physical system. (2022, October 16). IEEE Conference Publication. https://doi.org/DOI: 10.1109/MysuruCon55714.2022.9972679

Sohn, S.. (2019). A Hybrid Approach to Automatic De-identification of Electronic Medical Records. *Journal of the American Medical Informatics Association : JAMIA*.

Somashekhar, S. P.. (2018). Implementation of IBM Watson for Oncology in a Multispecialty Hospital in India: A Prospective, Multicenter, Observational Study. *Journal of Clinical Oncology*.

Steinhubl, S. R., Muse, E. D., & Topol, E. J. (2015). The emerging field of mobile health: Research methods, issues, and challenges. *Health Affairs*, *34*(5), 924–930. DOI: 10.1377/hlthaff.2015.0010

Sun, T. Q., & Medaglia, R. (2019). Mapping the challenges of artificial intelligence in the public sector: Evidence from public healthcare. *Government Information Quarterly*, *36*(2), 368–383. DOI: 10.1016/j.giq.2018.09.008

Ting, D. S., Liu, Y., Burlina, P., Xu, X., Bressler, N. M., & Wong, T. Y. (2018). AI for medical imaging goes deep. *Nature Medicine*, *24*, 539–540. DOI: 10.1038/s41591-018-0029-3 PMID: 29736024

Ting, D. S. W., Cheung, C. Y. Y., & Lim, G.. (2017). Development and validation of a deep learning system for diabetic retinopathy and related eye diseases using retinal images from multiethnic populations with diabetes. *Journal of the American Medical Association*, *318*(22), 2211–2223. DOI: 10.1001/jama.2017.18152 PMID: 29234807

Topol, E. J. (2019). High-performance medicine: The convergence of human and artificial intelligence. *Nature Medicine*, *25*(1), 44–56. DOI: 10.1038/s41591-018-0300-7 PMID: 30617339

Woebot Health. (2020). *AI in mental health: How Woebot delivers cognitive-behavioral therapy through AI-powered chat*. Woebot Health. https://woebothealth.com

World Health Organization. International Telecommunication Union, & World Intellectual Property Organization. (n.d.). *Global Initiative on AI for Health: Improving health outcomes through AI*. WHO, ITU, & WIPO. Retrieved March 25, 2025, from https://www.who.int/news-room/fact-sheets/detail/ai-for-health

Wubineh, B. Z., Deriba, F. G., & Woldeyohannis, M. M. (2024). Exploring the opportunities and challenges of implementing artificial intelligence in healthcare: A systematic literature review. *Urologic Oncology: Seminars and Original Investigations*, *42*(3), 48–56. DOI: 10.1016/j.urolonc.2023.11.019 PMID: 38101991

Yang, G. Z., Cambias, J., & Cleary, K.. (2022). Medical robotics—Regulatory, ethical, and legal considerations for increasing levels of autonomy. *Science Robotics*, *7*(66), eabl9514. Advance online publication. DOI: 10.1126/scirobotics.abl9514 PMID: 33157870

Yuste, R.. (2017). Four ethical priorities for neurotechnologies and AI. *Nature*, *551*, 159. DOI: 10.1038/551159a PMID: 29120438

Zhavoronkov, A., Ivanenkov, Y. A., & Aliper, A.. (2019). Deep learning enables rapid identification of potent DDR1 kinase inhibitors. *Nature Biotechnology*, *37*(9), 1038–1040. DOI: 10.1038/s41587-019-0224-x PMID: 31477924

Chapter 11
Revolutionizing Health Management Through Federated Learning and AI

A. Arulmurugan
https://orcid.org/0000-0001-7267-2074
Vel Tech Rangarajan Dr. Sagunthala R&D Institute of Science and Technology, India

Dhinakaran Damodaran
https://orcid.org/0000-0002-3183-576X
Vel Tech Rangarajan Dr. Sagunthala R&D Institute of Science and Technology, India

J. Jeno Jasmine
https://orcid.org/0000-0003-1369-5895
Vel Tech Rangarajan Dr. Sagunthala R&D Institute of Science and Technology, India

S. Edwin Raja
https://orcid.org/0000-0002-2948-9669
Vel Tech Rangarajan Dr. Sagunthala R&D Institute of Science and Technology, India

A. Ramathilagam
https://orcid.org/0000-0002-2219-2870
P.S.R. Engineering College, Sivakasi, India

M. S. Girija
R.M.K. Engineering College, India

ABSTRACT

The integration of Artificial Intelligence (AI) and Internet of Things (IoT) technologies is transforming healthcare by enabling continuous, personalized health monitoring and proactive medical interventions. However, the sensitive nature of health data presents critical privacy and security challenges. This chapter explores the role of Federated Learning (FL) as a privacy-preserving machine learning paradigm that

DOI: 10.4018/979-8-3693-3864-3.ch011

enables collaborative model training across distributed healthcare data sources without compromising patient confidentiality. We examine the synergy between AI, IoT, and FL in applications such as chronic disease management, remote monitoring, and personalized treatment. Key privacy-enhancing techniques like differential privacy, homomorphic encryption, and secure aggregation are discussed alongside real-world use cases and FL architectures. The chapter also addresses infrastructure enablers including edge computing and 5G/6G connectivity, as well as the challenges of scalability, trust, and adversarial threats.

1. INTRODUCTION

Artificial Intelligence (AI) is a fairly recent occurrence in the healthcare industry, yet it has been an essential part of the business in recent years, serving as one of the factors in making the massive paradigm shift in how medical treatment used to be reactive and generalized to proactive, personalized, and data-driven. Medical workers are empowered to make faster and more accurate decisions that are evidence-based with the help of AI-based technologies, in particular, machine learning (ML), deep learning (DL), and natural language processing (NLP). The spectrum of uses of such applications is broad, consisting of uses in disease diagnosis, drug discovery, patient risk stratification, clinical workflow optimization, and population health management (Vizitiu et al., 2020). One of the most prominent areas of AI use is diagnostic support, in which algorithms trained on medical images, genomics data, or electronic health records (EHRs) may identify patterns and abnormalities that human clinicians can acknowledge with a certain delay. AI systems have demonstrated performance superior to or comparable to medical professionals in tasks such as the classification of skin lesions, detection of diabetic retinopathy, and radiographic interpretation. Lastly, there is an attempt to use predictive models to predict the course of chronic diseases such as diabetes, cardiovascular disease, and cancer, so that clinicians and patients can engage earlier and more productively to prevent the progression of the disease.

Outside the clinical sphere, AI is increasingly involved in the larger sphere of well-being and preventative health (Selva Kumar et al., 2025). The abundance of physiological and behavioral data is constantly produced by IoT-connected devices, including wearable fitness trackers, smartwatches, home health monitors, or other gadgets. AI algorithms process this data in real time to offer individual recommendations, identify deteriorating health at the early stages, and encourage healthy lifestyles. The apps have been found most useful in the management of aging populations, mental health promotion, and in assisting people with poor access to conventional health care services. Nevertheless, the deployment of AI in healthcare is not having an entirely smooth ride. One of the most serious issues is the gathering, storage, and utilization of personal sensitive health information (Liu et al., 2022). The conventional centralized AI models demand centralization of data on remote servers posing serious questions on privacy, security, and ethical concerns. As regulation and scrutiny intensify, and populations become more aware of data privacy, privacy-preserving AI methods become urgent, to ensure that the advantages of intelligent health systems can be realized without compromising the autonomy of the individual. When we are on the verge of technological advances and human-focused care, ethical and privacy-preserving AI is a necessity. Such a requirement preconditions the arrival of Federated Learning, a decentralized machine learning framework, as a potential solution to facilitate AI-based health management systems with a heavy emphasis on individual privacy and data security.

1.1 The Data-Driven Personalized Health Management Paradigm Shift

Healthcare is experiencing a radical shift as a combination of cutting-edge technologies, data everywhere, and the expanding need to provide patient-centered care are coming together. The old paradigms of health care that were largely reactive, generalized, and mostly based on clinical impression are slowly giving way to proactive, individualized, and evidence-based health care that considers the individual physiological, behavioral, and genetic peculiarities of a person. The combination of Artificial Intelligence (AI), Machine Learning (ML), Internet of Things (IoT) devices, and massive-scale health data analytics is the driving force behind this paradigm shift towards precision health management (Dhinakaran et al., 2025). Customized health care is not a vision of the future anymore. It is quickly moving beyond science fiction to become a reality due to the real-time gathering and crunching of data on a wide variety of sources electronic health records (EHRs), genomics, wearable sensors, mobile applications, and even social determinants of health. When properly utilized, these heterogeneous streams of data can enable AI models to build very personalized health profiles. The effect is a real-time and constantly evolving picture of the health condition of a person that can be used to deliver a personalized intervention that is capable of preventing the onset of disease, improving the effectiveness of treatment, and generally improving the quality of life.

Among the facilitators of such a shift is the availability of consumer-grade health monitoring technologies. Heart rate, sleep patterns, physical activity, stress levels, and other variables that were previously unmeasurable can now be tracked by wearable devices and smart home sensors to create a steady stream of data (Romiti et al., 2020). By examining this data, AI systems can identify even minor changes in an individual that are not normal to their baseline, and in many cases can predict adverse events or disease flare-ups before they are clinically visible. These capabilities become especially useful in the treatment of chronic conditions, especially diabetes, hypertension, and COPD, where early treatment can hugely lower hospitalization rates and healthcare expenditures. Patients are also gaining the power to become active participants in the running of their health due to this transformation (Harini et al., 2023). With customizable dashboards, push messaging to mobile devices, and an artificially intelligent recommendation engine, people are presented with insights that are specifically tailored to their lifestyle, routine, and health history. Consequently, healthcare is becoming patient-centric as opposed to provider-centric and this is causing a culture of engagement, prevention, and shared-decision making. However, the more personalized healthcare is data-intensive, the more it increases questions of data ownership, consent, and privacy. Such fine-grained personal data usage needs to be counterbalanced by strong data management and privacy-enhancing technologies, which is also where Federated Learning has a lot of potential. It is fully compatible with the vision of secure and personalized healthcare because it allows AI models to learn from distributed data sources, never transferring raw data.

1.2 The Growing Need for Privacy-Preserving Solutions

Due to the rise of digitization and data-driven healthcare, the amounts and sensitivity of patient data being gathered, processed, and stored are increasing unprecedentedly. Although the implementation of AI and IoT technologies into the health system opens the possibility of serious improvements in the field of diagnostics, treatment, and patient engagement, it also raises serious issues related to data privacy, security, and ethical application (Dhinakaran et al., 2025). Health data is one of the most sensitive types of personal information--it can identify very personal information about the physical and mental health of the individual, her or his lifestyle habits, and genetic tendencies. Accordingly, its abuse, misuse, violation, or illicit use may have serious consequences, such as discrimination, stigmatization, monetary loss, and loss of confidence in the healthcare system. A variety of high-profile data leaks and the rising awareness of the issue among people have made the weak point of traditional, centralized data management methods highly apparent. Centralized AI models have the tendency to send raw data collected in hospitals, wearable devices, and mobile apps to a remote server or cloud-based storage to be processed (Dey et al., 2018). Although this is effective in training models, it introduces a single point of failure, making the data vulnerable to hacking, data leakage, and Third parties. Besides, anonymized data may in some cases be re-identified with the help of auxiliary data, making traditional de-identification techniques incomplete.

Regulatory agencies and governments have reacted by imposing stringent data protection legislation, including the General Data Protection Regulation (GDPR) in the European Union and the Health Insurance Portability and Accountability Act (HIPAA) in the United States. These rules focus on data minimization, consent of the user, transparency, and accountability. Nevertheless, regulation cannot merely ensure this issue through compliance, as it is not sufficient to combat the fundamental risks of centralized data processing and black-box AI.

To address these challenges, there is a growing consensus around the need for privacy-preserving solutions that embed data protection directly into the architecture of AI systems. These include advanced techniques such as differential privacy, secure multiparty computation, homomorphic encryption, and—most notably—Federated Learning (FL). These approaches allow developers and researchers to extract value from health data while ensuring that individual privacy is not compromised. FL, in particular, is rapidly gaining traction as it offers a paradigm shift: enabling collaborative model training across multiple data sources without moving the data itself. This inherently reduces the attack surface and upholds user autonomy. As we move toward more connected and intelligent health ecosystems, adopting such privacy-aware technologies will be essential to maintain public trust and realize the full potential of AI in healthcare.

1.3 Chapter Objectives and Structure

With the healthcare scenario changing constantly, this chapter attempts to explore how Artificial Intelligence (AI) and the Internet of Things (IoT), along with privacy-preserving technologies, can have a compelling combination in building future-ready, ethical health management systems. As healthcare becomes more digitized and the use of connected health devices becomes mainstream, healthcare is moving towards continuous, data-driven, and personalized care delivery as opposed to reactive, episodic care-based models. Although this evolution is largely promising in terms of the outcomes in patient care and system optimizations, it is associated with the emergence of critical issues regarding data privacy, security, and ethical implementation of AI. This chapter discusses how intelligent healthcare solutions can be realized with the consideration of user privacy and using the maximum potential of distributed health data with the help of emerging techniques, especially Federated Learning (FL). The key goal of the presented chapter is to provide a coherent and cohesive grasp of how FL, together with the other assisting technologies, including edge computing and secure communication schemes, is transforming AI-based health monitoring and management. It starts with a background exploration of how AI and IoT are making possible real-time, personalized health interventions, composed of wearable sensors, mobile apps, and interconnected devices. The story next moves into a more detailed discussion of the privacy risk posed by the centralized data gathering in the traditional machine learning model, and how this is an issue that desperately needs a privacy-preserving solution in the medical field.

The main body of the chapter is devoted to the presentation of Federated Learning which is a novel paradigm enabling machine learning models to be trained on decentralized data sources without moving sensitive data to a central server. The structure further details the technicalities behind the concept of FL, contrasts it with conventional ML and shows how it can be applied to healthcare settings where data is extremely sensitive and usually siloed. It also argues about the communication infrastructure needed to enable FL, and what role 5G/6G, edge devices, and secure aggregation protocols play. Complementary privacy-enhancing methods, such as differential privacy and homomorphic encryption, are also introduced as integral components of a robust, privacy-centric AI framework. Finally, the chapter offers a critical perspective on open challenges, future directions, and ethical considerations that must be addressed to fully realize the vision of AI-powered, privacy-respecting healthcare. Through a mix of conceptual insight, practical use cases, and forward-looking analysis, this chapter provides a roadmap for researchers, developers, and policymakers committed to building trustworthy and intelligent health systems.

2. AI AND IOT IN HEALTH MONITORING

Artificial Intelligence (AI) and the Internet of Things (IoT) are converging to transform how health is tracked, evaluated, and controlled in either a clinical or real-world setting. Collectively, these technologies are helping to transform the way care has traditionally been delivered in a sporadic fashion (assessing a patient at regular intervals) to one that is more continuous and real-time focused, aimed at early diagnosis, customized treatment, and long-term health (Dhinakaran et al., 2023). AI can offer the intelligence to make sense of massive, continuous flows of health-relevant data, and IoT can enable easy data acquisition with an increasingly large ecosystem of interconnected instruments. The combination of the two areas enables the health systems to be more responsive, personal, and reachable, especially to the patients with chronic ailments or those in rural and underserved areas. The need to constantly monitor health has never been as high as the global healthcare landscape transforms to be able to handle an aging population and a continuously increasing prevalence of lifestyle-related diseases. Health solutions powered by AI and IoT respond to this requirement with scalable, non-invasive, and cost-efficient tools that can be used either in the clinical environment or at home (Yan et al., 2019). By helping to alleviate the load on the healthcare infrastructure, those systems also help individuals manage their health by encouraging them to become active participants in the process. This paradigm is setting the basis of predictive, preventive, and participatory healthcare, occasionally dubbed as P4 medicine.

2.1 Role of IoT Devices in Continuous Health Tracking (Wearables, Smart Devices)

The proliferation of Internet of Things (IoT) devices—particularly wearable sensors and smart home health technologies—has been instrumental in enabling continuous, real-time health monitoring outside traditional clinical environments as shown in Fig. 1. These devices are designed to collect physiological, behavioral, and environmental data seamlessly, without requiring active input from the user. From fitness bands and smartwatches to smart scales, biosensors, and ambient monitoring systems, IoT-enabled health technologies are transforming the way individuals track and manage their well-being daily.

Figure 1. Role of IoT Devices in Continuous Health Tracking

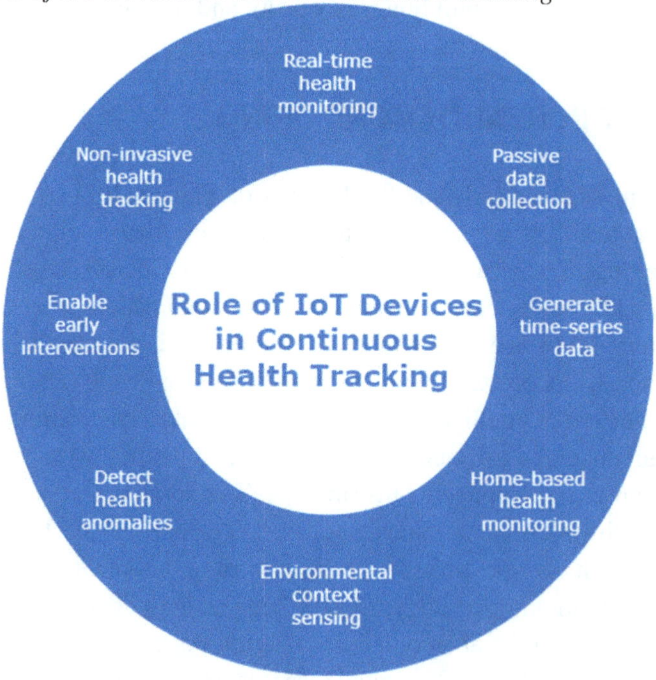

One of the most embraced tools in this ecosystem is the wearable devices. Widely used devices like smartwatches and fitness trackers are able to detect heart rate, respiratory rate, physical activity, caloric expenditure, sleep patterns, and blood oxygen saturation (SpO 2). Higher-level medical-grade wearables such as continuous glucose monitors (CGMs) or wearable ECG patches are essential in chronic condition management of diabetes and cardiovascular diseases (Al Alkeem et al., 2015). The devices are non-invasive and user-friendly with support for long-term monitoring and providing a continuous flow of time-series data. This would allow a dynamic and changing perspective of the health condition of an individual as opposed to the point-in-time data that is collected during regular medical check-ups. In addition to wearables, smart home health devices are also taking an important role. Examples are smart thermometers, connected weight scales, digital blood pressure monitors, and intelligent medication dispensers. Such devices would be especially helpful with geriatric patients, or with patients who are bedridden or recovering at home after an operation. By becoming a part of a connected health infrastructure, these devices can offer contextual information on the environment in which a patient lives, including the quality of air, the ambient temperature, or the activity rates- all of which are frequently ignored in a conventional health examination, yet can have a drastic effect on the health outcome (Bond et al., 2018).

The real value of IoT devices lies in their ability to deliver actionable insights when combined with AI. Data collected from these devices is often analyzed locally on edge devices or remotely through cloud platforms using machine learning algorithms. These algorithms detect patterns, anomalies, and trends that may indicate early signs of illness or deteriorating health conditions (Dhinakaran et al., 2025). For example, sudden drops in daily activity levels, irregular heart rhythms, or interrupted sleep patterns can be flagged for medical review. These insights enable timely interventions, better chronic disease management, and reduced hospital admissions, thus enhancing overall patient outcomes.

2.2 Integration of AI for Predictive and Personalized Healthcare

With the ever-growing and increasing complexity of health data, Artificial Intelligence (AI) has become an invaluable asset in transforming raw information into actionable insights that power personalized and predictive healthcare (Rahman et al., 2021). When applied to contemporary health systems, AI can strengthen decision-making abilities by means of identifying patterns, correlations, and premonitory signs that could be lost on human clinicians. Such capabilities are moving healthcare delivery beyond a reactive system (i.e., treating diseases once their symptoms manifest) to a proactive, preventive, and highly personalized system that focuses on promoting wellness and managing risks as well as customizing treatments to the individual patient profile (Dhinakaran et al., 2025). Predictive healthcare uses AI algorithms taught with large quantities of data, such as electronic health records (EHRs), genomics, wearable device data, imaging data, and environmental data to make predictions about future health outcomes. These models can pick out people who are likely to develop chronic diseases like diabetes, hypertension, or cardiovascular disorders long before the actual symptoms of the disease appear. To give some examples, using trends in daily heart rate variability, sleep quality, and activity level measured by wearable sensors, AI systems can identify small deviations that could indicate stress, fatigue, or the beginning of an infection. Predictive models have also been used to determine risks of hospital readmission, indicate non-compliance with medications, or predict disease progression; all of which can improve timely interventions and effective resource planning.

Also, it is worth mentioning the significance of AI in the sphere of personalized healthcare, meaning that treatment programs and lifestyle suggestions are based on the genetic composition, previous health history, behavioral patterns, and even likes and dislikes of a particular person (Rahman et al., 2020). AI could help clinicians to propose the most effective treatments, anticipate reactions to drugs, and suggest lifestyle changes that would be appropriate and acceptable in the particular circumstances of each patient. One application of AI in oncology, for example, is attempting to match patients to targeted treatments using tumor genomics and response data to treatment. AI-powered chatbots and mobile applications in the field of mental health have been used to make interventions more personalized, depending on the mood patterns and engagement behavior of the users. AI's ability to continuously learn and adapt from real-time data enables it to refine recommendations over time, creating a closed-loop feedback system that supports continuous improvement in patient care (Alghanim et al., 2017). When deployed alongside IoT devices, AI transforms passive monitoring into intelligent, actionable guidance, fostering a more engaged and empowered patient experience. However, the full potential of predictive and personalized healthcare depends on responsible AI practices, including fairness, transparency, and robust privacy protection—principles that are foundational to the privacy-preserving models discussed in the following sections.

2.3 Real-World Use Cases (e.g., Chronic Disease Management, Elderly Care)

The integration of AI and IoT technologies into healthcare has already begun to reshape how specific populations and conditions are managed, with chronic disease management and elderly care emerging as two of the most impactful real-world applications as shown in Fig. 2. These domains illustrate the transformative potential of continuous monitoring, predictive analytics, and personalized interventions when backed by privacy-conscious technologies.

Figure 2. Real-world use cases

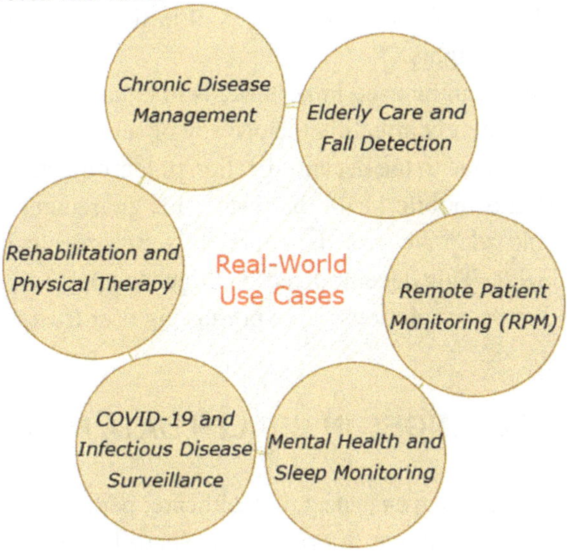

The management of chronic diseases is one of the most urgent and resource-dependent tasks of healthcare systems in the modern world. Chronic diseases like diabetes, high blood pressure, asthma, and heart ailments need constant supervision, prompt treatment, and good compliance of patients to medical regimens. IoT devices, including continuous glucose monitors, smart inhalers, wearable ECGs, and blood pressure cuffs, coupled with AI-powered systems, allow the collection and analysis of data in real time. Machine learning algorithms can identify potential complications, or abnormal glucose patterns or arrhythmias, in advance and issue alerts to the patient and provider (Almalki & Soufiene, 2021). As an example, AI models can process the patterns of insulin use among type-1 diabetes patients to either readjust the doses or suggest dietary adjustments, exposing the patient to the minimum risk of hypo- or hyperglycemic events. This initiative helps decrease hospital visits, increases life quality, and helps sustain disease management.

In elderly care, where the aspect of constant monitoring and safety is most needed, AI and IoT systems have transformed the way aging people are taken care of both in assisted living centers and at home (Dhinakaran et al., 2025). Fall detectors, motion sensors, smart pill dispensers, and voice-activated assistants are wearable devices that can analyze the level of activity, detect a fall, remind a patient to take medications, and even analyze behavioral changes that could beognitive decline. Behavioral patterns can also be taught to AI algorithms as deviations that indicate an emerging health problem or a mental health issue, such as limited mobility, abnormal sleep, or a lack of food consumption. Such technologies can assist in improving patient safety, with the additional effect of reducing the pressure on the caregivers and medical staff due to automation of basic monitoring processes and delivery of actionable insights.

Federated Learning can be used in both fields to enhance the predictive power of models without negatively affecting the privacy of sensitive patient information (Shrestha et al., 2016). Due to the decentralization of learning across hospital beds, household devices, and mobile health hardware, FL guarantees that models will be more accurate and adaptive over the course of time - meanwhile, patient data never leaves the device. This decentralized intelligence approach is key to scaling personalized care across populations while preserving user trust and data integrity.

3. PRIVACY CHALLENGES IN HEALTH DATA MANAGEMENT

With the growing data-driven aspect of healthcare, personal health information (PHI) poses a considerable threat to privacy and security. Not only is health data incredibly sensitive, but it is also very personal, spanning biometric and genetic information, behavioral data, mental health, and lifestyle choices (Karunarathne et al., 2021). This predisposes health data as an ideal target to be abused, compromised, and spied on-bringing urgent questions of confidentiality, trust, and ethical responsibility with regard to how digital health technologies are designed and implemented. As incredible as the value of AI and IoT systems are in predictive care and individualized interventions, they gather enormous quantities of fine-grained data typically with little or no reflections on how that data might be used. In the absence of effective privacy technologies, such systems will involuntarily subject persons to privacy infringements, discrimination, and exploitation (Dhinakaran et al., 2025). Therefore, privacy is a technical issue, but above all, it is a foundation of ethical management of health data, which has a direct influence on the adoption and effectiveness of smart healthcare systems.

Regulatory Landscape and Sensitivity of Health Data: Health data is assumed to be among the most sensitive forms of personal information as it can be used to obtain very intimate details about the state of a person, both physically and mentally. The social stigma, financial damage, insurance discrimination, and loss of trust in healthcare service providers may be caused by a leak or misuse of this data (Almalawi et al., 2022). In order to curb these risks, there are a number of privacy laws that are set around the world. The Health Insurance Portability and Accountability Act (HIPAA) in the United States provides strict guidelines on the protection and confidentiality of patient health data with particular emphasis on consent, control of access to the data, and notification in the event of a breach. European Union countries have a more comprehensive privacy regime in the General Data Protection

Regulation (GDPR), which incorporates the right to be forgotten, data portability, and explicit consent to process data. Both frameworks mandate that organizations adopt responsible data practices, but the technical implementation of these principles often remains challenging in real-world, data-rich environments.

Risks of Centralized Data Collection and Sharing: Traditional AI systems often rely on centralized architectures where data from multiple sources—hospitals, wearables, apps—is aggregated to a central server for training. While this approach can optimize algorithm performance, it creates a single point of vulnerability. Centralized data repositories are attractive targets for cyberattacks, and a breach could expose sensitive information at scale. Moreover, centralized systems inherently increase the risk of surveillance, profiling, and unauthorized third-party access. Even anonymized datasets are susceptible to re-identification attacks when combined with auxiliary information, posing further challenges to privacy preservation.

Need for Privacy-by-Design Approaches: To address these risks, there is a growing recognition that privacy must be embedded into the architecture of health technologies from the outset—a principle known as privacy by design (Guo et al., 2021). Rather than treating privacy as an afterthought or a compliance checkbox, systems must be engineered to minimize data collection, limit data access, and secure data transmission by default. Techniques like data minimization, encryption, secure multi-party computation, differential privacy, and Federated Learning exemplify this approach. By keeping data local and training models across distributed nodes, federated systems reduce the attack surface and help preserve user autonomy. This paradigm shift toward privacy-aware AI frameworks is essential not only for regulatory compliance but also for building long-term trust in digital healthcare innovations.

4. FEDERATED LEARNING

As privacy concerns escalate in the era of AI-driven healthcare, traditional centralized machine learning approaches are proving inadequate in protecting sensitive patient information. The need for models that can learn from distributed health data—without requiring that data to be moved or shared—has led to the emergence of Federated Learning (FL) as a transformative solution. Introduced by Google in 2017, FL is a machine learning paradigm designed to train algorithms across decentralized devices or servers holding local data samples, without exchanging the actual data itself. This privacy-preserving architecture aligns perfectly with the demands of modern healthcare, where data is typically siloed across hospitals, clinics, wearable devices, and home health systems. Federated Learning enables collaborative model development across these data silos, offering a powerful balance between data utility and data privacy. By bringing the algorithm to the data instead of the data to the algorithm, FL significantly reduces the risk of data exposure, while still enabling robust and personalized model training.

4.1 What is Federated Learning (FL)?

Federated Learning (FL) is a distributed machine learning algorithm such that the model training takes place on a number of devices or nodes that store local data. Rather than each device sending its raw data to a central server, each device trains a local copy of the model on its local data and only sends the updated model parameters (e.g. gradients or weights) to a central aggregator. These local updates are then aggregated, usually with methods such as Federated Averaging, to create a global model that backs the cumulative knowledge of all the participants without ever seeing their personal information. This approach is especially targeting the cases in which the privacy of data, regulation, or bandwidth restrictions make the centralization of data impossible (Sengan et al., 2022). In healthcare, FL can enable training AI models in a collaborative fashion across multiple hospitals, wearable devices, and health apps, enabling better diagnosis, risk prediction, or treatment suggestions, all with the guarantee that sensitive patient data never leaves the local setting.

FL allows horizontal, vertical, and federated transfer learning based on the data distribution among the participants. It also enables asynchronous training, where the devices can play a role at different times, improving scalability and feasibility. FL also enhances its capacity to provide accurate AI insights in a privacy-preserving, regulation-compliant, and scalable way via secure aggregation, encryption, and differential privacy. Federated Learning (FL) is a privately-aware, powerful technique of collaborative machine learning that moves the model training procedure out of centralized data centers and onto the edge, where the information exists. The security and performance of FL are determined by the well-coordinated system architecture that includes a few fundamental components and a clear training process. These fundamental aspects are crucial to comprehend how FL can scale the training of large models whilst safeguarding sensitive information, particularly in domains regarded as sensitive, such as healthcare.

4.2 Core Components of FL

1. **Client Devices (or Nodes):** These are decentralized endpoints that hold local data and perform local model training. In healthcare, clients can be hospitals, mobile phones, smartwatches, wearable sensors, or remote patient monitoring systems.

2. **Global Model:** A shared machine learning model initialized by the central server and distributed to all clients for local training. This model evolves over multiple training rounds.
3. **Local Models and Updates:** Each client trains the global model using its own data and produces local updates (e.g., gradients or weights) without exposing raw data.
4. **Federated Aggregator (Server):** The central server collects model updates from participating clients and aggregates them—commonly using Federated Averaging—to produce an improved global model.
5. **Communication Protocol:** A secure and efficient communication channel is required for sharing model parameters, especially in bandwidth-limited or resource-constrained settings.
6. **Privacy Enhancing Technologies (PETs):** FL often incorporates differential privacy, secure multi-party computation (SMPC), or homomorphic encryption to ensure that model updates cannot be reverse-engineered to extract sensitive data.

Figure 3. Workflow of Federated Learning (FL)

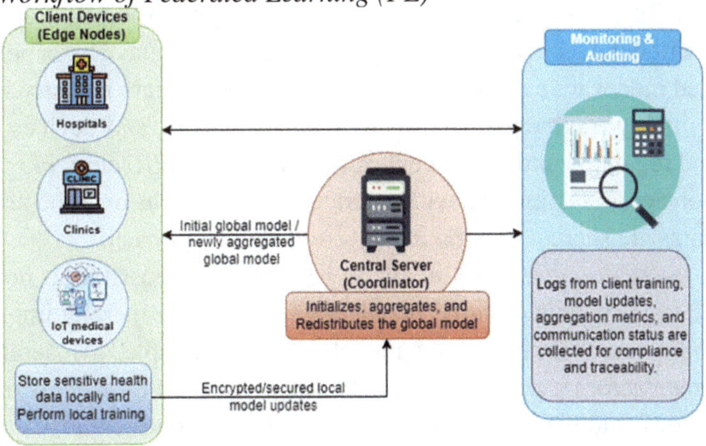

The workflow of Federated Learning (FL) is structured around a collaborative and iterative process that maintains data privacy throughout. It begins with the initialization phase, where a central server creates and distributes a global machine-learning model to a selected group of client devices as shown in Fig. 3. In the local training phase, each client independently trains this model using its private dataset over several epochs, generating updated model parameters such as weights or gradients. Rather than transmitting raw data, clients then enter the model update transmission phase, sending their encrypted or masked updates back to the central server. In the aggregation phase, the server combines the received updates—typically using techniques like Federated Averaging—to refine the global model. This iterative process is repeated over multiple communication rounds, with the updated global model being redistributed to clients for further local training, allowing the system to progressively improve its performance. Finally, in the deployment phase, the fully trained model is deployed either globally for general use or personalized locally to cater to the specific needs of individual clients or institutions. This entire workflow enables effective collaborative learning while ensuring that sensitive data remains decentralized and secure.

4.3 Advantages of FL for Healthcare Data

Federated Learning (FL) proposes a revolutionary model of analyzing healthcare data, as it provides a solution to one of the most paramount issues of the contemporary digital health infrastructure the privacy of patients. The conventional machine learning algorithms require the consolidation of data to a central depository, not only does this approach evoke serious ethical and legal issues but it also exposes the data to greater possibility of breach (Selvaraj et al., 2025). Conversely, FL enables healthcare facilities, wearables, and mobile health apps to jointly train powerful AI models without ever exchanging unprocessed patient data. The benefits of this decentralized model are especially applicable to the healthcare industry where data tends to be highly fragmented (between hospitals, clinics, and devices owned by patients) and regulated under stringent rules (HIPAA, GDPR, etc.). FL also allows collaboration across institutions without transferring data, as only the anonymized model updates are shared, making it a data-sovereign approach.

Among the main advantages of FL in healthcare, is possible to note the opportunity to train models on large populations of patients, thereby improving the generalizability and fairness of AI models. As an example, a federated model trained on data across a range of hospitals can be exposed to patients of different ages, ethnicities, and medical backgrounds, resulting in more inclusive diagnostic and prediction models (Puiu et al., 2021). Moreover, FL decreases the latency and bandwidth consumption since the model parameters that are sent are lightweight instead of huge datasets. FL also enables personalized medicine, since it enables local refinement of models to match specific patient attributes or local institutional processes, without sacrificing the advantage of global knowledge pooling. Such a trade-off between personalization and generalization is important to developing not just accurate but also contextually relevant AI systems. Also, by combining FL with other privacy-preserving technologies like differential privacy and secure multi-party computation, it is possible to enhance further its ability to protect sensitive health data. In general, FL is one of the key innovations to develop AI in healthcare safely, ethically, and at scale.

4.4 Comparison With Traditional Centralized Machine Learning

While traditional centralized machine learning (ML) has been instrumental in developing intelligent systems, it presents several limitations when applied to sensitive domains like healthcare. In centralized ML, data from various sources—such as hospitals, clinics, wearable devices, and apps—is collected and transmitted to a central server where model training occurs. Although this approach allows for the training of highly accurate models with large datasets, it comes with significant challenges, particularly in terms of privacy, data security, regulatory compliance, and scalability (Dhinakaran et al., 2025). Centralized models inherently increase the risk of data breaches and unauthorized access, since aggregating all data in a single location creates a high-value target for cyberattacks. This is especially problematic in healthcare, where patient records contain deeply personal and often irreplaceable information. Additionally, transmitting large volumes of medical data (e.g., imaging, EHRs) to a central server can be bandwidth-intensive and inefficient, especially in low-resource settings.

In contrast, Federated Learning (FL) offers a privacy-first alternative that mitigates these risks by keeping data localized. FL enables model training directly on edge devices or institutional servers where data is originally generated or stored. Only encrypted model updates are shared with a central aggregator, significantly reducing the exposure of sensitive information. From a compliance perspective, this decentralized approach aligns more effectively with privacy regulations such as HIPAA and GDPR, which restrict cross-border and cross-institutional data sharing. Moreover, FL can leverage data diversity more effectively than centralized systems (Liu et al., 2022). In traditional ML, institutions may be reluctant to share data due to legal or competitive concerns, leading to biased models trained on homogeneous datasets. FL overcomes this by allowing each institution or device to contribute to the model without relinquishing data control—resulting in more generalizable and fair models. In essence, while centralized ML remains useful in many scenarios, FL provides a more secure, ethical, and collaborative paradigm—one that is particularly well-suited for the complex, sensitive, and distributed nature of healthcare data.

5. FEDERATED LEARNING FOR AI-POWERED HEALTH MANAGEMENT

The convergence of artificial intelligence (AI) and healthcare has opened new frontiers in how medical services are delivered, diagnosed, and personalized. However, the full potential of AI in health management is often hindered by the fragmented nature of healthcare data, stringent privacy regulations, and ethical concerns surrounding the sharing of sensitive medical information. Federated Learning (FL) emerges as a pivotal enabler in this context, allowing AI models to be trained collaboratively across multiple decentralized sources without transferring or exposing raw patient data. This privacy-preserving framework is not only compliant with data protection laws like HIPAA and GDPR but also supports a more inclusive and representative model training process across diverse populations and healthcare settings. As a result, FL paves the way for powerful, scalable, and secure AI-powered health management systems.

5.1 Applications in Medical Diagnosis, Remote Monitoring, and Treatment Personalization

FL has demonstrated huge potential in many areas of AI-enabled health management, particularly medical diagnosis, remote patient monitoring, and individual treatment planning. Medical diagnosis FL allows training collaborative models in a scenario involving multiple hospitals and diagnostic centers without affecting patient privacy. As an illustration, radiology images, like chest X-rays or brain MRIs, can be used to learn a federated model to detect diseases in radiology images when distributed across institutions. This enables the model to be more generalizable across populations and imaging machines, diagnostic bias is avoided and the accuracy is increased particularly in uncommon or underrepresented conditions. In remote health monitoring, FL helps to create smart systems capable of processing data on wearable devices, home sensors, and mobile health applications on the fly. The continuous monitoring of patients with chronic conditions like diabetes, hypertension, or heart disease can be done, and federated AI models can predict complications like arrhythmias or glucose imbalances without requiring raw biometric data to be uploaded to the cloud. Not only does this decrease latency and bandwidth consumption, but it also conserves patient autonomy and privacy.

Moreover, FL allows treating personalization (without data sharing between institutions) because the models can fit the idiosyncratic health patterns of specific patients or groups, their genetic histories, and responses to treatments. Federated models can optimize personalized medicine, therapy design, and rehabilitation protocols, learning local data but enjoying the global trends. It is this combination of localized intelligence and collaborative learning that makes FL an important tool for developing responsive, ethical, and effective AI-driven healthcare systems.

5.2 Federated Learning Architectures in Healthcare

Federated Learning (FL) can be implemented in several architectural forms, each suited to different healthcare scenarios depending on data distribution, institutional structure, and computational infrastructure. Understanding these architectures is essential for designing FL systems that are both effective and privacy-preserving in real-world medical environments.

Figure 4. Horizontal Federated Learning (HFL)

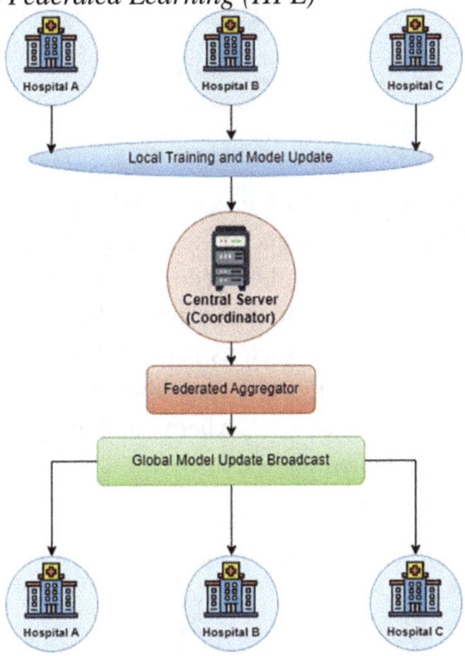

Horizontal Federated Learning (HFL): Horizontal FL is the most common architecture in healthcare settings where institutions (e.g., hospitals or clinics) share the same type of data features (such as medical images, vital signs, or electronic health records) but from different patient populations as shown in Fig. 4. For example, multiple hospitals may have records of patient demographics and lab results with similar schema, but each hospital treats different patients. HFL allows these institutions to collaboratively train a global model without centralizing data, improving generalizability while maintaining data locality. This architecture is ideal for disease classification, clinical risk prediction, and population-level health analytics.

Figure 5. Vertical Federated Learning (VFL)

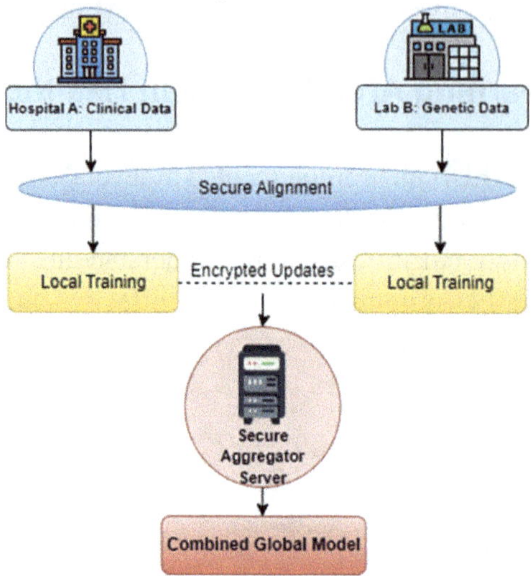

Vertical Federated Learning (VFL): Vertical FL applies when different organizations possess complementary datasets for the same group of patients. For instance, a hospital may hold clinical data, while a genomic lab has sequencing data for the same patients. VFL allows these entities to train models together by aligning their data based on common identifiers, such as patient IDs, using privacy-preserving matching protocols as shown in Fig. 5. This architecture enables richer feature sets for applications like precision medicine, where combining molecular and clinical data can significantly improve outcomes.

Figure 6. Federated Transfer Learning (FTL)

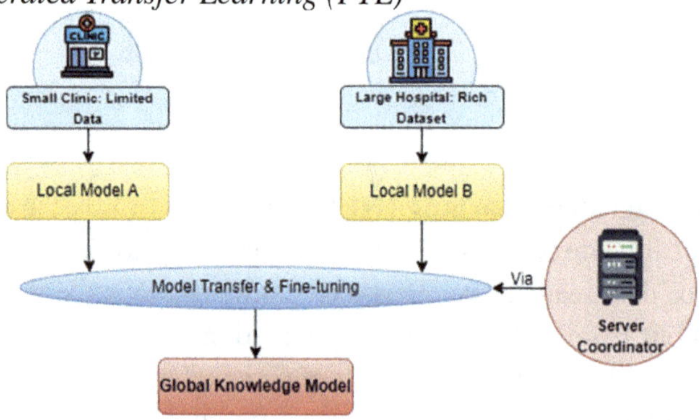

Federated Transfer Learning (FTL): In cases where data overlaps are minimal in both samples and features, Federated Transfer Learning becomes applicable as shown in Fig. 6. This is especially useful when a well-trained model from a resource-rich institution needs to be adapted to a smaller clinic with limited data. FTL enables knowledge transfer from the global model to the local environment, refining the model without exposing sensitive data or requiring large-scale local training.

Cross-device vs. Cross-silo FL: Healthcare FL can also be categorized as cross-device (e.g., millions of wearables contributing to a model) or cross-silo (e.g., collaboration among a few large hospitals). Each scenario requires different communication and security protocols, depending on computational power, connectivity, and privacy expectations. In practice, selecting the right FL architecture depends on institutional goals, data characteristics, and privacy requirements. By aligning the architecture with the use case, FL can unlock powerful, compliant, and collaborative health solutions.

5.3 Case Studies or Prototype Systems

Several case studies and prototype systems have demonstrated the practical potential of Federated Learning (FL) in healthcare. These implementations showcase how FL can effectively bridge the gap between privacy, data utility, and AI innovation in medical settings.

Federated Tumor Segmentation (FeTS) Challenge: One of the most prominent demonstrations of FL in healthcare is the Federated Tumor Segmentation (FeTS) initiative. Conducted by researchers from the University of Pennsylvania and Intel, this project used FL to train AI models on brain tumor MRI scans distributed across over 30 international healthcare institutions. Each institution trained the model locally on its data, contributing to a robust global model capable of identifying and segmenting gliomas without sharing any raw imaging data. This project highlighted how FL could enable large-scale, multi-institutional collaborations without compromising patient confidentiality.

NVIDIA Clara: NVIDIA's Clara Federated Learning platform has been used in pilot projects across hospitals to train AI models for tasks like chest X-ray analysis, COVID-19 diagnosis, and pathology image interpretation. Clara enables healthcare institutions to develop shared models while preserving local data privacy using a modular and scalable FL infrastructure. The platform supports integration with privacy-enhancing technologies like differential privacy and homomorphic encryption, making it a practical choice for real-world healthcare environments.

Google's FL for Mobile Health: Google has implemented FL on edge devices such as smartphones and wearables to support applications like heart rate prediction and activity tracking. These models are trained locally on devices, ensuring user data never leaves the device. The system incorporates privacy-preserving techniques like Secure Aggregation to further safeguard user information. Though not limited to clinical settings, this approach is particularly relevant for remote health monitoring and preventive care systems.

Prototype for Diabetes Monitoring: Researchers have also developed FL-based prototypes for diabetes management, where federated models predict blood glucose levels using data from continuous glucose monitors (CGMs) and fitness trackers. These systems have shown promising results in predicting hypoglycemic events while keeping sensitive metabolic data on-device.

These case studies underline the versatility and promise of FL across a spectrum of healthcare use cases—from hospital-based diagnostics to personal health management—offering a secure, collaborative path forward for AI in medicine.

6. COMMUNICATION AND INFRASTRUCTURE CONSIDERATIONS

As Federated Learning (FL) transitions from research to real-world deployment in healthcare, the importance of communication and computational infrastructure becomes increasingly evident. Unlike traditional centralized learning approaches, FL involves a dynamic network of decentralized participants—ranging from hospital systems to mobile devices—that must coordinate model training without compromising speed, privacy, or reliability (Dhinakaran et al., 2023). This decentralized training paradigm places significant demands on communication networks and edge computing capabilities. Effective FL deployment in healthcare, particularly in time-sensitive scenarios such as emergency diagnostics or intensive care monitoring, hinges on real-time data processing, minimal latency, and secure transmission of model updates. This section explores how emerging technologies like 5G/6G and edge computing can empower FL, while also addressing the challenges related to network latency, bandwidth limitations, and communication security.

Role of 5G/6G and Edge Computing in Enabling FL and Real-Time AI Inference: The advent of 5G and emerging 6G communication technologies provides the high-speed, low-latency backbone required for large-scale FL deployments. These networks enable ultra-reliable and fast communication between edge devices and central servers, reducing training round durations and enabling real-time decision-making. Paired with edge computing, FL can move computation closer to data sources—such as wearable health monitors, bedside sensors, or imaging equipment—allowing immediate inference and response. For instance, an edge-enabled federated system in an ambulance can analyze patient vitals in real-time and synchronize with hospital systems before arrival. Such integration improves response time, minimizes the need for cloud reliance, and supports privacy preservation by processing sensitive data locally.

Network Latency, Bandwidth, and Synchronization Challenges: While 5G and edge computing enhance FL infrastructure, practical implementation still faces significant network challenges. Synchronizing model updates across numerous, often heterogeneous, clients can result in asynchronous training delays, communication dropouts, and resource contention. Variations in internet connectivity, especially in rural or under-resourced healthcare settings, may lead to straggler effects—where slower nodes hinder overall training progress. Moreover, frequent transmission of high-dimensional model updates can cause bandwidth bottlenecks, particularly in deep learning models with large parameter sets. To address these issues, techniques such as adaptive client selection, model update compression, and partial aggregation are employed to reduce communication overhead while maintaining model performance.

Security Mechanisms in FL Communication: Ensuring the security and integrity of communication in FL is critical, especially when handling sensitive patient data. One of the key approaches is Secure Aggregation, which enables the central server to aggregate model updates without accessing individual contributions. Additionally, Differential Privacy (DP) introduces calibrated noise to model updates before transmission, obscuring identifiable patterns while maintaining statistical utility. Advanced cryptographic techniques like Homomorphic Encryption (HE) and Secure Multi-party Computation (SMPC) offer even stronger protection by allowing encrypted computations without exposing raw data. These security mechanisms ensure that even if communication channels are compromised, sensitive medical information remains confidential and tamper-resistant.

7. ENSURING DATA PRIVACY AND MODEL SECURITY

In healthcare, where patient trust and regulatory compliance are paramount, preserving the confidentiality and integrity of medical data is not just a technical requirement—it is a legal and ethical obligation. Federated Learning (FL), by design, improves privacy by keeping raw data localized. However, even in FL systems, model updates shared between clients and servers can potentially leak sensitive information if not properly protected. Adversaries may exploit these updates to reconstruct patient data, infer membership information, or corrupt the learning process through poisoning attacks. To safeguard against these risks, FL systems must integrate advanced privacy-enhancing technologies and robust security mechanisms that reinforce data protection at every stage of training and communication. This section explores the core techniques used to enhance data privacy and model security in FL-based healthcare systems.

7.1 Techniques for Enhancing Privacy in FL

Differential Privacy (DP): Differential Privacy is one of the most widely adopted methods for protecting user-level data during FL. It works by injecting calibrated noise into model updates or gradients before they are shared with the central server as shown in Fig. 7. This noise prevents the server—or any eavesdropper—from confidently inferring whether a specific individual's data influenced the model. DP can be applied at the client-side (local DP) or at the aggregator level (global DP), with each approach offering trade-offs between utility and privacy. In healthcare, DP ensures that sensitive characteristics such as disease status, medication usage, or genetic markers remain private even when aggregated models are released or audited.

Figure 7. Techniques for Enhancing Privacy in FL

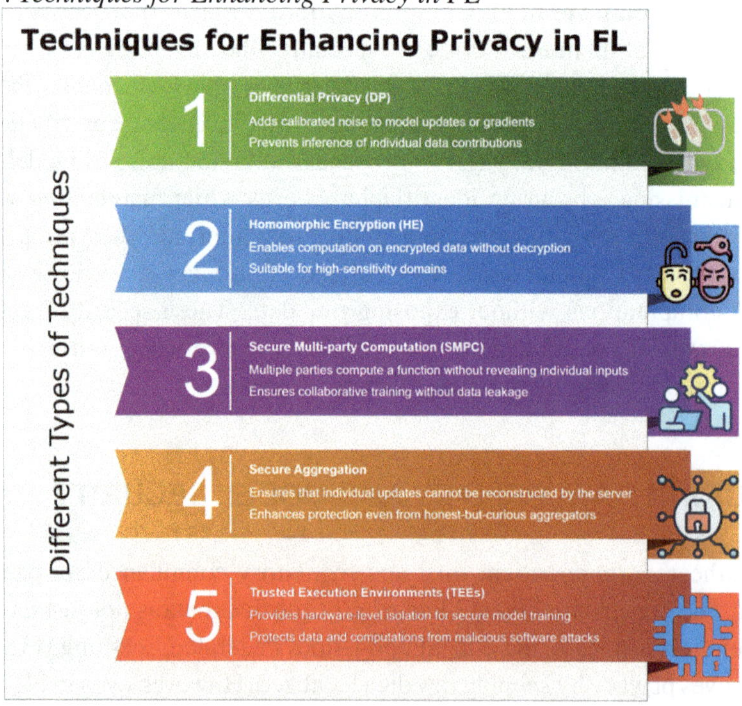

Homomorphic Encryption (HE): Homomorphic Encryption enables computations to be performed directly on encrypted data, eliminating the need to decrypt sensitive information during the training process. In the context of FL, clients encrypt their model updates before sending them to the server, which can then perform aggregation (e.g., weighted averaging) without ever accessing plaintext data. This technique significantly increases security, particularly when servers or intermediaries are not fully trusted (Bond et al., 2018). Though HE introduces computational overhead, its ability to preserve both functionality and privacy makes it attractive for high-stakes domains like oncology, genomics, and mental health. Other Techniques: Beyond DP and HE, several other methods are being integrated into FL to enhance privacy. Secure Multi-party Computation (SMPC) enables multiple parties to jointly compute a function over their inputs without revealing them to each other. Secure Aggregation ensures that individual updates cannot be isolated, even by the server, while Trusted Execution Environments (TEEs) offer hardware-level protections to secure data during computation. By combining these privacy-enhancing technologies, FL can be made significantly more resilient to privacy leakage, meeting both regulatory standards and ethical expectations in healthcare AI applications.

7.2 Handling Adversarial Threats and Model Poisoning

In Federated Learning (FL) systems, particularly those used in healthcare, the decentralized nature of training introduces new vulnerabilities to adversarial threats and model poisoning. Unlike traditional centralized systems where data and training are tightly controlled, FL relies on distributed participants—some of which may be compromised or malicious. One common threat is model poisoning, where a participant manipulates their local training data or gradients to intentionally degrade the performance of the global model. In a healthcare setting, such manipulation could lead to catastrophic misdiagnoses, such as misclassifying a malignant tumor as benign. Moreover, adversaries may attempt backdoor attacks, embedding hidden behaviors in the model that trigger incorrect outputs under specific conditions. FL is also susceptible to adversarial examples—carefully crafted inputs designed to mislead the model without appearing abnormal to humans.

To defend against these risks, several techniques have been developed. Robust aggregation methods, such as Krum or trimmed mean, reduce the influence of any single client's update by detecting and mitigating outliers. Anomaly detection algorithms can monitor gradient patterns for irregularities, while client reputation systems assign trust scores to participants based on historical behavior. Additionally, adversarial training—the practice of including adversarial examples in the training process—can increase model resilience. Post-hoc tools like SHAP or LIME help audit model decisions and reveal hidden biases or triggers, enhancing transparency. Ultimately, protecting FL-based health models requires a multi-layered security approach that combines secure communication, privacy-preserving techniques, behavioral monitoring, and model validation. Given the high stakes of medical decision-making, ensuring robustness against adversarial manipulation is essential to maintaining trust, accuracy, and patient safety in AI-powered health management systems.

7.3 Auditing and Transparency in FL-Based Systems

In privacy-sensitive domains like healthcare, auditing and transparency are critical for building trust and accountability in Federated Learning (FL)-based systems. Unlike centralized models, where data and training pipelines can be thoroughly inspected, FL's decentralized nature introduces challenges in monitoring and interpreting the learning process. Each participant trains a model on local data, and only model updates—not raw data—are shared. This limited visibility makes it difficult to track data provenance, identify harmful biases, or verify compliance with ethical standards and regulatory frameworks. As a result, FL systems must incorporate robust auditing mechanisms to ensure fairness, detect anomalies, and provide explainable insights to clinicians, regulators, and patients alike. One core approach to enhancing transparency is the use of model interpretability tools such as SHAP (SHapley Additive exPlanations), LIME (Local Interpretable Model-agnostic Explanations), or attention mechanisms that highlight influential features. These tools can be applied post-training to explain predictions made by the federated model, helping clinicians understand why certain diagnostic or treatment suggestions are made. In addition, training logs, update traces, and model versioning can be maintained to audit the contributions of different clients, monitor convergence trends, and trace the evolution of the global model over time.

FL systems can also implement federated audit trails that securely record metadata—such as timestamped participation records, update magnitudes, and differential privacy levels—without compromising patient privacy. These trails are particularly useful in verifying compliance with legal mandates like HIPAA or GDPR, as they provide proof that sensitive data was never shared or exposed. To further enhance trust, third-party auditing frameworks can be integrated, allowing external bodies to validate model behavior, robustness, and fairness without accessing private data. Finally, transparency must extend to stakeholders through clear communication and documentation. Medical professionals and data custodians should be informed of how FL works, what data is used locally, what privacy measures are in place, and what risks remain. By embedding transparency and auditing into the architecture of FL systems, healthcare institutions can better align with ethical AI principles, mitigate the risk of hidden biases, and ultimately foster greater confidence in AI-powered health technologies.

8. FUTURE DIRECTIONS AND CHALLENGES

As Federated Learning (FL) continues to evolve, its potential to revolutionize healthcare through secure, intelligent, and decentralized AI becomes increasingly apparent. However, alongside these opportunities lie critical challenges that must be addressed to ensure long-term impact and ethical adoption. One of the most pressing concerns is the ethical implication and trust associated with AI-driven health systems. Healthcare decisions are deeply personal, and any system that influences diagnosis, treatment, or patient management must be explainable, fair, and accountable. Establishing trust in FL requires not only strong privacy and security assurances but also mechanisms that allow patients, clinicians, and regulators to understand how models reach their conclusions. Issues like algorithmic bias, unequal access to technology, and the opacity of complex AI models raise questions about fairness and informed consent. Therefore, embedding ethical governance and human-in-the-loop practices will be essential to align FL technologies with medical standards and societal values.

Another key challenge is the scalability and standardization of FL in healthcare. Most successful FL implementations to date have been limited to pilot studies or proof-of-concept systems. Scaling FL to nationwide or global networks of hospitals, clinics, and personal devices introduces significant interoperability, infrastructure, and coordination challenges. Data heterogeneity across institutions—caused by differences in electronic health record (EHR) formats, medical imaging modalities, or patient demographics—can impair model performance. To address this, there is a growing need for standardized FL frameworks, shared ontologies, and regulatory guidelines that ensure consistency, fairness, and reproducibility across deployments. Establishing collaborative standards among medical AI developers, healthcare providers, and policymakers will be critical to accelerate adoption and trust.

Finally, open research problems in FL must be tackled to unlock its full potential in personalized medicine. A key technical dilemma is the trade-off between personalization and generalization. While global models trained through FL are designed to generalize across populations, personalized health care often demands models that adapt to individual patient contexts. Balancing these competing goals—without sacrificing accuracy, privacy, or equity—remains an active area of research. Other unsolved challenges include adaptive client selection in dynamic environments, fairness-aware FL algorithms, minimizing communication costs, and improving model robustness against real-world non-IID (non-independent and identically distributed) data. There is also an opportunity to explore cross-silo FL involving collaboration across healthcare institutions, and cross-device FL, where edge devices like wearables participate at scale.

9. CONCLUSION

As healthcare systems around the world undergo digital transformation, the convergence of Artificial Intelligence (AI), Internet of Things (IoT), and privacy-enhancing technologies presents a powerful opportunity to reshape the future of patient care. This chapter explored the critical role of Federated Learning (FL) in realizing a vision of health management that is not only intelligent and personalized but also privacy-conscious by design. We began by recognizing the paradigm shift toward data-driven, individualized health monitoring, powered by a growing ecosystem of wearable devices and smart sensors. These IoT tools, when paired with AI, enable real-time analytics, early disease detection, and treatment recommendations that adapt to individual physiological patterns. However, these innovations come with the inherent risk of exposing sensitive medical information—raising serious privacy, security, and ethical concerns. Traditional centralized machine learning architectures, which rely on aggregating data at a central location, are increasingly ill-suited to meet the regulatory and societal demands of modern healthcare systems.

Federated Learning offers a compelling alternative. By allowing models to be trained across decentralized data silos without transferring raw data, FL preserves data sovereignty, enhances security, and aligns with global privacy frameworks such as HIPAA and GDPR. Through real-world applications in chronic disease management, elderly care, remote diagnostics, and treatment personalization, we've seen how FL can empower both patients and providers without compromising confidentiality. We also examined the technical workflows of FL, its integration with secure communication infrastructure (e.g., 5G/6G and edge computing), and the layered security mechanisms such as differential privacy, homomorphic encryption, and robust aggregation that fortify the system against threats like model poisoning and adversarial attacks.

Despite its promise, FL is not a silver bullet. Significant challenges remain in terms of scalability, interoperability, trust, and standardization. The trade-offs between personalization and generalization, the need for cross-institutional collaboration, and the development of ethical, explainable AI frameworks are all open areas of research. As we look ahead, we issue a call to action for researchers, technologists, clinicians, policymakers, and ethicists to work together in shaping the next generation of health AI systems. Only through multidisciplinary collaboration and responsible innovation can we unlock the full potential of FL and ensure that future health technologies are inclusive, transparent, and worthy of the public trust. The future of well-being depends not just on smarter algorithms, but on designing systems that respect privacy, ensure security, and place human values at their core.

REFERENCES

Al Alkeem, E., Yeun, C. Y., & Zemerly, M. J. (2015). Security and privacy framework for ubiquitous healthcare IoT devices. In *Proceedings of the 10th IEEE International Conference for Internet Technology and Secured Transactions (ICITST)* (pp. 70–75). London, UK.

Alghanim, A. A., Rahman, S. M. M., & Hossain, M. A. (2017). Privacy analysis of smart city healthcare services. In *Proceedings of the 2017 IEEE International Symposium on Multimedia (ISM)* (pp. 394–398). Taichung, Taiwan.

Almalawi, A., Khan, A. I., Alsolami, F., Abushark, Y. B., Alfakeeh, A. S., & Mekuriyaw, W. D. (2022). Analysis of the exploration of security and privacy for healthcare management using artificial intelligence: Saudi hospitals. *Computational Intelligence and Neuroscience, 4048197.* Advance online publication. DOI: 10.1155/2022/4048197 PMID: 36156966

Almalki, F. A., & Soufiene, B. O. (2021). EPPDA: An efficient and privacy-preserving data aggregation scheme with authentication and authorization for IoT-based healthcare applications. *Wireless Communications and Mobile Computing, 5594159.* Advance online publication. DOI: 10.1155/2021/5594159

Bond, R., Novotny, T., Andrsova, I., Koc, L., Sisakova, M., Finlay, D., & Malik, M. (2018). Automation bias in medicine: The influence of automated diagnoses on interpreter accuracy and uncertainty when reading electrocardiograms. *Journal of Electrocardiology, 51*(6S), S6–S11. PMID: 30122457

Dey, D., Slomka, P., Leeson, P., Comaniciu, D., Shrestha, S., Sengupta, P., & Marwick, T. (2018). Artificial intelligence in cardiovascular imaging: JACC state-of-the-art review. *Journal of the American College of Cardiology, 73*(11), 1317–1335. PMID: 30898208

Dhinakaran, D., Edwin Raja, S., Velselvi, R., & Purushotham, N. (2025). Intelligent IoT-driven advanced predictive maintenance system for industrial applications. *SN Computer Science, 6*, 151. DOI: 10.1007/s42979-025-03695-x

Dhinakaran, D., Gopalakrishnan, S., Selvaraj, D., Girija, M. S., & Prabaharan, G. (2025). Mining privacy-preserving association rules using transaction hewer allocator and facile hash algorithm in multi-cloud environments. *MethodsX, 14*, 103317. DOI: 10.1016/j.mex.2025.103317 PMID: 40331027

Dhinakaran, D., Jagadish Kumar, N., Ponnuviji, N. P., & Praveen Kumar, B. (2025). Safeguarding confidentiality and privacy in cloud-enabled healthcare systems with SpectraSafe encryption and dynamic k-anonymity algorithm. *Expert Systems with Applications*, *279*, 127584. DOI: 10.1016/j.eswa.2025.127584

Dhinakaran, D., Prabaharan, G., Valarmathi, K., Sankar, S. U., & Sugumar, R. (2025). Safeguarding privacy by utilizing SC-DℓDA algorithm in cloud-enabled multi-party computation. *KSII Transactions on Internet and Information Systems*, *19*(2), 635–656. DOI: 10.3837/tiis.2025.02.014

Dhinakaran, D., Ramani, R., Edwin Raja, S., & Selvaraj, D. (2025). Enhancing security in electronic health records using an adaptive feature-centric polynomial data security model with blockchain integration. *Peer-to-Peer Networking and Applications*, *18*, 7. DOI: 10.1007/s12083-024-01883-9

Dhinakaran, D., Selvaraj, D., Dharini, N., Raja, S. E., & Priya, C. S. L. (2023). Towards a novel privacy-preserving distributed multiparty data outsourcing scheme for cloud computing with quantum key distribution. *International Journal of Intelligent Systems and Applications in Engineering*, *12*(2), 286–300.

Dhinakaran, D., Srinivasan, L., Gopalakrishnan, S., & Anish, T. P. (2025). An efficient data mining technique and privacy preservation model for healthcare data using improved darts game optimizer-based weighted deep neural network and hybrid encryption. *Biomedical Signal Processing and Control*, *100*(C), 107168. DOI: 10.1016/j.bspc.2024.107168

Guo, C., Tian, P., & Choo, K.-K. R. (2021). Enabling privacy-assured fog-based data aggregation in e-healthcare systems. *IEEE Transactions on Industrial Informatics*, *17*(3), 1948–1957. DOI: 10.1109/TII.2020.2995228 PMID: 37981962

Harini, M., Dhinakaran, D., & Prabhu, D. (2023). Leveraging blockchain for transparency in agriculture supply chain management using IoT and machine learning. In *2023 World Conference on Communication & Computing (WCONF)* (pp. 1–6). Raipur, India. https://doi.org/DOI: 10.1109/WCONF58270.2023.10235156

Karunarathne, S. M., Saxena, N., & Khan, M. K. (2021). Security and privacy in IoT smart healthcare. *IEEE Internet Computing*, *25*(4), 37–48. DOI: 10.1109/MIC.2021.3051675

Liu, Y., Yu, J., Fan, J., Vijayakumar, P., & Chang, V. (2022). Achieving privacy-preserving DSSE for intelligent IoT healthcare system. *IEEE Transactions on Industrial Informatics*, *18*(3), 2010–2020. DOI: 10.1109/TII.2021.3100873

Puiu, A., Vizitiu, A., Nita, C., Itu, L. M., Sharma, P., & Comaniciu, D. (2021). Privacy-preserving and explainable AI for cardiovascular imaging. *Studies in Informatics and Control*, *30*, 21–32.

Rahman, M. A., Hossain, M. S., Islam, M. S., Alrajeh, N. A., & Muhammad, G. (2020). Secure and provenance enhanced Internet of health things framework: A blockchain managed federated learning approach. *IEEE Access : Practical Innovations, Open Solutions*, *8*, 205071–205087. PMID: 34192116

Rahman, M. A., Hossain, M. S., Showail, A. J., Alrajeh, N. A., & Alhamid, M. F. (2021). A secure, private, and explainable IoHT framework to support sustainable health monitoring in a smart city. *Sustainable Cities and Society*, *72*, 103083.

Romiti, S., Vinciguerra, M., Saade, W., Cortajarena, I. A., & Greco, E. (2020). Artificial intelligence (AI) and cardiovascular diseases: An unexpected alliance. *Cardiology Research and Practice*, *5*, 1–8. PMID: 32676206

Selva Kumar, V., Mohan Raj, K. R., Gopalakrishnan, S., Vennila, G., Dhinakaran, D., & Kavitha, P. (2025). Adaptive distributed honeypot detection network for enhanced cybersecurity against DoS and DDoS attacks. *Results in Engineering*, *26*, 105521. DOI: 10.1016/j.rineng.2025.105521

Selvaraj, D., Jeno, J., Ramani, R., Dhinakaran, D., & Prabaharan, G. (2025). AFCP data security model for EHR data using blockchain. *Journal of Cybersecurity and Information Management*, *15*(1), 22–33. DOI: 10.54216/JCIM.150103

Sengan, S., Khalaf, O. I., Vidya Sagar, P., Sharma, D. K., Arokia Jesu Prabhu, L., & Hamad, A. A. (2022). Secured and privacy-based IDS for healthcare systems on e-medical data using machine learning approach. [IJRQEH]. *International Journal of Reliable and Quality E-Healthcare*, *11*(3), 1–11. DOI: 10.4018/IJRQEH.289175

Shrestha, N. M., Alsadoon, A., Prasad, P. W. C., Hourany, L., & Elchouemi, A. (2016). Enhanced e-health framework for security and privacy in healthcare system. In *2016 Sixth International Conference on Digital Information Processing and Communications (ICDIPC)* (pp. 75–79). Beirut, Lebanon. https://doi.org/DOI: 10.1109/ICDIPC.2016.7470795

Vizitiu, A., Nita, C. I., Puiu, A., Suciu, C., & Itu, L. (2020). Applying deep neural networks over homomorphic encrypted medical data. *Computational and Mathematical Methods in Medicine*, *4*, 1–26. PMID: 32351612

Yan, Y., Zhang, J., Zang, G., & Pu, J. (2019). The primary use of artificial intelligence in cardiovascular diseases: What kind of potential role does artificial intelligence play in future medicine? *Journal of Geriatric Cardiology : JGC*, *16*(8), 585–591. PMID: 31555325

Chapter 12

The Impact of Artificial Intelligence on Human Cognition and Thinking Processes

V. Devaki

https://orcid.org/0000-0002-6091-3173

JECRC University, Jaipur, India

ABSTRACT

The research explores the impact of AI on human cognition, highlighting both the potential benefits and concerns associated with AI technologies. AI systems, such as machine learning and neural networks, have shown remarkable capabilities in tasks like data analysis and problem-solving. However, there are concerns that certain cognitive skills may be diminished as AI takes over traditionally human domains. The lack of transparency in AI algorithms and the possibility of biased algorithms raise ethical and cognitive concerns, impacting how much people trust information and decisions driven by AI. This study underscores the critical role of responsible AI development, transparency, and education in mitigating cognitive drawbacks and maximizing the benefits of AI integration. Maintaining a harmonious equilibrium between human and artificial intelligence requires implementing strategies such as continuous learning programs for human-AI collaboration and incorporating ethical guidelines in AI development.

DOI: 10.4018/979-8-3693-3864-3.ch012

INTRODUCTION

In the rapidly evolving landscape of technology, Artificial Intelligence (AI) stands out as a pivotal branch of computer science, meticulously designed to replicate and simulate the nuances of human intelligence. This fascinating field encompasses a wide array of functionalities, including machine learning, natural language processing, and problem-solving abilities, all aimed at enabling machines to perform tasks that traditionally required human thought and reasoning. As AI technologies become increasingly sophisticated, they are not merely tools but rather integral components of our daily lives, influencing how we think and behave.To fully grasp the implications of AI on the human mind, it is essential to first understand the intricacies of human cognitive functions. These functions encompass a diverse range of mental abilities, including perception, understanding, reasoning, memory, and learning—all of which interact seamlessly to enable us to navigate complex environments, make informed decisions, and acquire new skills. The interplay between these cognitive processes forms the foundation of our intelligence and our ability to adapt to new experiences (Yongjun Xu et al, 2021; Zhang and Tao, 2020; Truong and Papagiannidi; 2022; Levy; Papadopoulou, 2024; Neuroscience; Sample, 2024). This study aims to investigate the multifaceted relationship between AI and human cognition, highlighting the ways in which AI systems not only influence our cognitive functions but also actively reshape them. By examining both the positive outcomes—such as enhanced learning, improved decision-making, and increased efficiency—and the potential drawbacks, including diminished critical thinking skills and reliance on technology, this exploration seeks to provide a comprehensive understanding of how AI is transforming our cognitive landscape. Ultimately, we will uncover the profound implications of this technological evolution, prompting necessary reflections on the future of human intelligence in an age increasingly dominated by intelligent machines.

The profound impact of artificial intelligence (AI) on various aspects of human life continues to grow rapidly, shaping our world in unprecedented ways. This transformative technology is revolutionizing industries, streamlining operations, and affecting everyday activities in countless ways (Bernard, 2021). By analyzing medical imagery such as X-rays, MRIs, and CT scans, AI algorithms can provide faster and more accurate diagnoses. Furthermore, AI can evaluate vast amounts of data to identify potential medication candidates and predict molecular interactions. This has enormous implications for personalized medicine, as AI can analyze patient data to tailor treatment plans and predict disease risks. In short, AI is playing an increasingly critical role in shaping our world, and its potential applications are limited only by our imaginations. As we continue to harness the power of AI, we can expect to see even more profound changes in the ways we live, work, and interact with one another (Dignum, 2019; Hasnain 2023; Sampe; Levy, 2024). Artificial intelligence (AI) is revolutionizing various sectors, bringing about exciting advancements that promise to make our lives easier and better.

The transformative impact of AI is evident in various sectors; for instance, AI-powered personalized medication algorithms have reduced treatment errors by 30% in clinical trials, enhancing patient outcomes and reducing healthcare costs. In the healthcare industry, AI is helping medical practitioners provide personalized treatment programs based on patients' data. Statistical analysis shows that AI algorithms have successfully predicted illness risks with an accuracy rate of over 90%, leading to timely interventions and improved patient outcomes. The integration of AI in transportation has introduced advanced safety features like collision detection systems and predictive maintenance algorithms, ensuring a 40% reduction in accidents and enhancing overall travel safety. AI optimizes traffic flow, predicts congestion, and enhances urban transportation. In the finance industry, AI algorithms are driving high-speed trading decisions based on market trends and data analysis. For instance, AI algorithms have identified fraudulent transactions with 98% accuracy, saving financial institutions millions in potential losses and safeguarding customer assets. In education, AI is helping to personalize the learning experience for students. By integrating instructional content with individual learning styles, preferences, and abilities, AI is improving student engagement and outcomes. Overall, AI is transforming various sectors and opening up new possibilities for innovation and growth. As we continue to embrace this technology, we can look forward to even more exciting advancements in the future (Tschopp & Ruef, 2017; Dhar, P. 2020; Hasnain, 2023; Financial News; Sample; Papadopoulou, 2024; Levy; Neoroscience; 2024).

The rise of artificial intelligence (AI) has been a game-changer in various fields, from healthcare to finance, transportation, and beyond. AI has transformed the way we do things, from increasing efficiency and productivity to creating entirely new products and services. However, the increasing use of AI also raises ethical, legal, and social concerns that need to be addressed (Kelly, J.E. 2015; Scherer, 2016). One of the most significant challenges posed by AI is the question of responsibility. With the increasing use of unmanned vehicles, the question arises: who is responsible if an autonomous car strikes a pedestrian? Current laws and regulations do not address this issue, and it is up to AI developers to determine how to address such situations. Similarly, in the case of global robotic weapon battles, who would be responsible for the actions of these machines? These questions require careful consideration and discussion to ensure that AI is developed and used responsibly. Another concern is the potential for AI to surpass human intelligence and control. While this scenario may seem far-fetched, the idea of machines becoming smarter than humans is not impossible. The development of super-intelligent machines that can operate autonomously could pose a significant threat to humanity. Therefore, it is crucial to ensure that AI is developed in a way that prioritizes human values and safety. As AI continues to advance, it is essential to consider the potential unintended consequences that may arise. Innovations in technology often lead to unexpected outcomes, and AI is no exception. For example, the increasing use of AI in decision-making processes could result in biased decisions that discriminate against certain groups. Therefore, we must be vigilant about ensuring that AI is developed in a way that promotes fairness and equality. (Scherer, 2016; Yongjun et al., 2021).

OBJECTIVES

The study aims to investigate the multifaceted relationship between AI and human cognition, highlighting the ways in which AI systems not only influence our cognitive functions but also actively reshape them. By examining both the positive outcomes—such as enhanced learning, improved decision-making, and increased efficiency—and the potential drawbacks, including diminished critical thinking skills and reliance on technology.

i. To determine how AI technologies affect human cognitive capacities such as information retrieval, memory, problem-solving, and decision-making.
ii. To determine if AI facilitates or obstructs independent analysis and assessment; study how AI-generated insights affect critical thinking processes.

THEORETICAL BACKGROUND

Artificial intelligence (AI) is a term used to describe the ability of machines to perform tasks that would normally require human intervention. AI has been a topic of great interest and importance in recent years, as it has the potential to revolutionize numerous industries and change the way we live our lives. The concept of AI dates back to antiquity, with philosophers and scientists pondering the possibility of creating machines that could think and reason like humans (Ruef, M. 2017; Tschopp, M. andRuef, M. 2017; Hasnain, 2023). However, it wasn't until the 20th century that significant progress was made in the field of AI. The development of computers and digital technology led to breakthroughs in computing power, algorithms, and data availability, which enabled researchers to develop more sophisticated AI systems. Today, AI is used in a wide range of applications, from self-driving cars and virtual assistants to medical diagnosis and financial analysis.

One of the key areas of research in the field of AI is its impact on cognition and thinking. AI systems are designed to replicate, automate, or enhance human-like behavior and intelligence, which raises important questions about the nature of human cognition and the potential consequences of relying on machines for decision-making. Some researchers argue that AI has the potential to augment human intelligence, providing us with new tools and insights that can help us solve complex problems and make more informed decisions. Others are concerned about the potential risks of AI, particularly in areas such as cybersecurity and privacy. There are also concerns about the impact of AI on the job market as machines become increasingly capable of performing tasks that were previously done by humans Hasnain (2023). As AI continues to advance and become more integrated into our daily lives, researchers need to study its impact on cognition and thinking and develop ethical guidelines and best practices for its use.

AI has progressed through several stages:

Figure 1. AI has evolved through several stages

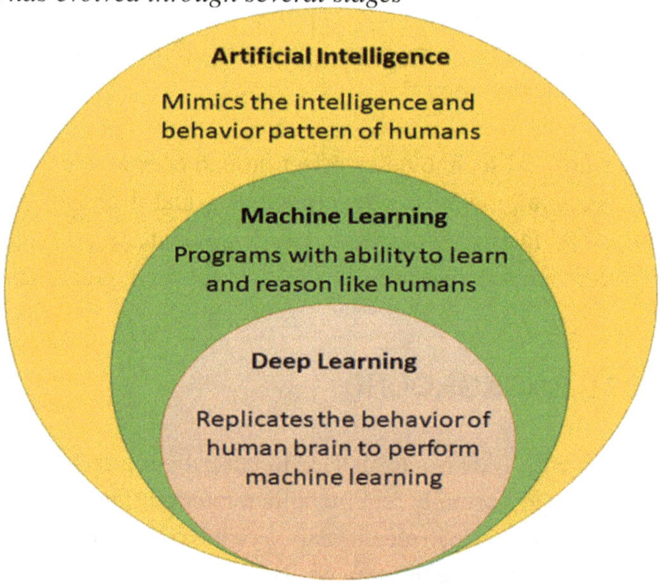

AI has evolved significantly over several decades, marked by advancements in its approaches and technologies. The initial phase, known as algebraic AI, took place from the 1950s to the 1980s and focused on creating rule-based systems that could solve specific problems. However, this approach had its limitations, as it lacked consistency and failed to learn from data. The Age of Machine Learning emerged in the 1980s and continues to this day, marking a significant shift in AI development. This epoch has witnessed the creation of machines that can derive information from data through the use of advanced algorithms. The algorithms utilized in machine learning enable computers to recognize patterns, make predictions, and improve performance based on prior experiences. Overall, the evolution of AI has come a long way, and the advancements made in machine learning have paved the way for the development of even more advanced AI systems in the future. The evolution of artificial intelligence (AI) has been an exciting journey spanning decades.

In the 1950s, the concept of AI was first introduced, and researchers developed rule-based systems to simulate human reasoning. However, this approach had its limitations, and it was not until the 1980s that significant progress was made with the creation of neural networks, decision trees, and other technologies. The field of deep learning emerged in the 2010s, and it revolutionized the way we process complex data such as images, audio, and text. Deep learning employs artificial neural networks with multiple layers to process and analyze information. This period witnessed phenomenal discoveries in image processing and other areas. Today, AI has become an integral part of our lives, with applications in mobile devices, AI-powered assistants, financial services, healthcare, and more. Artificial neural networks have advanced to the point where they can comprehend and create human language, identify objects in photographs and videos, and even make decisions on their own. The progress made so far is remarkable, and we can expect even more exciting developments in the future. Many scholars believe that one of the primary goals of AI research should be to comprehend the nature of learning and implement the ability to learn in machines. This is because learning is so closely tied to intelligent behavior, and advancements in AI research provide us with new insights and powerful tools to study it. (McCarthy, 1983; Schank, 1983). In his insightful theory of thinking, The Society of Mind (Minsky, 1985), he posits that "acquiring knowledge is making useful changes in our minds." Essentially, learning is all about making positive changes that enhance our cognitive abilities and help us become more intelligent. By understanding this process and replicating it in machines, we can create AI that is capable of learning and growing just like humans do. This is a fascinating area of research that has the potential to revolutionize the way we think about artificial intelligence and its role in society.

UNDERSTANDING COGNITIVE FUNCTIONS

Human cognition is a complex interplay of several essential components, each contributing uniquely to our understanding and interaction with the world (Yongjun Xu et al, 2021; Zhang and Tao, 2020; Truong and Papagiannidi; 2022; Hasnain 2023; Neuroscience; Levy, Finanical; Sample, 2024)

i. Perception: This refers to the intricate process through which we interpret and make sense of the sensory information we receive from our surroundings. It encompasses the detection of stimuli through our five senses and the subsequent integration of that information into a coherent understanding of the world around us.
ii. Attention: Attention is the mental mechanism that allows us to concentrate on specific pieces of information while intentionally sidelining distractions. It plays a crucial role in how we prioritize our cognitive resources, enabling us to navigate complex environments and focus on what is most relevant.
iii. Memory: Memory can be viewed as the mental library where we store and retrieve information over time. It includes various types—such as short-term and long-term memory—and is fundamental to learning, allowing us to recall past experiences, facts, and skills that shape our identity and inform our decisions.
iv. Problem-Solving: This cognitive function involves a series of mental processes aimed at identifying solutions to obstacles or challenges we encounter. It requires critical thinking, creativity, and logic, enabling us to analyze situations, generate potential solutions, and implement strategies to overcome difficulties.
v. Decision-Making: Decision-making is the cognitive process in which we weigh various options and make choices based on the information available to us. It involves assessing risks and benefits, considering potential outcomes, and sometimes relying on heuristics—mental shortcuts that simplify decision-making.

Cognitive biases are systematic patterns of deviation from norm or rationality in judgment, often leading to illogical conclusions or decisions. These biases can significantly influence human thought processes, introducing errors in perception, memory, and reasoning. For instance, confirmation bias leads individuals to favor information that confirms their existing beliefs while disregarding conflicting data. Similarly, availability heuristic may cause people to overestimate the importance of information that is readily available or recent in their memory. Such biases not only impact decision-making but can also create barriers to critical thinking and objective analysis, reinforcing the need for self-awareness and strategies to mitigate their influence in our cognitive processes.

How Artificial Intelligence Affects Cognition and Thought Processes is Crucial for Several Reasons

Artificial intelligence (AI) has the potential to enhance human cognitive capacities through cognitive augmentation, which involves data processing, decision-making, and problem-solving. This can lead to increased human efficacy and productivity. Critical thinking, a fundamental component of good decision-making, is closely related to cognitive processes. Understanding AI's impact on cognitive processes can help people, educators, and legislators prepare for the future. AI is rapidly transforming our lives, from self-driving cars to virtual assistants. However, ethical concerns arise as we increasingly rely on AI for decision-making. To ensure successful collaborations, it is crucial to understand how people use AI tools and how AI enhances human cognitive abilities. Exploring how AI affects cognitive functions can provide valuable insights into the skills required in an AI-dominated future. Educators can use this information to develop courses that prioritize abilities specific to human cognition (Shi and Li, 2018; Zhang and Tao, 2020; Hasnain, 2023). AI's influence extends beyond individual experiences and can transform society, from social structures to employment positions and economic models. To make well-informed decisions that maximize AI's benefits while preserving essential qualities of human intelligence and critical thought, we must have a thorough grasp of these ramifications. Understanding the impact of AI on cognition and thought processes is crucial for progress and development in the technological age.

Figure 2. The domain structure of the cognitive process

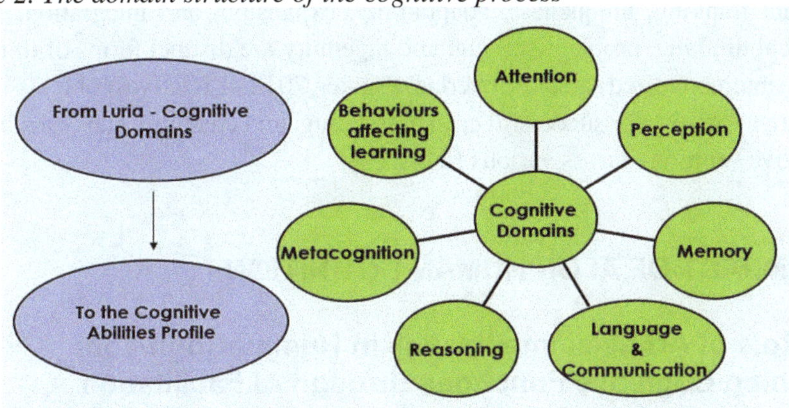

Adapted from Alexander Luria's concepts (1980)

The cognitive process comprises several components, including perception, attention, memory, language processing, reasoning, problem-solving, decision-making, creativity, and meta-cognition. These processes are interconnected and form the basis of human thinking, learning, problem-solving, and decision-making. Perception involves the brain's acquisition and interpretation of sensory information, attention involves prioritizing and analyzing information, memory stores and retrieves information over time, reasoning involves deriving conclusions and logical inferences, problem-solving involves identifying and evaluating solutions, decision-making involves selecting one option, creativity generates unique ideas, and meta-cognition involves self-correction Yongjun Xu et al, 2021; Zhang andTao, 2020; Truong and Papagiannidi; 2022; Neuroscience; Elana; Levy; Sample, 2024). Understanding these processes provides insights into how individuals receive information, adapt to new situations, and engage in complex mental tasks.

Various Aspects of Thinking: Critical Thinking, Problem-Solving, and Creativity

Critical thinking involves objectively examining and evaluating information to arrive at well-reasoned conclusions. It involves breaking down complex information, assessing its credibility, and drawing logical conclusions. Critical thinkers approach information with skepticism and aim to arrive at well-reasoned conclusions. Problem-solving involves identifying and resolving challenges through rational and creative approaches. Key characteristics of problem-solving include problem recognition, analysis, solution generation, evaluation, and execution (Zhang andTao, 2020; Truong andPapagiannidis, 2022). Ingenuity involves creating fresh ideas and solutions and incorporating new perspectives. Key components of creativity include divergent thinking, uniqueness, adaptability, expansion, and integration. While analytical thinking, problem-solving, and ingenuity are distinct forms of thinking, they are interconnected and often overlap. (Pinker, 2018). Effective problem-solving skills are necessary for successful critical thinking, and creativity can contribute to innovative solutions across various fields.

THE IMPACT OF AI ON HUMAN COGNITION

The Role of Artificial Intelligence in Human Cognition: Enriching Cognitive Functions through AI Facilitation

AI systems have an extraordinary capability to store, analyze, and process vast amounts of information, which significantly enhances memory and improves the efficiency of information retrieval. These sophisticated technologies function as external memory banks, enabling individuals to effortlessly access and recall data with remarkable speed and precision. By leveraging advanced algorithms and machine learning techniques, AI systems can not only store information but also categorize and retrieve it in ways that align with users' specific needs. This capability transforms the way we interact with information, allowing for seamless integration into daily decision-making processes and enhancing overall productivity. Furthermore, with constant advancements in natural language processing and other AI fields, these systems continue to evolve, becoming increasingly adept at understanding context and delivering relevant information tailored to individual preferences. The incorporation of AI in data analysis transforms decision-making processes (Hasnain, 2023; Levy; Papadopoulou, 2024; Neuorscience; Sample, 2024) . By sifting through large datasets, AI tools reveal patterns and insights that may not be immediately apparent, leading to more informed and strategic choices. By providing tools and technologies that complement and extend our natural cognitive processes, AI has the potential to significantly enhance human cognitive capacities. These AI-driven technologies can assist with tasks such as data analysis, pattern recognition, decision-making, and information retrieval, leading to more informed and efficient outcomes (Shi and Li, 2018).

Specimens of AI-Powered Tools:

i. AI algorithms can analyze vast amounts of data to generate valuable insights that assist in decision-making processes (Decision Support Systems).
ii. AI-driven data analysis tools can help identify patterns, trends, and correlations in large datasets. This is particularly beneficial in scientific research, medical diagnostics, and business intelligence.
iii. AI-assisted solutions can act as external memory boosters helping individuals remember important knowledge by providing instant access to relevant data, notes, and resources.
iv. AI systems can utilize spaced repetition techniques to deliver information at appropriate intervals, thereby improving long-term memory.
v. AI-powered language learning applications offer real-time feedback on pronunciation and grammar, accelerating the learning process.

AI-powered cognitive training programs offer a variety of workouts and activities designed to enhance memory, concentration, and problem-solving skills. Through AI-driven simulations and interactive experiences, learners can gain a deeper understanding of subjects by actively exploring them. While AI holds great potential for improving cognitive abilities, it is crucial to strike a balance between AI-assisted activities and the preservation of critical thinking, creativity, and human judgment. As these technologies continue to advance, it is important to address ethical concerns surrounding data confidentiality, bias, and the potential over-reliance on AI tools.

Analyzing the Potential for Cognitive Decline

The increasing reliance on AI tools raises significant concerns regarding the gradual erosion of individual cognitive skills. As people become more dependent on these technologies for essential tasks such as remembering important information, making decisions, or solving complex problems, there is a risk that their own mental faculties may begin to weaken. This over-dependence can create a cycle where individuals, feeling less confident in their cognitive abilities, may choose to rely even more on AI, further hindering their mental development (Hasnain, 2023; Financial Time; Levy; Papadopoulou, 2024; Neuroscience; Sample, 2024). Furthermore, as tasks traditionally managed by humans become increasingly delegated to AI systems, the complexity of these tasks may lead to diminished problem-solving capabilities among individuals. When AI handles intricate and challenging issues on behalf of users, it could result in a significant loss of the mental agility and critical thinking skills that are crucial for navigating real-world challenges independently. Over time, this could foster a generation that is less equipped to think creatively or approach problems with the necessary analytical mindset, ultimately impacting both personal growth and societal innovation. With readily available solutions at their fingertips, individuals may find themselves stunted in their cognitive development, potentially stifling innovative thought and the ability to evaluate situations from multiple perspectives. This raises important questions about the long-term effects on human cognition in an increasingly AI-driven world.

The Significance of Critical Thinking: AI's Role in Automating Routine Tasks and Liberating Cognitive Resources

Artificial intelligence (AI) has revolutionized various aspects of human life, particularly through its ability to automate tasks. One of the key advantages of AI is its capacity to handle repetitive and mundane jobs, which has significant implications for freeing up cognitive resources in individuals (Furber, F. 2016). This phenomenon has had a transformative impact on numerous fields and disciplines.

1. Routine Task Automation refers to the utilization of AI technologies, such as machine learning and robots, to effectively perform activities that follow established routines. AI can automate tasks that involve minimal cognitive involvement, such as data input, document categorization, inventory management, and basic customer support queries (Stone, P. et al., 2016). This automation leads to increased productivity, reduced errors, and faster performance.
2. The allocation of cognitive resources is limited, including memory, attention, and problem-solving abilities (Hasnain, 2023; Elena, 2024; Financial Time; Levy; Papadopoulou, 2024; Neuroscience; Sample, 2024). When individuals are relieved of repetitive tasks through AI automation, they can redirect their cognitive assets toward higher-level tasks that require critical thinking and decision-making. This enables experts to allocate their cognitive resources to tasks that genuinely require human expertise. Moreover, with the liberation of cognitive resources, individuals can engage in more in-depth problem-solving.

They can analyze complex challenges, identify patterns, and explore innovative solutions (Yongjun Xu et al, 2021; Zhang andTao, 2020; Truong and Papagiannidi; 2022; Levy; Elana; Neuroscience,Sample, 2024). Furthermore, creativity and innovation heavily rely on cognitive resources.

a) Individuals can focus on higher-level tasks that demand critical thinking and decision-making when they are freed from repetitive duties. This allows experts to dedicate their cognitive abilities to tasks that genuinely necessitate human expertise.
b) Higher Resolving issues: Individuals can participate in more profound problem-solving now that their cognitive resources are no longer tied up in regular routines. They can analyze difficult challenges, recognize structures, and explore novel solutions.
c) Innovation and creation: Creativity and invention require cognitive resources. Individuals have greater mental space to produce fresh ideas and approaches when mundane jobs are offloaded to AI, which contributes to organizational innovation.
d) Reduced Mental Exhaustion: Reduced Mental Exhaustion: Consistently engaging in mundane tasks can lead to mental fatigue and weariness. By automating these tasks, AI reduces the cognitive load, promoting better psychological well-being and enhancing long-term thinking abilities.

3. Impact in Various Industries: The significance of AI in automating everyday processes extends to a wide range of industries, such as manufacturing, finance, healthcare, customer service, and education. Robots equipped with AI can automate assembly line jobs, resulting in increased productivity and accuracy. AI algorithms in healthcare assist with tasks like medical image processing and administrative work, allowing medical professionals to focus more on patient care.
4. Ethical Considerations: While the role of AI in relieving cognitive burden offers significant benefits, ethical concerns arise. The potential for job losses due to automation necessitates the need for individuals to upgrade their skills and adapt to new work environments. Additionally, relying too heavily on AI for managerial decisions without human supervision may lead to unforeseen consequences. On the whole, AI's ability to automate basic tasks represents an evolutionary shift that frees up cognitive resources for higher-level thinking, problem-solving, and innovation.

IMPACT OF AI-GENERATED INSIGHTS ON THINKING CRITICALLY AND DECISION-MAKING

The utilization of artificial intelligence (AI) has become a powerful tool for generating suggestions and insights through statistical analysis. These insights from AI have the potential to significantly influence how critical thinking and decision-making occur in different fields. While they offer advantages such as speed and impartiality, these technologies also raise concerns about reliability, biases, and human supervision. (Bughin, Hazan and Ramaswamy, et al. 2017; Elena, 2024; Financial Time; Levy; Papadopoulou, 2024; Neuroscience; Sample, 2024)

- Enhancing Efficiency and Data Processing: AI can rapidly analyze vast datasets, uncovering connections and patterns that humans may overlook. This accuracy in data analysis provides executives with a more comprehensive and holistic view of the situation, empowering them to make decisions with increased confidence.
- Challenging Assumptions and Biases: AI-generated insights have the potential to challenge human assumptions and biases by promoting alternative perspectives. This can enhance critical thinking by enabling decision-makers to address biased ideas and consider options they may have otherwise overlooked.
- Lessening Cognitive Stack: Addressing Moral, Cultural, and Economic Concerns: While reaping the benefits of expanding automation, it is crucial to address the moral, cultural, and economic concerns that arise. The effort to tackle these concerns must be equal to the effort put into harnessing the advantages of automation across various sectors.

AI-generated insights have the potential to alleviate the cognitive burden on decision-makers by providing significant data and analysis. This allows decision-makers to shift their focus towards evaluating the implications and consequences of their choices, rather than spending excessive time gathering and processing information.

Impediments and Ethical Contemplation

AI algorithms can contain biases, which can impact the accuracy and relevance of the information they generate. It is crucial to address these biases to ensure the accuracy of AI-generated insights. Blind trust and a need for relevant understanding are also essential for AI to make informed decisions. Integrating human and AI commitments is essential for making informed decisions. Human supervision is essential for ethical, legal, or social decisions (Yongjun Xu et al, 2021; Zhang andTao, 2020; Truong and Papagiannidi; 2022; Sample; Levy; Elana, 2024). AI-generated insights can enhance critical thinking skills by examining how AI arrives at conclusions and identifying potential biases. Ultimately, AI can significantly impact human thinking and decision-making by improving efficiency and presenting new ideas based on scientific evidence.

Exploring Potential Challenges: Over-dependence on AI Input

The inclusion of artificial intelligence (AI) and the way it works in presenting ideas and information generates an array of possible obstacles, among which is the danger of excessive reliance on AI-generated suggestions. When artificial intelligence (AI) can assist with making decisions, depending heavily on its suggestions may have adverse implications and degrade critical human cognitive skills (Zhang andTao, 2020;Hasnain 2023;; Elena, 2024; Financial Time; Levy; Papadopoulou, 2024; Neuroscience; Sample, 2024). The reliance on AI for decision-making may lead to a decline in intellectual thinking, insufficient validation, failure to consider context and complexity, ethical and moral considerations, and suppression of innovative thinking. This could result in blindness to AI's authenticity, deception, and wrong choices. Additionally, AI may overlook ethical and moral considerations, leading to decisions without social accountability. Therefore, it is crucial to balance the benefits of AI with the potential drawbacks.

EMOTIONAL AND SOCIAL COGNITION

Investigating AI's Role in Shaping Interpersonal Relationships and Communication Patterns

Artificial intelligence (AI) is increasingly shaping interpersonal relationships and communication patterns, influencing how individuals engage emotionally and socially. AI-driven technologies, such as chat-bots, virtual assistants, and recommendation systems, are altering human interactions by mediating conversations, personalizing content, and even simulating empathy. These advancements raise questions about the impact on social cognition—how people perceive, interpret, and respond to others in digital environments. While AI enhances connectivity and provides emotional support, it also risks diminishing authentic human interaction, leading to potential challenges in empathy development and social skills (Hasnain, 2023; Elena, 2024; Levy; Papadopoulou, 2024; Neuroscience; Sample, 2024). Understanding AI's role in shaping emotional and social cognition is crucial for designing ethical and effective AI-driven communication tools that foster meaningful human connections.

As AI systems become more integrated into daily communication, their influence on emotional and social cognition grows increasingly complex. AI-powered chat-bots and virtual companions, such as Replika and Xiaoice, are designed to engage users in emotionally responsive conversations, sometimes offering companionship and mental health support. Social media algorithms shape users' perceptions by curating content that reinforces certain beliefs and emotional responses, potentially affecting social cognition by fostering echo chambers or amplifying emotional polarization. In professional settings, AI-driven communication tools like automated email respondents and sentiment analysis software influence workplace interactions by setting the tone for digital communication. While these advancements offer benefits such as increased accessibility, personalized interaction, and enhanced efficiency, they also raise ethical and psychological concerns. Over-reliance on AI for emotional support may weaken real-world social bonds, reducing the depth and authenticity of human relationships (Hasnain, 2023; Elena, 2024; Financial Time; Levy; Papadopoulou, 2024; Neuroscience; Sample, 2024). Additionally, AI's limitations in understanding nuanced human emotions can lead to misinterpretations, affecting decision-making and emotional well-being. As AI continues to evolve, it is crucial to examine its role in shaping emotional intelligence, empathy, and social behavior, ensuring that technology complements rather than replaces genuine human connection.

Assessing AI's Influence on Empathy and Emotional Intelligence

Artificial Intelligence (AI) is playing an increasingly prominent role in shaping human emotional intelligence and empathy, raising critical questions about its long-term impact. AI-driven tools, such as emotion recognition software, sentiment analysis systems, and virtual companions, are designed to interpret and respond to human emotions. These technologies are widely used in mental health support, customer service, and social interactions, offering personalized responses based on emotional cues (Yongjun Xu et al, 2021; Zhang and Tao, 2020; Truong and Papagiannidi; 2022; Hasnain, 2023). While AI can enhance emotional awareness by providing real-time feedback and training individuals in recognizing emotions, its effectiveness in fostering genuine empathy remains debatable.

One of the key concerns is whether AI can truly understand and express empathy or if it merely simulates empathetic responses based on data-driven patterns. Unlike human empathy, which involves deep emotional connection and subjective experience, AI operates on algorithms that predict and mirror human emotions without actual comprehension. This raises ethical questions about the authenticity of AI-mediated interactions, especially in fields such as therapy, education, and social work, where emotional intelligence plays a vital role. Moreover, excessive reliance on AI for emotional engagement may reduce human-to-human interactions, potentially weakening individuals' ability to develop and practice genuine empathy.

On the other hand, AI can serve as a valuable tool for improving emotional intelligence by helping individuals develop self-awareness and communication skills. AI-powered coaching platforms, for instance, provide users with feedback on their tone, facial expressions, and language, allowing them to refine their interpersonal skills. Additionally, AI-driven simulations in healthcare and education enable professionals to practice responding to emotionally charged situations, ultimately strengthening their empathy in real-world scenarios (Yongjun Xu et al, 2021; Zhang andTao, 2020; Truong and Papagiannidi; 2022; Sample, 2024). As AI continues to evolve, its role in shaping emotional intelligence and empathy must be carefully examined. While AI offers promising applications in enhancing emotional awareness and training, it is essential to ensure that these technologies complement rather than replace human emotional connections. Ethical considerations, transparency in AI design, and a balanced approach to AI-human interactions will be crucial in determining whether AI contributes positively or disrupts the fundamental aspects of human empathy and emotional intelligence.

Exploring Challenges Presented by AI in Social Contexts

The integration of AI in social contexts presents a range of challenges that can significantly impact the fabric of interpersonal relationships and societal dynamics. One of the primary concerns is the potential for AI to disrupt authentic human connections by mediating interactions in ways that may appear superficial or inauthentic. For example, AI-powered social platforms often prioritize engagement through algorithms that can inadvertently create echo chambers or amplify misinformation, thereby deepening social divides and reinforcing existing biases (Hasnain, 2023; Elena, 2024; Financial Time; Levy; Papadopoulou, 2024; Neuroscience; Sample, 2024). Privacy is another critical issue, as the extensive use of AI to analyze behavioral data raises concerns about surveillance and data misuse, potentially eroding public trust. Additionally, over-reliance on AI for social interactions might diminish opportunities for individuals to develop crucial interpersonal skills and genuine empathy, ultimately weakening the social cohesion necessary for resilient communities. Addressing these challenges requires a balanced approach that includes transparent ethical frameworks, robust data protection policies, and a continuous evaluation of AI's societal impact to ensure that technology serves to enhance, rather than compromise, human social experiences.

ANALYSIS OF AI'S INFLUENCE ON LEARNING

Artificial Intelligence (AI) has the potential to profoundly transform the educational landscape by addressing the diverse needs and preferences of students. By integrating adaptive technologies into the learning process, educators can develop highly personalized educational experiences tailored to each individual's unique learning style, pace, and preferences. For instance, AI-powered platforms can analyze students' performance in real-time, allowing teachers to identify areas of strength and weakness. This enables the implementation of targeted interventions that support struggling learners while also challenging advanced students. Moreover, these technologies can offer personalized content recommendations, ensuring that students engage with materials that resonate with their interests and abilities (Hasnain, 2023; Elena, 2024; Levy, 2024). Incorporating AI not only enhances instructional strategies but also fosters a more inclusive environment where learners of all backgrounds can thrive. By moving away from a one-size-fits-all approach, educational systems can cultivate a more effective, engaging, and supportive learning atmosphere that ultimately leads to improved outcomes for all students.

Adaptive Learning Technologies

Adaptive learning technologies harness advanced, data-driven algorithms to evaluate individual student performance with precision and personalize educational content to meet unique needs. For example, platforms such as Dream-box Learning and Smart Sparrow dynamically adjust the difficulty and complexity of lessons in real-time, providing immediate, contextual feedback that aligns with each learner's specific skill level. This capability allows educators to gain insights into each student's understanding, identifying areas of difficulty and strength more effectively. By pinpointing gaps in comprehension, these technologies can recommend targeted resources and tailored exercises that address students' individual learning styles and paces. This personalized approach not only promotes deeper mastery of subjects but also encourages greater student engagement, as learners are continuously challenged at levels that are suitable for their development (Hasnain, 2023; Levy; Sample, 2024). Moreover, as students take ownership of their educational journey—tracking their own progress and achievements—they often experience heightened motivation and confidence, ultimately fostering a more positive attitude toward learning as a lifelong endeavor.

Risks of Artificial Intelligence in the Field of Education

Artificial Intelligence (AI) has undoubtedly revolutionized various industries, including education. However, along with its benefits, there are inherent risks associated with the integration of AI in educational settings. One significant concern is the potential loss of human interaction in the learning process. While AI can provide personalized learning experiences, it may lack the empathy and understanding that human educators offer. This could result in a disconnect between students and their learning environment, impacting their overall academic and emotional development. Moreover, the reliance on AI systems in education raises concerns about data privacy and security (Levy, 2024). As AI algorithms collect and analyze massive amounts of student data, there is a heightened risk of data breaches and misuse. Safeguarding sensitive information and ensuring compliance with privacy regulations become paramount challenges for educational institutions adopting AI technologies. Another risk posed by AI in education is the perpetuation of biases and inequalities. AI systems are only as unbiased as the data they are trained on, which can reflect societal prejudices and stereotypes (Truong and Papagiannidis, 2022; Elena, 2024; Levy, 2024). This can lead to discriminatory outcomes in areas such as student assessments, admissions processes, and resource allocation. Addressing these biases requires constant monitoring, evaluation, and adjustment of AI algorithms to promote fairness and equity in educational practices. while AI offers immense potential to enhance learning experiences and outcomes in education, it is crucial to acknowledge and mitigate the risks it brings. By fostering a balance between technological advancement and human-centered approaches, educators can harness the benefits of AI while safeguarding against its potential pitfalls. Embracing a thoughtful and responsible integration of AI in education is essential to ensure equitable, inclusive, and effective learning environments for all students.

CONCLUSION

The field of artificial intelligence (AI) has made significant progress in recent years, thanks to the combination of AI systems with cognitive psychology. This combination has allowed for the development of machines that can replicate human cognition, learn and think like humans, and identify the skills required to perform various day-to-day activities. However, it is important to note that AI still has a long way to go before it can fully replicate the complete spectrum of human intellectual capacities. While AI has surpassed certain specialized duties and sectors, it still falls short of humans' broad cognitive abilities and flexibility. Human cognitive ability includes a wide range of competencies, such as creativity, abstract mental processing, behavioral intelligence, and decision-making based on ethics, which are yet to be fully attained by artificially intelligent machines. Thus, it is evident that humans and artificial agents will collaborate in the inevitable future regarding intellectual activity. The working relationships between humans and AI are already taking place in various tasks related to cognition, which is leading to the prompt incorporation of AI into human brain functions. This incorporation of AI into human brain functions is rapidly expanding and transforming the way we live and work. The integration of AI into various industries, such as healthcare, education, and manufacturing, is revolutionizing the way these sectors function, providing greater efficiency and accuracy in their operations (Truong and Papagiannidi, 2022; Hasnain, 2023; Levy, 2024). Furthermore, the use of AI in the field of healthcare is particularly noteworthy. AI systems are being used to diagnose and treat various diseases, including cancer, in ways that were not possible before. AI is also being used to improve patient outcomes by providing personalized medical care and reducing the chances of medical errors.

The combination of AI systems with cognitive psychology is advancing the field of artificial intelligence, and the future of AI-human collaboration is promising. While there is still much work to be done before AI can fully replicate human cognitive abilities, the progress that has been made thus far is impressive. The integration of AI into various industries is transforming the way we live and work, and the possibilities for the future are endless. How people connect and engage with information is a crucial aspect of modern society. To understand how this collaborative labor is organized, it is necessary to have a framework of concepts and theories that have been proven through extensive research. Exploring the interplay between artificial cognition and human interaction is crucial in various contexts, such as email communication and social media trends. Understanding how these interactions are organized requires a solid framework built on proven concepts and research. Whether it's in healthcare, business, or education, each context demands unique approaches. By shifting the focus from intelligence to cognition in the study of human-machine communication, researchers and practitioners can effectively design cognitive systems without relying on the unrealistic notion of artificial general intelligence. However, it is important to note that there are certain limitations to this approach. While computers can certainly emulate the reasoning of superior humans, they are not capable of replicating the full range of human cognitive processes. As a result, we must hold off on the false assumption of artificial general intelligence becoming a reality and instead focus on creating systems that are optimized for collaboration and cooperation between humans and machines.

REFERENCES

Bernard, M. (2021). What's the impact of artificial intelligence and technology on society? Available at: https://bernardmarr.com/whats-the-impact-of-artificial-intelligence-and-technology-on-society/

. Bughin J., Hazan E., and Ramaswamy S. et al. (2017). Artificial intelligence: the next digital frontier? Information security and communications privacy.

Dhar, P. (2020). The Carbon Impact of Artificial Intelligence. *Nature Machine Intelligence*, *2*, 423–425.

Dignum, V. (2019). *Responsible Artificial Intelligence: How to Develop and Use AI Responsibly. Artificial Intelligence: Foundations, Theory, and Algorithms, Springer.* International Publishing.

Elena, P. A. P. (2024). The Impact of Artificial Intelligence on Psychological and Cognitive Development. Retrieved from https://elenapap.com/en/the-impact-of-artificial-intelligence-on-psychological-and-cognitive-development?utm

Furber, F. (2016). *Artificial Intelligence vs. the Human Brain*. Huffington.

. Hasnain (2023). Artificial Intelligence Relationship with Human Cognitive Power.

Kelly, J. E. (2015). Computing, cognition, and the future of knowing How Humans and machines are forging a new age of Understanding. White Paper, IBM Research

Levy, S. (2024). AI will understand humans better than humans do. WIRED. Retrieved from https://www.wired.com/story/plaintext-ai-will-understand-humans-better-than-humans-do

. Minsky, M. (1985). The Society of Mind. Simon andSchuster.

Neuroscience News. (2024). How AI is reshaping human thought and decision-making. Retrieved from https://neurosciencenews.com/ai-human-decision-thought-28911/

Papadopoulou, E. (2024). The impact of artificial intelligence on psychological and cognitive development. Retrieved from https://elenapap.com/en/the-impact-of-artificial-intelligence-on-psychological-and-cognitive-development

Pinker, S. (2018). *Enlightenment Now: A Manifesto for Science, Reason, Humanism, and Progress*. Allen Lane.

Ruef, M. (2017). Artificial Intelligence: A Model for Humanity, SCIP AG. https://www.scip.ch/?labs.20180104

Sample, I. (2024). AI can change belief in conspiracy theories, study finds. The Guardian. Retrieved from https://www.theguardian.com/science/2024/sep/12/ai-can-change-belief-in-conspiracy-theories-study-finds

. Scherer, M.U. (2016). Regulating Artificial Intelligence Systems: Risks, Challenges, Competencies, and Strategies. Harvard Journal of Law andTechnology, 29, 48.

Shi, Y., & Li, C. (2018). "Exploration of computer emotion decision based on artificial intelligence," in *Proceedings of the 2018 International Conference on Virtual Reality and Intelligent Systems (ICVRIS)* (Hunan: IEEE), 293–295. Available at: https://doi.org/DOI: 10.1109/ICVRIS.2018.00078

Stone, P.. (2016). *Artificial Intelligence and Life in 2030. One Hundred Year Study on Artificial Intelligence: Report of the 2015–2016 Study Panel*. Stanford University.

Truong, Y., & Papagiannidis, S. (2022). Artificial Intelligence as an Enabler for Innovation: A Review and Future Research Agenda. *Technological Forecasting and Social Change*, *183*, 121852.

Tschopp, M. & Ruef, M. (2017). Development of an Artificial Intelligence Quotient. Available at: https://www.iaiqs.org/

Xu, Y.. (2021). Artificial intelligence is a powerful paradigm for scientific research. *The Innovation*, *2*(4), 100179. DOI: 10.1016/j.xinn.2021.100179 PMID: 34877560

Xu, Y.. (2024). *2021; Zhang andTao, 2020; Truong and Papagiannidi; 2022*. Sample.

Zhang, J., & Tao, D. J. (2020). Empowering things with intelligence: A survey of the progress, challenges, and opportunities in the artificial intelligence of things. *IEEE Internet of Things Journal*, *8*, 7789–7817.

Compilation of References

AbuKhousa, E., Mohamed, N., & Al-Jaroodi, J. (2012). e-Health cloud: Opportunities and challenges. *Future Internet*, *4*(3), 621–645.

Aghdam, Z. N., Rahmani, A. M., & Hosseinzadeh, M. (2021). The role of the Internet of Things in healthcare: Future trends and challenges. *Computer Methods and Programs in Biomedicine*, *199*, 105903. PMID: 33348073

Ahanger, T. A., Tariq, U., Nusir, M., Aldaej, A., Ullah, I., & Sulman, A. (2022). A novel IoT–fog–cloud-based healthcare system for monitoring and predicting COVID-19 outspread. *The Journal of Supercomputing*, *78*(2), 1783–1806. PMID: 34177116

Ahmed, A., Shahzad, A., Naseem, A., Ali, S., & Ahmad, I. (2025). Evaluating the effectiveness of data governance frameworks in ensuring security and privacy of healthcare data: A quantitative analysis of ISO standards, GDPR, and HIPAA in blockchain technology. *PLoS One*, *20*(5), e0324285. PMID: 40408373

Ahmed, I., Ahmad, A., & Jeon, G. (2021). An IoT-based deep learning framework for early assessment of COVID-19. *IEEE Internet of Things Journal*, *8*(21), 15855–15862. DOI: 10.1109/JIOT.2020.3034074 PMID: 35782174

AI Global Healthcare Initiative. (n.d.). *AI Global Healthcare Initiative: Revolutionizing patient care and medical innovation*. AI Global Healthcare Initiative. Retrieved March 25, 2025, from https://healthcareproducts.org/ai/aighi

Akhila, S., Rani, D. M., Divyashree, D., & Varshini, S. S. (2016). Smart stick for blind using Raspberry Pi. [IJERT]. *International Journal of Engineering Research & Technology (Ahmedabad)*, *4*(22).

Akhil, P., Akshara, R., Athira, R., Kumar, S., Thamotharan, M., & Christila, S. D. (2022). Smart blind walking stick with integrated sensor. *Materials Proceedings*, *12*. Advance online publication. DOI: 10.3390/materproc2022010012

Akhtar, F., Li, J., Pei, Y., Imran, A., Rajput, A., Azeem, M., & Wang, Q. (2019). Diagnosis and prediction of large-for-gestational-age fetus using the stacked generalization method. *Applied Sciences (Basel, Switzerland)*, *9*(20), 4317.

Akseer, R., Connolly, M., Cosby, J., Frost, G., Kanagarajah, R. R., & Lim, S. H. E. (2021). Clinician–patient relationships after two decades of a paradigm of patient-centered care. *International Journal of Healthcare Management*, *14*(3), 888–897.

Al Alkeem, E., Yeun, C. Y., & Zemerly, M. J. (2015). Security and privacy framework for ubiquitous healthcare IoT devices. In *Proceedings of the 10th IEEE International Conference for Internet Technology and Secured Transactions (ICITST)* (pp. 70–75). London, UK.

Alaba, F. A., Othman, M., Hashem, I. A. T., & Alotaibi, F. (2017). Internet of Things security: A survey. *Journal of Network and Computer Applications*, *88*, 10–28.

Alabi, M. (2023). Data Governance and Quality: Ensuring Data Reliability and Trustworthiness. *ResearchGate, October*.

Albarrak, M. M., Zakaria, N., & Meo, S. A. (2024). The role of mobile health applications (mHealth apps) in reshaping the body weight for better healthcare: A cross-sectional study. *Pakistan Journal of Medical Sciences*, *40*(9), 1930–1936. DOI: 10.12669/pjms.40.9.9064 PMID: 39416646

Alghanim, A. A., Rahman, S. M. M., & Hossain, M. A. (2017). Privacy analysis of smart city healthcare services. In *Proceedings of the 2017 IEEE International Symposium on Multimedia (ISM)* (pp. 394–398). Taichung, Taiwan.

Ali, I., Sabir, S., & Ullah, Z. (2019). Internet of things security, device authentication and access control: a review. *arXiv preprint arXiv:1901.07309*.

Almalawi, A., Khan, A. I., Alsolami, F., Abushark, Y. B., Alfakeeh, A. S., & Mekuriyaw, W. D. (2022). Analysis of the exploration of security and privacy for healthcare management using artificial intelligence: Saudi hospitals. *Computational Intelligence and Neuroscience*, *4048197*. Advance online publication. DOI: 10.1155/2022/4048197 PMID: 36156966

Almalki, F. A., & Soufiene, B. O. (2021). EPPDA: An efficient and privacy-preserving data aggregation scheme with authentication and authorization for IoT-based healthcare applications. *Wireless Communications and Mobile Computing*, *5594159*. Advance online publication. DOI: 10.1155/2021/5594159

Ambarkar, S. S., & Shekokar, N. (2020). Toward smart and secure IoT based healthcare system. *Internet of things, smart computing and technology: A roadmap ahead*, pp.283-303.

Amin, J., Sharif, M., Raza, M., Saba, T., & Anjum, M. A. (2019). Brain tumor detection using statistical and machine learning method. *Computer Methods and Programs in Biomedicine*, *177*, 69–79. DOI: 10.1016/j.cmpb.2019.05.016 PMID: 31319962

Amin, J., Sharif, M., Yasmin, M., & Fernandes, S. L. (2020). A distinctive approach in brain tumor detection and classification using MRI. *Pattern Recognition Letters*, *139*, 118–127. DOI: 10.1016/j.patrec.2020.07.014

Amin, S. U., & Hossain, M. S. (2021). Edge intelligence and Internet of Things in healthcare: A survey. *IEEE Access : Practical Innovations, Open Solutions*, *9*, 45–59. DOI: 10.1109/ACCESS.2020.3045115

An IoT-based heart healthcare platform for the Sultanate of Oman. (2022, October 27). IEEE Conference Publication. https://doi.org/DOI: 10.1109/MA-JICC56935.2022.9994183

Antwi, E., Amoakoh-Coleman, M., Vieira, D. L., Madhavaram, S., Koram, K. A., Grobbee, D. E., & Klipstein-Grobusch, K. (2020). Systematic review of prediction models for gestational hypertension and preeclampsia. *PLoS One*, *15*(4), e0230955. PMID: 32315307

Anwar, S. M., Majid, M., Qayyum, A., Awais, M., Alnowami, M., & Khan, M. K. (2018). Medical image analysis using convolutional neural networks: A review. *Journal of Medical Systems*, *42*, 1–13. DOI: 10.1007/s10916-018-1045-1 PMID: 30298337

Archip, A., ... (2016). An IoT based system for remote patient monitoring. In *2016 17th International Carpathian Control Conference (ICCC)*. IEEE.

Arisdakessian, S., Wahab, O. A., Mourad, A., Otrok, H., & Guizani, M. (2023). A survey on IoT intrusion detection: Federated learning, game theory, social psychology, and explainable AI as future directions. *IEEE Internet of Things Journal*, *10*(5), 4059–4092. DOI: 10.1109/JIOT.2022.3203249

Asiri, A. A., Shaf, A., Ali, T., Aamir, M., Irfan, M., Alqahtani, S., & Mehdar, K. M.. (2023). Brain tumor detection and classification using fine-tuned CNN with ResNet50 and U-Net model: A study on TCGA-LGG and TCIA dataset for MRI applications. *Life (Chicago, Ill.)*, *13*(7), 1449. DOI: 10.3390/life13071449 PMID: 37511824

Asiri, A. A., Shaf, A., Ali, T., Pasha, M. A., Aamir, M., Irfan, M., & Alqahtani, S.. (2023). Advancing brain tumor classification through fine-tuned vision transformers: A comparative study of pre-trained models. *Sensors (Basel)*, *23*(18), 7913. DOI: 10.3390/s23187913 PMID: 37765970

Aslam, U., & Jack, W. (2025). The Convergence of IoT and AI in Healthcare: Revolutionizing Real-Time Patient Monitoring and Predictive Diagnostics.

Ateriya, N., Saraf, A., Meshram, V. P., & Setia, P. (2018). Telemedicine and virtual consultation: The Indian perspective. *The National Medical Journal of India*, *31*(4), 215–218. DOI: 10.4103/0970-258X.258220 PMID: 31134926

Australian Institute of Digital Health. (2023). Roadmap recommendations for safe, ethical, sustainable, and personalised AI in healthcare.

Awaisi, K. S., Hussain, S., Ahmed, M., Khan, A. A., & Ahmed, G. (2020). Leveraging IoT and fog computing in healthcare systems. *IEEE Internet of Things Magazine*, *3*(2), 52–56.

Awotunde, J. B., Jimoh, R. G., Folorunso, S. O., Adeniyi, E. A., Abiodun, K. M., & Banjo, O. O. (2021). Privacy and security concerns in IoT-based healthcare systems. In *The Fusion of Internet of Things, Artificial Intelligence, and Cloud Computing in Health Care* (pp. 105–134). Springer International Publishing.

Azimi, I., Rahmani, A. M., Liljeberg, P., & Tenhunen, H. (2017). Internet of things for remote elderly monitoring: A study from user-centered perspective. *Journal of Ambient Intelligence and Humanized Computing*, *8*(2), 273–289.

Badža, M. M., & Barjaktarović, M. Č. (2020). Classification of brain tumors from MRI images using a convolutional neural network. *Applied Sciences (Basel, Switzerland)*, *10*(6), 1999. DOI: 10.3390/app10061999

Baker, S. B., Xiang, W., & Atkinson, I. (2017). Internet of things for smart healthcare: Technologies, challenges, and opportunities. *IEEE Access : Practical Innovations, Open Solutions*, *5*, 26521–26544.

Baldini, G., Botterman, M., Neisse, R., & Tallacchini, M. (2018). Ethical design in the internet of things. *Science and Engineering Ethics*, *24*, 905–925. PMID: 26797878

Balouch, F. A., Wafa, K. M., & Ahmad, A. (2022). Internet of Things (IoT), its application area and combination with GPS. *Galaxy International Interdisciplinary Research Journal*, *10*(1), 725–734.

Banerjee, A., Shit, M., Muhuri, S. S., Adhikari, S., Himanshee, S., & Mohapatra, H. (2025) Revolutionizing Healthcare from Inside: Leveraging Expanded Reality with Ingestible Sensors. In *Embedded Artificial Intelligence* (pp. 227-251). Chapman and Hall/CRC Press.

Barry, A. F.. (2022). Physical activity, cardiorespiratory fitness, and cardiovascular health: A clinical practice statement of the American Society for Preventive Cardiology Part II. *American Journal of Preventive Cardiology*, *12*, 100425. PMID: 36281325

Beale, S. S., & Berris, P. (2017). Hacking the Internet of Things: Vulnerabilities, dangers, and legal responses. *Duke L. & Tech. Rev.*, *16*, 161.

Berlin, G., Darino, L., Greenfield, M., Starikova, I., & JGI/Tom Grill/Getty Images. (2019). Women in the healthcare industry. https://hbanet.org/sites/default/files/2023-06/Women-in-the-healthcare-industry_Aug.2019.pdf

Bernabé, O., Acevedo, E., Acevedo, A., Carreño, R., & Gómez, S. (2021). Classification of eye diseases in fundus images. *IEEE Access : Practical Innovations, Open Solutions*, *9*, 101267–101276. DOI: 10.1109/ACCESS.2021.3094649

Bernard, M. (2021). What's the impact of artificial intelligence and technology on society? Available at: https://bernardmarr.com/whats-the-impact-of-artificial-intelligence-and-technology-on-society/

Bertl, M., Ross, P., & Draheim, D. (2023). Systematic AI support for decision-making in the healthcare sector: Obstacles and success factors. *Health Policy and Technology*, *12*(3), 100748.

Bharadwaj, H. K., Agarwal, A., Chamola, V., Lakkaniga, N. R., Hassija, V., Guizani, M., & Sikdar, B. (2021). A review on the role of machine learning in enabling IoT based healthcare applications. *IEEE Access : Practical Innovations, Open Solutions*, *9*, 38859–38890.

Bhatia, M., & Kumari, S. (2022). A novel IoT-fog-cloud-based healthcare system for monitoring and preventing encephalitis. *Cognitive Computation*, *14*(5), 1609–1626.

Bhosale, K. S., Nenova, M., & Iliev, G. (2021). A study of cyber attacks: In the healthcare sector. In *2021 Sixth Junior Conference on Lighting (Lighting)* (pp. 1-6). IEEE.

Bhuiyan, M. N., Rahman, M. M., Billah, M. M., & Saha, D. (2021). Internet of things (IoT): A review of its enabling technologies in healthcare applications, standards protocols, security, and market opportunities. *IEEE Internet of Things Journal*, *8*(13), 10474–10498.

Bisio, I., Garibotto, C., Lavagetto, F., & Sciarrone, A. (2019). When eHealth meets IoT: A smart wireless system for post-stroke home rehabilitation. *IEEE Wireless Communications*, *26*(6), 24–29.

Boeren, E. (2019). Understanding Sustainable Development Goal (SDG) 4 on "quality education" from micro, meso and macro perspectives. *International Review of Education*, *65*(2), 277–294. DOI: 10.1007/s11159-019-09772-7

Bond, R., Novotny, T., Andrsova, I., Koc, L., Sisakova, M., Finlay, D., & Malik, M. (2018). Automation bias in medicine: The influence of automated diagnoses on interpreter accuracy and uncertainty when reading electrocardiograms. *Journal of Electrocardiology*, *51*(6S), S6–S11. PMID: 30122457

Botzel, K., Tronnier, V., & Gasser, T. (2014, March 28). The differential diagnosis and treatment of tremor. *Deutsches Ärzteblatt International*, *111*(13), 225–235. DOI: 10.3238/arztebl.2014.0225 PMID: 24739887

Brundage, M., ... (2018). The malicious use of artificial intelligence. *arXiv preprint arXiv:1802.07228*. https://arxiv.org/abs/1802.07228

Butpheng, C., Yeh, K. H., & Xiong, H. (2020). Security and privacy in IoT-cloud-based e-health systems—A comprehensive review. *Symmetry*, *12*(7), 1191.

Butun, I., Österberg, P., & Song, H. (2019). Security of the Internet of Things: Vulnerabilities, attacks, and countermeasures. *IEEE Communications Surveys and Tutorials*, *22*(1), 616–644.

Bzai, J.. (2022). Machine learning-enabled Internet of Things (IoT): Data, applications, and industry perspective. *Electronics (Basel)*, *11*, 2676.

Caciquinho, P. O., & Arruda, K. M. (2025). The power of learning culture as an instrument to effective implementation of social justice. *Journal of Social and Labor Relations Law*, *11*(1), 33–42. https://publicacoes.udf.edu.br/index.php/relacoes-sociais-trabalhista/article/view/571

Cao, C., Liu, F., Tan, H., Song, D., Shu, W., Li, W., Zhou, Y., Bo, X., & Xie, Z. (2018). Deep learning and its applications in biomedicine. *Genomics, Proteomics & Bioinformatics*, *16*(1), 17–32. DOI: 10.1016/j.gpb.2018.01.001 PMID: 29522900

Castaneda, C., Nalley, K., Mannion, C., Bhattacharyya, P., Blake, P., Pecora, A., & Suh, K. S. (2015). Clinical decision support systems for improving diagnostic accuracy and achieving precision medicine. *Journal of Clinical Bioinformatics*, *5*(1), 4. PMID: 25834725

Chacko, A., & Hayajneh, T. (2018). Security and privacy issues with IoT in healthcare. *EAI Endorsed Transactions on Pervasive Health and Technology, 4*(14).

Chan, H.-P., Samala, R. K., Hadjiiski, L. M., & Zhou, C. (2020). Deep learning in medical image analysis. In *Deep Learning in Medical Image Analysis: Challenges and Applications* (pp. 3–21). Springer. https://doi.org/DOI: 10.1007/978-3-030-33128-3_1

Chan, M., Estève, D., Escriba, C., & Campo, E. (2008). A review of smart homes—Present state and future challenges. *Computer Methods and Programs in Biomedicine, 91*(1), 55–81. PMID: 18367286

Chen, H., Hailey, D., Wang, N., & Yu, P. (2014). A review of data quality assessment methods for public health information systems. *International Journal of Environmental Research and Public Health, 11*(5), 5170–5207. PMID: 24830450

Chen, X., Wang, X., Zhang, K., Fung, K.-M., Thai, T. C., Moore, K., Mannel, R. S., Liu, H., Zheng, B., & Qiu, Y. (2022). Recent advances and clinical applications of deep learning in medical image analysis. *Medical Image Analysis, 79*, 102444. DOI: 10.1016/j.media.2022.102444 PMID: 35472844

Chi, H. R., de Fátima Domingues, M., Zhu, H., Li, C., Kojima, K., & Radwan, A. (2023). Healthcare 5.0: In the perspective of consumer Internet-of-Things-based fog/cloud computing. *IEEE Transactions on Consumer Electronics*.

Chin, M. H., Afsar-Manesh, N., Bierman, A. S., Chang, C., Colón-Rodríguez, C. J., Dullabh, P., Duran, D. G., Fair, M., Hernandez-Boussard, T., Hightower, M., & Ohno-Machado, L. (2023). Guiding principles to address the impact of algorithm bias on racial and ethnic disparities in health and health care. *JAMA Network Open, 6*(12), e2345050–e2345050. PMID: 38100101

Choudhary, A. (2024). Internet of Things: A comprehensive overview, architectures, applications, simulation tools, challenges, and future directions. *Discover Internet of Things, 4*, 31. DOI: 10.1007/s43926-024-00084-3

Cui, A., Costello, M., & Stolfo, S. (2013). When firmware modifications attack: A case study of embedded exploitation.

Cukic, V., Lovre, V., Dragisic, D., & Ustamujic, A. (2012). Asthma and chronic obstructive pulmonary disease (COPD) – Differences and similarities. *Materia Socio-Medica, 24*(2), 100–105. DOI: 10.5455/msm.2012.24.100-105 PMID: 23678316

Dada, E., Shani, A., & Adekunle, A. (2017). Smart walking stick for visually impaired people using ultrasonic sensors and Arduino. *IACSIT International Journal of Engineering and Technology, 9*, 3435–3447. DOI: 10.21817/ijet/2017/v9i5/170905302

Dadkhah, M., Mehraeen, M., Rahimnia, F., & Kimiafar, K. (2021). Use of Internet of Things for chronic disease management: An overview. *Journal of Medical Signals and Sensors*, *11*(2), 138–157. DOI: 10.4103/jmss.JMSS_13_20 PMID: 34268102

Dang, L. M., Piran, M. J., Han, D., Min, K., & Moon, H. (2019). A survey on Internet of Things and cloud computing for healthcare. *Electronics (Basel)*, *8*(7), 768. DOI: 10.3390/electronics8070768

Dasaka, S. (2024). Optimizing decision-making: Balancing intuition with evidence in digital experience design.

Dash, S. P. (2020). The impact of IoT in healthcare: Global technological change & the roadmap to a networked architecture in India. *Journal of the Indian Institute of Science*, *100*(4), 773–785. PMID: 33162693

Das, J., Ghosh, S., Mukherjee, A., Ghosh, S. K., & Buyya, R. (2022). RESCUE: Enabling green healthcare services using integrated IoT-edge-fog-cloud computing environments. *Software, Practice & Experience*, *52*(7), 1615–1642.

Das, S., & Goswami, R. S. (2023). Review, limitations, and future prospects of neural network approaches for brain tumor classification. *Multimedia Tools and Applications*, *82*, 1–43. DOI: 10.1007/s11042-023-14123-7

Davenport, T., & Kalakota, R. (2019). The potential for artificial intelligence in healthcare. *Future Healthcare Journal*, *6*(2), 94–98. PMID: 31363513

Deepak, S., & Ameer, P. M. (2021). Automated categorization of brain tumor from MRI using CNN features and SVM. *Journal of Ambient Intelligence and Humanized Computing*, *12*, 8357–8369. DOI: 10.1007/s12652-020-02756-0

DeepMind & BioNTech. (2023). Collaborating to develop AI lab assistants for healthcare research. DeepMind & BioNTech. Retrieved March 25, 2025, from https://www.deepmind.com/healthcare

Demiris, G., Rantz, M. J., Aud, M. A., Marek, K. D., Tyrer, H. W., Skubic, M., & Hussam, A. A. (2004). Older adults' attitudes towards and perceptions of 'smart home'technologies: A pilot study. *Medical Informatics and the Internet in Medicine*, *29*(2), 87–94. PMID: 15370989

Devarajan, J. P., Sreedharan, V. R., & Narayanamurthy, G. (2021). Decision making in health care diagnosis: Evidence from Parkinson's disease via hybrid machine learning. *IEEE Transactions on Engineering Management*, *70*(8), 2719–2731.

Dewangan, K., & Mishra, M. (2018). Review: Security of IOT Based Healthcare System. *CCET Journal of Science and Engineering Education*, *3*, 25–28.

Dey, D., Slomka, P., Leeson, P., Comaniciu, D., Shrestha, S., Sengupta, P., & Marwick, T. (2018). Artificial intelligence in cardiovascular imaging: JACC state-of-the-art review. *Journal of the American College of Cardiology*, *73*(11), 1317–1335. PMID: 30898208

Dhar, P. (2020). The Carbon Impact of Artificial Intelligence. *Nature Machine Intelligence*, *2*, 423–425.

Dhaygude, R., & Waghmare, S. (2023). Innovative solutions for visual impairment: Design and implementation of a real-time assistance system. *Journal of Data Acquisition and Processing*, *38*, 3188. DOI: 10.5281/zenodo.98549777

Dhermain, F. G., Hau, P., Lanfermann, H., Jacobs, A. H., & van den Bent, M. J. (2010). Advanced MRI and PET imaging for assessment of treatment response in patients with gliomas. *Lancet Neurology*, *9*(9), 906–920. DOI: 10.1016/S1474-4422(10)70164-1 PMID: 20705518

Dhinakaran, D., Edwin Raja, S., Velselvi, R., & Purushotham, N. (2025). Intelligent IoT-driven advanced predictive maintenance system for industrial applications. *SN Computer Science*, *6*, 151. DOI: 10.1007/s42979-025-03695-x

Dhinakaran, D., Gopalakrishnan, S., Selvaraj, D., Girija, M. S., & Prabaharan, G. (2025). Mining privacy-preserving association rules using transaction hewer allocator and facile hash algorithm in multi-cloud environments. *MethodsX*, *14*, 103317. DOI: 10.1016/j.mex.2025.103317 PMID: 40331027

Dhinakaran, D., Jagadish Kumar, N., Ponnuviji, N. P., & Praveen Kumar, B. (2025). Safeguarding confidentiality and privacy in cloud-enabled healthcare systems with SpectraSafe encryption and dynamic k-anonymity algorithm. *Expert Systems with Applications*, *279*, 127584. DOI: 10.1016/j.eswa.2025.127584

Dhinakaran, D., Prabaharan, G., Valarmathi, K., Sankar, S. U., & Sugumar, R. (2025). Safeguarding privacy by utilizing SC-DℓDA algorithm in cloud-enabled multi-party computation. *KSII Transactions on Internet and Information Systems*, *19*(2), 635–656. DOI: 10.3837/tiis.2025.02.014

Dhinakaran, D., Ramani, R., Edwin Raja, S., & Selvaraj, D. (2025). Enhancing security in electronic health records using an adaptive feature-centric polynomial data security model with blockchain integration. *Peer-to-Peer Networking and Applications*, *18*, 7. DOI: 10.1007/s12083-024-01883-9

Dhinakaran, D., Selvaraj, D., Dharini, N., Raja, S. E., & Priya, C. S. L. (2023). Towards a novel privacy-preserving distributed multiparty data outsourcing scheme for cloud computing with quantum key distribution. *International Journal of Intelligent Systems and Applications in Engineering*, *12*(2), 286–300.

Dhinakaran, D., Srinivasan, L., Gopalakrishnan, S., & Anish, T. P. (2025). An efficient data mining technique and privacy preservation model for healthcare data using improved darts game optimizer-based weighted deep neural network and hybrid encryption. *Biomedical Signal Processing and Control*, *100*(C), 107168. DOI: 10.1016/j.bspc.2024.107168

Dhruv, P., & Naskar, S. (2020). Image classification using convolutional neural network (CNN) and recurrent neural network (RNN): A review. In *Machine Learning and Information Processing: Proceedings of ICMLIP 2019* (pp. 367–381). Springer. https://doi.org/DOI: 10.1007/978-981-15-4936-3_28

Dias, D., & Cunha, J. P. S. (2018). Wearable Health Devices—Vital Sign Monitoring, systems and Technologies. *Sensors (Basel)*, *18*(8), 2414. PMID: 30044415

Dickson, D. W. (2012). Parkinson's disease and parkinsonism: Neuropathology. *Cold Spring Harbor Perspectives in Medicine*, *2*(8), a009258. PMID: 22908195

Dignum, V. (2019). *Responsible Artificial Intelligence: How to Develop and Use AI Responsibly. Artificial Intelligence: Foundations, Theory, and Algorithms, Springer.* International Publishing.

Dineen Griffin, S.. (2019). Helping patients help themselves: A systematic review of self-management support strategies in primary health care practice. *PLoS One*, *14*(8), e0220116. PMID: 31369582

Dixon, D., Sattar, H., Moros, N., Kesireddy, S. R., Ahsan, H., Lakkimsetti, M., Fatima, M., Doshi, D., Sadhu, K., & Hassan, M. J. (2024). Unveiling the influence of AI predictive analytics on patient outcomes: A comprehensive narrative review. *Cureus*, *16*(5), e59954. DOI: 10.7759/cureus.59954 PMID: 38854327

Dixon, E., Anderson, J., & Lazar, A. (2022). Understanding how sensory changes experienced by individuals with a range of age-related cognitive changes can affect technology use. [TACCESS]. *ACM Transactions on Accessible Computing*, *15*(2), 1–33. PMID: 35919105

Domingo, M. C. (2012). An overview of the Internet of Things for people with disabilities. *journal of Network and Computer Applications, 35*(2), 584-596.

Edemekong, P. F.. (2024). Health Insurance Portability and Accountability Act. In *StatPearls* [Internet]. StatPearls Publishing.

Elena, P. A. P. (2024). The Impact of Artificial Intelligence on Psychological and Cognitive Development. Retrieved from https://elenapap.com/en/the-impact-of-artificial-intelligence-on-psychological-and-cognitive-development?utm

Esteva, A.. (2017). Dermatologist-Level Classification of Skin Cancer with Deep Neural Networks. *Nature*.

Farahani, B., Firouzi, F., & Chakrabarty, K. (2020). Healthcare iot. *Intelligent Internet of Things: From Device to Fog and Cloud*, 515-545.

Felici, M., & Pearson, S. (2014). Accountability for data governance in the cloud. In *Summer School on Accountability and Security in the Cloud* (pp. 3–42). Springer International Publishing.

Feng, X., Zhu, X., Han, Q. L., Zhou, W., Wen, S., & Xiang, Y. (2022). Detecting vulnerability on IoT device firmware: A survey. *IEEE/CAA Journal of Automatica Sinica, 10*(1), 25-41.

Fereidouni, H., Fadeitcheva, O., & Zalai, M. (2025). IoT and man-in-the-middle attacks. *Security and Privacy, 8*(2), e70016.

Filip, R., Gheorghita Puscaselu, R., Anchidin-Norocel, L., Dimian, M., & Savage, W. K. (2022). Global challenges to public health care systems during the COVID-19 pandemic: A review of pandemic measures and problems. *Journal of Personalized Medicine, 12*(8), 1295. DOI: 10.3390/jpm12081295 PMID: 36013244

Flaxman, S. R., Bourne, R. R., Resnikoff, S., Ackland, P., Braithwaite, T., Cicinelli, M. V., Das, A., Jonas, J. B., Keeffe, J., Kempen, J. H., & Leasher, J. (2017). Global causes of blindness and distance vision impairment 1990–2020: A systematic review and meta-analysis. *The Lancet. Global Health, 5*(12), e1221–e1234. DOI: 10.1016/S2214-109X(17)30393-5 PMID: 29032195

Flessa, S.. (2021). Innovations in health care – A conceptual framework. *International Journal of Environmental Research and Public Health, 18*(19), 10026. PMID: 34639328

Fox, R., Kitt, J., Leeson, P., Aye, C. Y., & Lewandowski, A. J. (2019). Preeclampsia: Risk factors, diagnosis, management, and the cardiovascular impact on the offspring. *Journal of Clinical Medicine, 8*(10), 1625. PMID: 31590294

Freckmann, G., Pleus, S., Grady, M., Setford, S., & Levy, B. (2019). Measures of accuracy for continuous glucose monitoring and blood glucose monitoring devices. *Journal of Diabetes Science and Technology, 13*(3), 575–583. PMID: 30453761

Furber, F. (2016). *Artificial Intelligence vs. the Human Brain*. Huffington.

FUTURE-AI Consortium. (n.d.). *FUTURE-AI Guidelines: Best practices for trustworthy AI in healthcare*. FUTURE-AI Consortium. Retrieved March 25, 2025, from https://www.futureaiguidelines.org

Garcia, C. A. (2022). *Creating New Value from Laboratory Testing and Services in Value-Based Healthcare: Investigating Data Monetization Strategies from Clinical Laboratories* (Doctoral dissertation, Massachusetts Institute of Technology).

Gargioni, L., Fogli, D., & Baroni, P. (2024). A systematic review on pill and medication dispensers from a human-centered perspective. *Journal of Healthcare Informatics Research*, *8*(2), 244–285. DOI: 10.1007/s41666-024-00161-w PMID: 38681758

Garovic, V. D., Dechend, R., Easterling, T., Karumanchi, S. A., McMurtry Baird, S., & Magee, L. A. (2022). Hypertension in pregnancy: Diagnosis, blood pressure goals, and pharmacotherapy: A scientific statement from the American Heart Association. *Hypertension*, *79*(2), e21–e41. PMID: 34905954

Gaur, L., Bhatia, U., Jhanjhi, N. Z., Muhammad, G., & Masud, M. (2023). Medical image-based detection of COVID-19 using deep convolution neural networks. *Multimedia Systems*, *29*(3), 1729–1738. DOI: 10.1007/s00530-023-01083-6 PMID: 33935377

Gaytan, J.C.T. (2022). A literature survey of security and privacy issues in internet of medical things. *International Journal of Computations, Information and Manufacturing (IJCIM), 2*(2).

Ghosh, A. M., Halder, D., & Hossain, S. A. (2016). May. Remote health monitoring system through IoT. In *2016 5th International Conference on Informatics, Electronics and Vision (ICIEV)* (pp. 921-926). IEEE.

Goh, A. C.. (2020). Early experience with the da Vinci single-port robotic system in urology. *Journal of Endourology*, *34*(1), 75–81. PMID: 31895594

Golas, S. B., et al. (2018). "Feasibility of Utilizing Real-Time Electronic Health Record Data to Predict Risk of 30-Day Hospital Readmissions Among Medicare Patients." Journal of Medical Internet Research.

Google Health. (2020). *AI for eye disease diagnosis: DeepMind's revolutionary work in diabetic retinopathy*. Google. https://health.google.com/ai

Gourisaria, M. K., Agrawal, R., Singh, V., Rautaray, S. S., & Pandey, M. (2022). AI and IoT Enabled Smart Hospital Management Systems. In *Data Science in Societal Applications: Concepts and Implications* (pp. 77–106). Springer Nature Singapore.

Goutham, V., Sameerunnisa, A., Babu, S., & Prakash, T. B. (2022). Brain tumor classification using EfficientNet-B0 model. In *2022 2nd International Conference on Advance Computing and Innovative Technologies in Engineering (ICACITE)* (pp. 2503–2509). IEEE. https://doi.org/DOI: 10.1109/ICACITE53721.2022.9772123

Goyal, S., Sharma, N., Bhushan, B., Shankar, A., & Sagayam, M. (2021). Iot enabled technology in secured healthcare: Applications, challenges and future directions. *Cognitive Internet of Medical Things for Smart Healthcare: Services and Applications*, pp.25-48.

Guan, Z., Li, H., Liu, R., Cai, C., Liu, Y., Li, J., Wang, X., Huang, S., Wu, L., Liu, D., Yu, S., Wang, Z., Shu, J., Hou, X., Yang, X., Jia, W., & Sheng, B. (2023). Artificial intelligence in diabetes management: Advancements, opportunities, and challenges. *Cell Reports Medicine*, *4*(10), 101213. DOI: 10.1016/j.xcrm.2023.101213 PMID: 37788667

Guo, C., Tian, P., & Choo, K.-K. R. (2021). Enabling privacy-assured fog-based data aggregation in e-healthcare systems. *IEEE Transactions on Industrial Informatics*, *17*(3), 1948–1957. DOI: 10.1109/TII.2020.2995228 PMID: 37981962

Gupta, A., Yadav, S., Shahid, S., & Venkanna, U. (2019). December. HeartCare: IoT based heart disease prediction system. In *2019 International Conference on Information Technology (ICIT)* (pp. 88-93). IEEE.

Gupta, S., & Gupta, M. (2021). Deep learning for brain tumor segmentation using magnetic resonance images. In *2021 IEEE Conference on Computational Intelligence in Bioinformatics and Computational Biology (CIBCB)* (pp. 1–6). IEEE. https://doi.org/DOI: 10.1109/CIBCB52658.2021.9577313

Gyrard, A., & Serrano, M. (2016). March. Connected smart cities: interoperability with SEG 3.0 for the internet of things. In *2016 30th International Conference on Advanced Information Networking and Applications Workshops (WAINA)* (pp. 796-802). IEEE.

Haleem, A., & Javaid, M.. (2021). Telemedicine for healthcare: Capabilities, features, barriers, and applications. *Sensors International*, *2*, 100117. PMID: 34806053

Hales, R., & Birdthistle, N. (2022). The Sustainable Development Goals – SDG#9 Industry, Innovation and Infrastructure. In Attaining the 2030 sustainable development goal of industry, innovation and infrastructure. https://doi.org/DOI: 10.1108/9781803825731

Haller, S., Badoud, S., Nguyen, D., Barnaure, I., Montandon, M.-L., Lovblad, K.-O., & Burkhard, P. R. (2013). Differentiation between Parkinson disease and other forms of Parkinsonism using support vector machine analysis of susceptibility-weighted imaging (SWI): Initial results. *European Radiology*, *23*(12), 12–19. DOI: 10.1007/s00330-012-2579-y PMID: 22797981

Hamdan, S.. (2020). Edge-computing architectures for Internet of Things applications: A survey. *Sensors (Basel)*, *20*, 6441. PMID: 33187267

Hanumantharaju, R., Shreenath, K. N., Sowmya, B. J., & Srinivasa, K. G. (2022). Fog based smart healthcare: A machine learning paradigms for IoT sector. *Multimedia Tools and Applications*, *81*(26), 37299–37318.

Harini, M., Dhinakaran, D., & Prabhu, D. (2023). Leveraging blockchain for transparency in agriculture supply chain management using IoT and machine learning. In *2023 World Conference on Communication & Computing (WCONF)* (pp. 1–6). Raipur, India. https://doi.org/DOI: 10.1109/WCONF58270.2023.10235156

Häußermann, S., Arendsen, L. J., & Pritchard, J. N. (2022). Smart dry powder inhalers and intelligent adherence management. *Advanced Drug Delivery Reviews*, *191*, 114580. PMID: 36273513

Hayyolalam, V., Aloqaily, M., Ozkasap, O., & Guizani, M. (2022). Edge-assisted solutions for IoT-based connected healthcare systems: A literature review. *IEEE Internet of Things Journal*, *9*(12), 9419–9443. DOI: 10.1109/JIOT.2021.3135200

Hazra, A., Adhikari, M., Amgoth, T., & Srirama, S. N. (2021). A comprehensive survey on interoperability for IIoT: Taxonomy, standards, and future directions. *ACM Computing Surveys*, *55*(1), 1–35.

Health, A. I. Partnership. (n.d.). *Empowering healthcare professionals to use AI effectively and equitably*. Health AI Partnership. Retrieved March 25, 2025, from https://www.healthaipartnership.org

He, J., Baxter, S. L., Xu, J., Xu, J., Zhou, X., & Zhang, K. (2019). The practical implementation of artificial intelligence technologies in medicine. *Nature Medicine*, *25*(1), 30–36. DOI: 10.1038/s41591-018-0307-0 PMID: 30617336

Hilty, D. M.. (2021). Sensor, wearable, and remote patient monitoring competencies for clinical care and training: Scoping review. *Journal of Technology in Behavioral Science*, *6*(2), 252–277. PMID: 33501372

Hollander, J. E., & Carr, B. G. (2020). Virtually perfect? Telemedicine for COVID-19. *The New England Journal of Medicine*, *382*(18), 1679–1681. PMID: 32160451

Hui, C. Y., McKinstry, B., Fulton, O., Buchner, M., & Pinnock, H. (2021). Patients' and clinicians' perceived trust in internet-of-things systems to support asthma self-management: Qualitative interview study. *JMIR mHealth and uHealth*, *9*(7), e24127. PMID: 34269684

Hustinx, R., & Fosse, P. (2010). PET in brain tumors. *PET Clinics*, *5*(2), 185–197. DOI: 10.1016/j.cpet.2010.02.002 PMID: 27157672

Inkster, B., Sarda, S., & Subramanian, V. (2018). Machine learning and mental health: A systematic review of algorithms and applications. *Psychological Medicine*, *48*(9), 1426–1448. DOI: 10.1017/S0033291718000932

Insilico Medicine. (2020). *AI-driven drug discovery: How AI accelerated the development of a fibrosis drug*. Insilico Medicine. https://www.insilico.com/ai-drug-discovery

Iqbal, S., Qureshi, A. N., Ullah, A., Li, J., & Mahmood, T. (2022). Improving the robustness and quality of biomedical CNN models through adaptive hyperparameter tuning. *Applied Sciences (Basel, Switzerland)*, *12*(22), 11870. DOI: 10.3390/app122211870

Istepanian, R. S., Hu, S., Philip, N. Y., & Sungoor, A. (2011). August. The potential of Internet of m-health Things "m-IoT" for non-invasive glucose level sensing. In *2011 annual international conference of the IEEE engineering in medicine and biology society* (pp. 5264-5266). IEEE.

Jaime, F. J., Muñoz, A., Rodríguez-Gómez, F., & Jerez-Calero, A. (2023). Strengthening privacy and data security in biomedical microelectromechanical systems by IoT communication security and protection in smart healthcare. *Sensors (Basel)*, *23*(21), 8944. PMID: 37960646

Jain, L., Murthy, H. V. S., Patel, C., & Bansal, D. (2018). Retinal eye disease detection using deep learning. In *Proceedings of the 14th International Conference on Information Processing (ICINPRO)* (pp. 1–6). IEEE. https://doi.org/DOI: 10.1109/ICINPRO43533.2018.9096838

Javaid, M., Haleem, A., Singh, R. P., Suman, R., Khan, S., & Rab, S. (2025). Adoption of Internet of Things for smart city-enabled smart hospitals. *Intelligent Hospital*, *1*(2), 100011. DOI: 10.1016/j.inhs.2025.100011

Javaid, M., & Khan, I. H. (2021). Internet of Things (IoT) enabled healthcare helps to take the challenges of COVID-19 pandemic. *Journal of Oral Biology and Craniofacial Research*, *11*(2), 209–214. PMID: 33665069

Javaid, M., & Khan, I. H. (2021). Internet of Things (IoT) enabled healthcare helps to take the challenges of COVID-19 Pandemic. *Journal of Oral Biology and Craniofacial Research, 11*(2), 209–214. PMID: 33665069

Jiang, F., Jiang, Y., Zhi, H., Dong, Y., Li, H., Ma, S., & Wang, Y. (2017). Artificial intelligence in healthcare: Past, present, and future. *Stroke and Vascular Neurology, 2*(4), 230–243. DOI: 10.1136/svn-2017-000101 PMID: 29507784

Joshitta, R. S. M., Arockiam, L., & Jeyanthi, N. (2017). Device authentication mechanism for IoT-enabled healthcare system. In *2017 International Conference on Algorithms, Methodology, Models and Applications in Emerging Technologies (ICAMMAET)* (pp. 1–6). IEEE.

Kakria, P., Tripathi, N. K., & Kitipawang, P. (2015). A real-time health monitoring system for remote cardiac patients using smartphone and wearable sensors. *International Journal of Telemedicine and Applications, 2015*(1), 373474. PMID: 26788055

Kang, H. S., & Exworthy, M. (2022). Wearing the future—Wearables to empower users to take greater responsibility for their health and care: Scoping review. *JMIR mHealth and uHealth, 10*(7), e35684. DOI: 10.2196/35684 PMID: 35830222

Karam, A.A. (2022). Investigating the importance of ethics and security on internet of medical things (IoMT). *International Journal of Computations, Information and Manufacturing (IJCIM), 2*(2).

Karunarathne, S. M., Saxena, N., & Khan, M. K. (2021). Security and privacy in IoT smart healthcare. *IEEE Internet Computing, 25*(4), 37–48. DOI: 10.1109/MIC.2021.3051675

Kashani, M. H., Madanipour, M., Nikravan, M., Asghari, P., & Mahdipour, E. (2021). A systematic review of IoT in healthcare: Applications, techniques, and trends. *Journal of Network and Computer Applications, 192*, 103164.

Kashyap, V., Kumar, A., Kumar, A., & Hu, Y. C. (2022). A systematic survey on fog and iot driven healthcare: Open challenges and research issues. *Electronics (Basel), 11*(17), 2668.

Kaur, D., Goel, S., Nijhawan, R., & Gupta, S. (2022). Analysis of brain tumor using pre-trained CNN models and machine learning techniques. In *2022 IEEE International Students' Conference on Electrical, Electronics and Computer Science (SCEECS)* (pp. 1–6). IEEE. https://doi.org/DOI: 10.1109/SCEECS54163.2022.9776670

Keesara, S., Jonas, A., & Schulman, K. (2020). COVID-19 and health care's digital revolution. *The New England Journal of Medicine, 382*(23), e82. DOI: 10.1056/NEJMp2005835 PMID: 32240581

Kelly, J. E. (2015). Computing, cognition, and the future of knowing How Humans and machines are forging a new age of Understanding. White Paper, IBM Research

Kelly, D., & Hammoudeh, M. (2018). Optimisation of the public key encryption infrastructure for the internet of things. In *Proceedings of the 2nd International Conference on Future Networks and Distributed Systems* (pp. 1-5).

Kelly, J. T., Campbell, K. L., Gong, E., & Scuffham, P. (2020). The Internet of Things: Impact and implications for health care delivery. *Journal of Medical Internet Research*, *22*(11), e20135. DOI: 10.2196/20135 PMID: 33170132

Khan, M. A. R., Shavkatovich, S. N., Nagpal, B., Kumar, A., Haq, M. A., Tharini, V. J., & Alazzam, M. B. (2022). Optimizing hybrid metaheuristic algorithm with cluster head to improve performance metrics on the IoT. *Theoretical Computer Science*, *927*, 87–97.

Khan, M. A., & Salah, K. (2018). IoT security: Review, blockchain solutions, and open challenges. *Future Generation Computer Systems*, *82*, 395–411.

Khan, M. M., Shah, N., Shaikh, N., Thabet, A., & Belkhair, S. (2024). Towards secure and trusted AI in healthcare: A systematic review of emerging innovations and ethical challenges. *International Journal of Medical Informatics*, •••, 105780. PMID: 39753062

Khan, M. S. I., Rahman, A., Debnath, T., Karim, M. R., Nasir, M. K., Band, S. S., Mosavi, A., & Dehzangi, I. (2022). Accurate brain tumor detection using deep convolutional neural network. *Computational and Structural Biotechnology Journal*, *20*, 4733–4745. DOI: 10.1016/j.csbj.2022.08.057 PMID: 36147663

Khan, M. S., Tafshir, N., Alam, K. N., Dhruba, A. R., Albraikan, A. A., & Almalki, F. A. (2022). Deep learning for ocular disease recognition: An inner-class balance. *Journal of Healthcare Engineering*, *2022*, 5007111. Advance online publication. DOI: 10.1155/2022/5007111 PMID: 35528343

Khezr, S., Moniruzzaman, M., Yassine, A., & Benlamri, R. (2019). Blockchain technology in healthcare: A comprehensive review and directions for future research. *Applied Sciences (Basel, Switzerland)*, *9*(9), 1736.

Kim, B., Park, J., & Suh, J. (2020). Transparency and accountability in AI decision support: Explaining and visualizing convolutional neural networks for text information. *Decision Support Systems*, *134*, 113302. DOI: 10.1016/j.dss.2020.113302

Kishor, A., Chakraborty, C., & Jeberson, W. (2021). Intelligent healthcare data segregation using fog computing with internet of things and machine learning. *International Journal of Engineering Systems Modelling and Simulation*, *12*(2-3), 188–194.

Knupp, R. J.. (2023). Analytical approaches to evaluating hypertensive disorders of pregnancy. *American Journal of Obstetrics & Gynecology MFM*, *5*(2), 100816. PMID: 36396039

Kolachalama, V. B., & Garg, P. S. (2018). Machine learning and medical education. *NPJ Digital Medicine*, *1*(1), 54. DOI: 10.1038/s41746-018-0061-1 PMID: 31304333

Kopetz, H., & Steiner, W. (2022). Internet of things. In *Real-time systems: design principles for distributed embedded applications* (pp. 325–341). Springer International Publishing.

Kora, P., Ooi, C. P., Faust, O., Raghavendra, U., Gudigar, A., Chan, W. Y., Meenakshi, K., Swaraja, K., Plawiak, P., & Acharya, U. R. (2022). Transfer learning techniques for medical image analysis: A review. *Biocybernetics and Biomedical Engineering*, *42*(1), 79–107. DOI: 10.1016/j.bbe.2021.12.004

Korte, M. (2020). The impact of the digital revolution on human brain and behavior: Where do we stand? *Dialogues in Clinical Neuroscience*, *22*(2), 101–111. PMID: 32699510

Kousalya, K., & Saranya, T. (2023). Improved the detection and classification of breast cancer using hyperparameter tuning. *Materials Today: Proceedings*, *81*, 547–552. DOI: 10.1016/j.matpr.2023.01.107

Kshatri, S. S., Chandrakar, M. K., Bhonsle, D., Nayak, M., Tamrakar, P., & Sharma, P. (2025). Smart Medication Dispensing: IoT Innovations in Drug Development. *The Impact of Algorithmic Technologies on Healthcare*, 255-277.

Kshatri, S. S., & Singh, D. (2023). Convolutional neural network in medical image analysis: A review. *Archives of Computational Methods in Engineering*, *30*(4), 2793–2810. DOI: 10.1007/s11831-022-09848-w

Kshetri, N. (2017). Can blockchain strengthen the internet of things? *IT Professional*, *19*(4), 68–72.

Kumar, N., Gupta, M., Gupta, D., & Tiwari, S. (2023). Novel deep transfer learning model for COVID-19 patient detection using X-ray chest images. *Journal of Ambient Intelligence and Humanized Computing*, *14*(1), 469–478. DOI: 10.1007/s12652-022-04655-2 PMID: 34025813

Kumar, Y.. (2021). Study of machine and deep learning classifications for IoT enabled healthcare devices. In *2021 International Conference on Technological Advancements and Innovations (ICTAI)*. IEEE.

Lakshmi, G. J., Ghonge, M., & Obaid, A. J. (2021). Cloud based iot smart healthcare system for remote patient monitoring. *EAI Endorsed Transactions on Pervasive Health and Technology*, *7*(28), e4–e4.

Latif, J., Xiao, C., Tu, S., Rehman, S. U., Imran, A., & Bilal, A. (2020). Implementation and use of disease diagnosis systems for electronic medical records based on machine learning: A complete review. *IEEE Access : Practical Innovations, Open Solutions*, *8*, 150489–150513.

Levy, S. (2024). AI will understand humans better than humans do. WIRED. Retrieved from https://www.wired.com/story/plaintext-ai-will-understand-humans-better-than-humans-do

Liang, W., Tadesse, G. A., Ho, D., Fei-Fei, L., Zaharia, M., Zhang, C., & Zou, J. (2022). Advances, challenges and opportunities in creating data for trustworthy AI. *Nature Machine Intelligence*, *4*(8), 669–677.

Liao, J., Li, X., Gan, Y., Han, S., Rong, P., Wang, W., Li, W., & Zhou, L. (2023). Artificial intelligence assists precision medicine in cancer treatment. *Frontiers in Oncology*, *12*, 998222. DOI: 10.3389/fonc.2022.998222 PMID: 36686757

Li, T., & Le, W. (2020). Biomarkers for Parkinson's disease: How good are they? *Neuroscience Bulletin*, *36*(2), 183–194. PMID: 31646434

Litjens, G., & Kooi, T., EhteshamiBejnordi, B., Setio, A. A. A., Ciompi, F., Ghafoorian, M., Van Der Laak, J. A. W. M., Van Ginneken, B., & Sánchez, C. I. (2017). A survey on deep learning in medical image analysis. *Medical Image Analysis*, *42*, 60–88. DOI: 10.1016/j.media.2017.07.005 PMID: 28778026

Liu, C., Nitschke, P., Williams, S. P., & Zowghi, D. (2020). Data quality and the Internet of Things. *Computing*, *102*(2), 573–599.

Liu, Y., Yu, J., Fan, J., Vijayakumar, P., & Chang, V. (2022). Achieving privacy-preserving DSSE for intelligent IoT healthcare system. *IEEE Transactions on Industrial Informatics*, *18*(3), 2010–2020. DOI: 10.1109/TII.2021.3100873

Liu, Z., Tong, L., Chen, L., Jiang, Z., Zhou, F., Zhang, Q., Zhang, X., Jin, Y., & Zhou, H. (2023). Deep learning based brain tumor segmentation: A survey. *Complex & Intelligent Systems*, *9*(1), 1001–1026. DOI: 10.1007/s40747-022-01015-4

Livongo. (2020). *AI in chronic disease management: Revolutionizing diabetes care with real-time monitoring*. Livongo Health. https://www.livongo.com

López, L., Green, A. R., Tan-McGrory, A., King, R. S., & Betancourt, J. R. (2011). Bridging the digital divide in health care: The role of health information technology in addressing racial and ethnic disparities. *Joint Commission Journal on Quality and Patient Safety*, *37*(10), 437–445. PMID: 22013816

Loyola-Gonzalez, O. (2019). Black-box vs. white-box: Understanding their advantages and weaknesses from a practical point of view. *IEEE Access : Practical Innovations, Open Solutions*, *7*, 154096–154113.

Lupton, D. (2013). The digitally engaged patient: Self-monitoring and self-care in the digital health era. *Social Theory & Health*, *11*, 256–270.

Luxton, D. D. (2014). Recommendations for the ethical use and design of artificial intelligent care providers. *Artificial Intelligence in Medicine*, *62*(1), 1–10. DOI: 10.1016/j.artmed.2014.06.004 PMID: 25059820

Maddali, R. (2024). Ai-Powered Data Security Frameworks For Regulatory Compliance (GDPR, CCPA, HIPAA). [IJETRM]. *International Journal of Engineering Technology Research & Management*, *8*(04).

Makhdoom, I., Abolhasan, M., Lipman, J., Liu, R. P., & Ni, W. (2018). Anatomy of threats to the internet of things. *IEEE Communications Surveys and Tutorials*, *21*(2), 1636–1675.

Maktoubian, J.. (2019). An IoT architecture for preventive maintenance of medical devices in healthcare organizations. *Health and Technology*, *9*, 233–243.

Malhotra, P., Gupta, S., Koundal, D., Zaguia, A., & Enbeyle, W. (2022). Deep neural networks for medical image segmentation. *Journal of Healthcare Engineering*, *2022*, 1–13. DOI: 10.1155/2022/9845752 PMID: 35310182

Mallik, P. (2021). Analysis of vulnerabilities in iot and its solutions. In *Managing Resources for Futuristic Wireless Networks* (pp. 157–177). IGI Global.

Marques, G., Pitarma, R. M., Garcia, N., & Pombo, N. (2019). Internet of things architectures, technologies, applications, challenges, and future directions for enhanced living environments and healthcare systems: A review. *Electronics (Basel)*, *8*(10), 1081.

Matthew, P.. (2025). A review of the state of the art for the Internet of Medical Things. *Sci*, *7*, 36.

Mavrogiorgou, A., Kiourtis, A., Perakis, K., Pitsios, S., & Kyriazis, D. (2019). IoT in healthcare: Achieving interoperability of high-quality data acquired by IoT medical devices. *Sensors (Basel)*, *19*(9), 1978. PMID: 31035612

Mayer, J., Jose, R., Kurgansky, G., Singh, P., Coletti, C., Devine, T., & Toma, M. (2023). Evaluating the feasibility of euler angles for bed-based patient movement monitoring. *Signals*, *4*(4), 788–799.

Mazalica, M., & Ivetic, D. (2021, October). Fog Computing architecture for IoT Smart traffic applications. In *International Conference* (p. 95).

Mazharuddin, H. (2025). Beyond the wrist: Wearables in healthcare. In *Digital Health* (pp. 63–73). Academic Press.

McLean, A. (2011). Ethical frontiers of ICT and older users: Cultural, pragmatic and ethical issues. *Ethics and Information Technology*, *13*(4), 313–326.

Merchant, R.. (2018). Impact of a digital health intervention on asthma resource utilization. *The World Allergy Organization Journal*, *11*(1), 28. PMID: 30524644

Mercurio, B., & Yu, R. (2022). *Regulating Cross-Border Data Flows: Issues, Challenges and Impact.* Anthem Press.

Mitchell-Box, K.. (2012). Fathers' thoughts on breastfeeding and implications for a theory-based intervention. *Journal of Obstetric, Gynecologic, and Neonatal Nursing : JOGNN*, *41*(6), E41–E50. PMID: 22861175

Mitchell, M.. (2019). Digital technology and the future of health systems. *Health Systems and Reform*, *5*(2), 113–120. PMID: 30908111

Mittelstadt, B. (2017). Ethics of the health-related internet of things: A narrative review. *Ethics and Information Technology*, *19*(3), 157–175.

Mohamed, K. S., & Mohamed, K. S. (2022). An introduction to IoT. *Bluetooth 5.0 Modem Design for IoT Devices*, 33-43.

Mohite, S., Patel, A., Patel, M., & Gaikwad (Mohite), V. (2018). *Smart walking stick for visually impaired people.* SSRN. https://doi.org/DOI: 10.2139/ssrn.3274784

Moore, A. A., Ellis, J. R., Dellavalle, N., Akerson, M., Andazola, M., Campbell, E. G., & DeCamp, M. (2025). Patient-facing chatbots: Enhancing healthcare accessibility while navigating digital literacy challenges and isolation risks—a mixed-methods study. *Digital Health*, *11*, 20552076251337321. PMID: 40308811

Muchuchuti, S., & Viriri, S. (2023). Retinal disease detection using deep learning techniques: A comprehensive review. *Journal of Imaging*, *9*(4), 84. DOI: 10.3390/jimaging9040084 PMID: 37103235

Mukherjee, A., Ghosh, S., Behere, A., Ghosh, S. K., & Buyya, R. (2021). Internet of Health Things (IoHT) for personalized health care using integrated edge-fog-cloud network. *Journal of Ambient Intelligence and Humanized Computing*, *12*(1), 943–959.

Mustacoglu, A. F., Catak, F. O., & Fox, G. C. (2020). Password-based encryption approach for securing sensitive data. *Security and Privacy*, *3*(5), e121.

Myszczynska, M. A., Ojamies, P. N., Lacoste, A. M., Neil, D., Saffari, A., Mead, R., & Ferraiuolo, L. (2020). Applications of machine learning to diagnosis and treatment of neurodegenerative diseases. *Nature Reviews. Neurology*, *16*(8), 440–456. PMID: 32669685

Nadhan, A. S., & Jacob, I. J. (2024). Enhancing healthcare security in the digital era: Safeguarding medical images with lightweight cryptographic techniques in IoT healthcare applications. *Biomedical Signal Processing and Control*, *88*, 105511.

Nandankar, P., Thaker, R., Mughal, S. N., Saidireddy, M., Linda, A., Kostka, J. E., & Nag, M. A. (2021). An iot based healthcare data analytics using fog and cloud computing. *Turk. J. Physiother. Rehabil*, *3*, 32.

Nasser, A. R., Hasan, A. M., Humaidi, A. J., Alkhayyat, A., Alzubaidi, L., Fadhel, M. A., & Duan, Y. (2021). Iot and cloud computing in health-care: A new wearable device and cloud-based deep learning algorithm for monitoring of diabetes. *Electronics (Basel)*, *10*(21), 2719.

National Academies of Sciences, Engineering, and Medicine. (2016). *Making eye health a population health imperative: Vision for tomorrow*. National Academies Press. https://doi.org/DOI: 10.17226/23471

Nayak, P., Mohapatra, S. K., & Sharma, S. C. M. (2022). Privacy and security issues in IoT cloud convergence of smart health care. In *Connected e-Health: Integrated IoT and Cloud Computing* (pp. 439–455). Springer International Publishing.

Nazir, S.. (2019). Internet of Things for healthcare using effects of mobile computing: A systematic literature review. *Wireless Communications and Mobile Computing*, *2019*, 1–20.

Neuroscience News. (2024). How AI is reshaping human thought and decision-making. Retrieved from https://neurosciencenews.com/ai-human-decision-thought-28911/

Noah, B., Keller, M. S., Mosadeghi, S., Stein, L., Johl, S., Delshad, S., Tashjian, V. C., Lew, D., Kwan, J. T., Jusufagic, A., & Spiegel, B. M. (2018). Impact of remote patient monitoring on clinical outcomes: An updated meta-analysis of randomized controlled trials. *NPJ Digital Medicine*, *1*(1), 20172. PMID: 31304346

O'donoghue, J., & Herbert, J. (2012). Data management within mHealth environments: Patient sensors, mobile devices, and databases. [JDIQ]. *Journal of Data and Information Quality*, *4*(1), 1–20.

Obermeyer, Z.. (2019). Dissecting racial bias in an algorithm used to manage the health of populations. *Science*, *366*(6464), 447–453. PMID: 31649194

Paganelli, A. I.. (2022). Real-time data analysis in health monitoring systems: A comprehensive systematic literature review. *Journal of Biomedical Informatics*, *127*, 104009. PMID: 35196579

Page, X., Bahirat, P., Safi, M. I., Knijnenburg, B. P., & Wisniewski, P. (2018). The internet of what? understanding differences in perceptions and adoption for the internet of things. *Proceedings of the ACM on Interactive, Mobile, Wearable and Ubiquitous Technologies*, *2*(4), 1–22.

Palm, E. (2020). Who cares? Moral obligations in formal and informal care provision in the light of ICT-based home care. In *The Ethical Challenges of Emerging Medical Technologies* (pp. 205–222). Routledge.

Palumbo, B., Bianconi, F., Nuvoli, S., Spanu, A., & Fravolini, M. L. (2021). Artificial intelligence techniques support nuclear medicine modalities to improve the diagnosis of Parkinson's disease and Parkinsonian syndromes. *Clinical and Translational Imaging*, *9*, 19–35.

Papadopoulou, E. (2024). The impact of artificial intelligence on psychological and cognitive development. Retrieved from https://elenapap.com/en/the-impact-of-artificial-intelligence-on-psychological-and-cognitive-development

Parihar, A.. (2024). Role of IoT in healthcare: Applications, security & privacy concerns. *Intelligent Pharmacy*, *2*(5), 707–714.

Paris, I. L. B. M., Habaebi, M. H., & Zyoud, A. M. (2023). Implementation of SSL/TLS Security with MQTT Protocol in IoT Environment. *Wireless Personal Communications*, *132*(1), 163–182.

Pattar, S., Buyya, R., Venugopal, K. R., Iyengar, S. S., & Patnaik, L. M. (2018). Searching for the IoT resources: Fundamentals, requirements, comprehensive review, and future directions. *IEEE Communications Surveys and Tutorials*, *20*(3), 2101–2132.

Peralta, G., Cid-Fuentes, R. G., Bilbao, J., & Crespo, P. M. (2019). Homomorphic encryption and network coding in iot architectures: Advantages and future challenges. *Electronics (Basel)*, *8*(8), 827.

Percival, J., & Hanson, J. (2006). Big brother or brave new world? Telecare and its implications for older people's independence and social inclusion. *Critical Social Policy, 26*(4), 888–909.

Pinker, S. (2018). *Enlightenment Now: A Manifesto for Science, Reason, Humanism, and Progress*. Allen Lane.

Poole, T. (2014). *Enhancing The Privacy Framework: An analysis of Privacy in Canadian and Brazilian health care* (Doctoral dissertation, Dalhousie University).

Popescul, D., & Georgescu, M. (2014). Internet of Things–some ethical issues. *The USV Annals of Economics and Public Administration, 13*(2 (18)), 208–214.

Poyner, I. K., & Sherratt, R. S. (2018). Privacy and security of consumer IoT devices for the pervasive monitoring of vulnerable people. In *Living in the Internet of Things: Cybersecurity of the IoT-2018* (pp. 1–5). IET.

Pradhan, B., Bhattacharyya, S., & Pal, K. (2021). IoT-based applications in healthcare devices. *Journal of Healthcare Engineering, 2021*, 1–18. PMID: 33791084

Puiu, A., Vizitiu, A., Nita, C., Itu, L. M., Sharma, P., & Comaniciu, D. (2021). Privacy-preserving and explainable AI for cardiovascular imaging. *Studies in Informatics and Control, 30*, 21–32.

Puustjärvi, J., & Puustjärvi, L. (2011). Automating remote monitoring and information therapy: An opportunity to practice telemedicine in developing countries. In *2011 IST-Africa Conference Proceedings* (pp. 1-9). IEEE.

Quinn, M., Forman, J., Harrod, M., Winter, S., Fowler, K. E., Krein, S. L., Gupta, A., Saint, S., Singh, H., & Chopra, V. (2019). Electronic health records, communication, and data sharing: Challenges and opportunities for improving the diagnostic process. *Diagnosis (Berlin, Germany), 6*(3), 241–248. PMID: 30485175

Quy, V. K., Hau, N. V., Anh, D. V., & Ngoc, L. A. (2022). Smart healthcare IoT applications based on fog computing: Architecture, applications and challenges. *Complex & Intelligent Systems, 8*(5), 3805–3815. PMID: 34804767

Rachim, V. P., & Chung, W. Y. (2016). Wearable noncontact armband for mobile ECG monitoring system. *IEEE Transactions on Biomedical Circuits and Systems, 10*(6), 1112–1118. PMID: 27214910

Raghav, Y. Y., Choudhary, S., Pandey, P., Singh, S., & Varshney, D. (2025). Smart Healthcare: Cloud-IoT Solutions for Enhanced Patient Well-Being. *African Journal of Biomedical Research, 28*(1), 14–28.

Raghu, M., Zhang, C., Kleinberg, J., & Bengio, S. (2019). Transfusion: Understanding transfer learning for medical imaging. *Advances in Neural Information Processing Systems, 32*. https://proceedings.neurips.cc/paper/2019/hash/32a9a0c1f0aaf8f7b6c5b2f4010a512c-Abstract.html

Rahman, M. A., Hossain, M. S., Islam, M. S., Alrajeh, N. A., & Muhammad, G. (2020). Secure and provenance enhanced Internet of health things framework: A blockchain managed federated learning approach. *IEEE Access : Practical Innovations, Open Solutions*, *8*, 205071–205087. PMID: 34192116

Rahman, M. A., Hossain, M. S., Showail, A. J., Alrajeh, N. A., & Alhamid, M. F. (2021). A secure, private, and explainable IoHT framework to support sustainable health monitoring in a smart city. *Sustainable Cities and Society*, *72*, 103083.

Rajpurkar, P., Irvin, J., Zhu, K., Yang, B., Mehta, H., Duan, T., Ding, D., Bagul, A., Langlotz, C., Shpanskaya, K., Lungren, M. P., & Ng, A. Y. (2017). *CheXNet: Radiologist-level pneumonia detection on chest X-rays with deep learning* (arXiv:1711.05225). arXiv. https://arxiv.org/abs/1711.05225

Rajpurkar, P.. (2017). "CheXNet: Radiologist-Level Pneumonia Detection on Chest X-Rays with Deep Learning." arXiv:1711.05225.

Rangarajan, D., Rangarajan, A., Reddy, C. K. K., & Doss, S. (2025). Exploring the Next-Gen Transformations in Healthcare Through the Impact of AI and IoT. In *Intelligent Systems and IoT Applications in Clinical Health* (pp. 73–98). IGI Global.

Rathee, G., Sharma, A., Saini, H., Kumar, R., & Iqbal, R. (2020). A hybrid framework for multimedia data processing in IoT-healthcare using blockchain technology. *Multimedia Tools and Applications*, *79*(15), 9711–9733.

Rayes, B., Ardissino, M., Slob, E. A., Patel, K. H. K., Girling, J., & Ng, F. S. (2023). Association of hypertensive disorders of pregnancy with future cardiovascular disease. *JAMA Network Open*, *6*(2), e230034. PMID: 36800181

Ray, P. P., Dash, D., Salah, K., & Kumar, N. (2020). Blockchain for IoT-based healthcare: Background, consensus, platforms, and use cases. *IEEE Systems Journal*, *15*(1), 85–94.

Reddy, S., Fox, J., & Purohit, M. P. (2019). Artificial intelligence-enabled healthcare delivery. *Journal of the Royal Society of Medicine*, *112*(1), 22–28. DOI: 10.1177/0141076818815510 PMID: 30507284

Reel, P. S.. (2022). Machine learning for classification of hypertension subtypes using multi-omics: A multi-centre, retrospective, data-driven study. *EBioMedicine*, *84*, 104258. PMID: 36179553

Rehiman, K.R. and Veni, S. (2016). A secure authentication infrastructure for IoT enabled smart mobile devices-An initial prototype. *Indian journal of science and technology, 9*(9), pp.0974-6846.

Rejeb, A., Rejeb, K., Treiblmaier, H., Appolloni, A., Alghamdi, S., Alhasawi, Y., & Iranmanesh, M. (2023). The Internet of Things (IoT) in healthcare: Taking stock and moving forward. *Internet of Things : Engineering Cyber Physical Human Systems*, *22*, 100721.

Romiti, S., Vinciguerra, M., Saade, W., Cortajarena, I. A., & Greco, E. (2020). Artificial intelligence (AI) and cardiovascular diseases: An unexpected alliance. *Cardiology Research and Practice*, *5*, 1–8. PMID: 32676206

Rothschild, J. M., Keohane, C. A., Cook, E. F., Orav, E. J., Burdick, E., Thompson, S., Hayes, J., & Bates, D. W. (2005). A controlled trial of smart infusion pumps to improve medication safety in critically ill patients. *Critical Care Medicine*, *33*(3), 533–540. PMID: 15753744

Ruef, M. (2017). Artificial Intelligence: A Model for Humanity, SCIP AG. https://www.scip.ch/?labs.20180104

Ruiz, M. N., García, J. M., & Fernández, B. M. (2009). Body temperature and its importance as a vital constant. *Revista de Enfermeria (Barcelona, Spain)*, *32*(9), 44–52. PMID: 19839238

Saarikko, T.. (2017). The Internet of Things: Are you ready for what's coming? *Business Horizons*, *60*(5), 667–676.

Saeedi, S., Rezayi, S., & Keshavarz, H., & NiakanKalhori, S. R. (2023). MRI-based brain tumor detection using convolutional deep learning methods and chosen machine learning techniques. *BMC Medical Informatics and Decision Making*, *23*(1), 16. DOI: 10.1186/s12911-022-02093-2 PMID: 36691030

Safdar, Z., Farid, S., Qadir, M., Asghar, K., Iqbal, J., & Hamdani, F. K. (2020). A novel architecture for internet of things based E-health systems. *Journal of Medical Imaging and Health Informatics*, *10*(10), 2378–2388.

Sagu, A., & Gill, N. S. (2020). Machine learning techniques for securing IoT environment. [IJITEE]. *International Journal of Innovative Technology and Exploring Engineering*, •••, 9.

Sahoo, N., Lin, H. W., & Chang, Y. H. (2019). Design and implementation of a walking stick aid for visually challenged people. *Sensors (Basel)*, *19*(1), 130. DOI: 10.3390/s19010130 PMID: 30609745

Saini, R., Semwal, P., & Jaware, T. H. (2022). Brain tumor classification using VGG-16 and MobileNetV2 deep learning techniques on magnetic resonance images (MRI). In *International Conference on Soft Computing and its Engineering Applications* (pp. 300–313). Springer Nature Switzerland. https://doi.org/DOI: 10.1007/978-3-031-17191-2_26

Sakib, S., Miah, M. A. S., & Acharjee, U. K.. (2022). Deep learning models for magnetic cardiography edge sensors implementing noise processing and diagnostics. *IEEE Access : Practical Innovations, Open Solutions*, *10*, 2656–2668. DOI: 10.1109/ACCESS.2021.3138976

Samaila, M. G., Neto, M., Fernandes, D. A., Freire, M. M., & Inácio, P. R. (2018). Challenges of securing Internet of Things devices: A survey. *Security and Privacy*, *1*(2), e20.

Sample, I. (2024). AI can change belief in conspiracy theories, study finds. The Guardian. Retrieved from https://www.theguardian.com/science/2024/sep/12/ai-can-change-belief-in-conspiracy-theories-study-finds

Sarangi, A. K., Mohapatra, A. G., Mishra, T. C., & Keswani, B. (2021). Healthcare 4.0: A voyage of fog computing with iot, cloud computing, big data, and machine learning. *Fog Computing for Healthcare 4.0 Environments: Technical, Societal, and Future Implications*, 177-210.

Sarki, R., Ahmed, K., Wang, H., & Zhang, Y. (2020). Automatic detection of diabetic eye disease through deep learning using fundus images: A survey. *IEEE Access : Practical Innovations, Open Solutions*, *8*, 151133–151149. DOI: 10.1109/ACCESS.2020.3015258

Sarrab, M., & Alshohoumi, F. (2021). Assisted-fog-based framework for IoT-based healthcare data preservation. [IJCAC]. *International Journal of Cloud Applications and Computing*, *11*(2), 1–16.

Sattigeri, S. K., Harshith, N., Gowda, D. N., Ullas, K. A., & Aditya, M. S. (2022). Eye disease identification using deep learning (Vol. 9).

Satwik Mamidi. (2022). Electronic health record (EHR) systems integration. *Journal of Health Statistics Reports*. https://doi.org/DOI: 10.47363/JHSR/2022(1)E107

Satyender, S. D. (2025). Smart Implants: The Role of Biocompatible Sensors in Personalized Medicine and Remote Monitoring. *Siddhanta's International. Journal of Science and Technology*, *1*(1), 25–45.

Seh, A. H., Zarour, M., Alenezi, M., Sarkar, A. K., Agrawal, A., Kumar, R., & Ahmad Khan, R. (2020). May. Healthcare data breaches: Insights and implications. [MDPI.]. *Health Care*, *8*(2), 133. PMID: 32414183

Selva Kumar, V., Mohan Raj, K. R., Gopalakrishnan, S., Vennila, G., Dhinakaran, D., & Kavitha, P. (2025). Adaptive distributed honeypot detection network for enhanced cybersecurity against DoS and DDoS attacks. *Results in Engineering*, *26*, 105521. DOI: 10.1016/j.rineng.2025.105521

Selvaraj, D., Jeno, J., Ramani, R., Dhinakaran, D., & Prabaharan, G. (2025). AFCP data security model for EHR data using blockchain. *Journal of Cybersecurity and Information Management*, *15*(1), 22–33. DOI: 10.54216/JCIM.150103

Selvaraj, S., & Sundaravaradhan, S. (2020). Challenges and opportunities in IoT healthcare systems: A systematic review. *SN Applied Sciences*, *2*(1), 139.

Sengan, S., Khalaf, O. I., Vidya Sagar, P., Sharma, D. K., Arokia Jesu Prabhu, L., & Hamad, A. A. (2022). Secured and privacy-based IDS for healthcare systems on e-medical data using machine learning approach. [IJRQEH]. *International Journal of Reliable and Quality E-Healthcare*, *11*(3), 1–11. DOI: 10.4018/IJRQEH.289175

Shah, S. T. U., Yar, H., Khan, I., Ikram, M., & Khan, H. (2019). Internet of things-based healthcare: recent advances and challenges. *Applications of Intelligent Technologies in Healthcare*, pp.153-162.

Shah, H. A., Saeed, F., Yun, S., Park, J.-H., Paul, A., & Kang, J.-M. (2022). A robust approach for brain tumor detection in magnetic resonance images using finetuned EfficientNet. *IEEE Access : Practical Innovations, Open Solutions*, *10*, 65426–65438. DOI: 10.1109/ACCESS.2022.3184028

Shahid, J., Ahmad, R., Kiani, A. K., Ahmad, T., Saeed, S., & Almuhaideb, A. M. (2022). Data protection and privacy of the internet of healthcare things (IoHTs). *Applied Sciences (Basel, Switzerland)*, *12*(4), 1927.

Shamayleh, A.. (2020). IoT based predictive maintenance management of medical equipment. *Journal of Medical Systems*, *44*(4), 72. PMID: 32078712

Shastri, S., Kour, P., Kumar, S., Singh, K., Sharma, A., & Mansotra, V. (2021). A nested stacking ensemble model for predicting districts with high and low maternal mortality ratio (MMR) in India. *International Journal of Information Technology : an Official Journal of Bharati Vidyapeeth's Institute of Computer Applications and Management*, *13*, 433–446.

Shen, D., Wu, G., & Suk, H.-I. (2017). Deep learning in medical image analysis. *Annual Review of Biomedical Engineering*, *19*, 221–248. DOI: 10.1146/annurev-bioeng-071516-044442 PMID: 28301734

Shermock, S. B., Shermock, K. M., & Schepel, L. L. (2023). Closed-loop medication management with an electronic health record system in U.S. and Finnish hospitals. *International Journal of Environmental Research and Public Health*, *20*, 6680. DOI: 10.3390/ijerph20176680 PMID: 37681820

Shin, H. W., Hong, S. W., & Youn, Y. C. (2022). Clinical aspects of the differential diagnosis of Parkinson's disease and parkinsonism. *Journal of Clinical Neurology (Seoul, Korea)*, *18*(3), 259. PMID: 35589315

Shi, Y., & Li, C. (2018). "Exploration of computer emotion decision based on artificial intelligence," in *Proceedings of the 2018 International Conference on Virtual Reality and Intelligent Systems (ICVRIS)* (Hunan: IEEE), 293–295. Available at: https://doi.org/DOI: 10.1109/ICVRIS.2018.00078

Shortliffe, E. H., & Sepúlveda, M. J. (2018). Clinical decision support in the era of artificial intelligence. *Journal of the American Medical Association*, *320*(21), 2199–2200. DOI: 10.1001/jama.2018.17163 PMID: 30398550

Shrestha, N. M., Alsadoon, A., Prasad, P. W. C., Hourany, L., & Elchouemi, A. (2016). Enhanced e-health framework for security and privacy in healthcare system. In *2016 Sixth International Conference on Digital Information Processing and Communications (ICDIPC)* (pp. 75–79). Beirut, Lebanon. https://doi.org/DOI: 10.1109/ICDIPC.2016.7470795

Silva, G. F. S.. (2022). Machine learning for hypertension prediction: A systematic review. *Current Hypertension Reports*, *24*(11), 523–533. PMID: 35731335

Singal, V., & Tomar, S. (2022). Patient data: Solving ownership question. *Pharmaceutical Commerce, 17*(6).

Singh, V., Paul, R., Mehra, D., Gupta, A. G., Sharma, V. D., Jain, S., Agarwal, C., Garg, A., Gujral, S. S., Balakrishnan, M., Paul, K., Rao, P. V., & Manocha, D. (2010). *"Smart" cane for the visually impaired: Design and controlled field testing of an affordable obstacle detection system.*

Smart healthcare in IoT using convolutional based cyber physical system. (2022, October 16). IEEE Conference Publication. https://doi.org/DOI: 10.1109/MysuruCon55714.2022.9972679

Sohn, S.. (2019). A Hybrid Approach to Automatic De-identification of Electronic Medical Records. *Journal of the American Medical Informatics Association : JAMIA*.

Somashekhar, S. P.. (2018). Implementation of IBM Watson for Oncology in a Multispecialty Hospital in India: A Prospective, Multicenter, Observational Study. *Journal of Clinical Oncology*.

Steinhubl, S. R., Muse, E. D., & Topol, E. J. (2015). The emerging field of mobile health: Research methods, issues, and challenges. *Health Affairs*, *34*(5), 924–930. DOI: 10.1377/hlthaff.2015.0010

Stephen, M., & Kolachala, R. (2025). Revolutionizing Healthcare: IoT Powered Telemedicine Advancements. In *Scalable Modeling and Efficient Management of IoT Applications* (pp. 59-86). IGI Global.

Stone, P.. (2016). *Artificial Intelligence and Life in 2030. One Hundred Year Study on Artificial Intelligence: Report of the 2015–2016 Study Panel*. Stanford University.

Stowe, S., & Harding, S. (2010). Telecare, telehealth and telemedicine. *European Geriatric Medicine*, *1*(3), 193–197.

Subbiah, S., Ramya, S., Krishna, G. P., & Nayagam, S. (2019). Smart cane for visually impaired based on IoT. In *2019 3rd International Conference on Computing and Communications Technologies (ICCCT)* (pp. 50–53). IEEE. https://doi.org/ DOI: 10.1109/ICCCT2.2019.8824893

Sun, T. Q., & Medaglia, R. (2019). Mapping the challenges of artificial intelligence in the public sector: Evidence from public healthcare. *Government Information Quarterly*, *36*(2), 368–383. DOI: 10.1016/j.giq.2018.09.008

Sun, Y., Lo, F. P. W., & Lo, B. (2019). Security and privacy for the internet of medical things enabled healthcare systems: A survey. *IEEE Access : Practical Innovations, Open Solutions*, *7*, 183339–183355.

Supriya, S., & Padaki, S. (2016). December. Data security and privacy challenges in adopting solutions for IOT. In *2016 IEEE International Conference on Internet of Things (iThings) and IEEE Green Computing and Communications (GreenCom) and IEEE Cyber, Physical and Social Computing (CPSCom) and IEEE Smart Data (SmartData)* (pp. 410-415). IEEE.

Szegedy, C., Liu, W., Jia, Y., Sermanet, P., Reed, S., Anguelov, D., Erhan, D., Vanhoucke, V., & Rabinovich, A. (2015). Going deeper with convolutions. In *Proceedings of the IEEE Conference on Computer Vision and Pattern Recognition* (pp. 1–9). https://doi.org/DOI: 10.1109/CVPR.2015.7298594

Tahir, M., Badriyah, T., & Syarif, I. (2018). Neural networks algorithm to inquire previous preeclampsia factors in women with chronic hypertension during pregnancy in childbirth process. In *2018 International Electronics Symposium on Knowledge Creation and Intelligent Computing (IES-KCIC)* (pp. 51–55). IEEE.

Tan, M., & Le, Q. (2019). EfficientNet: Rethinking model scaling for convolutional neural networks. In *International Conference on Machine Learning* (pp. 6105–6114). PMLR.

Thakur, A., Singh, R., & Gehlot, A. (2018). Smart blind stick for obstacle detection and navigation system. *International Journal of Engineering Research & Technology (Ahmedabad)*, *5*, 216–221.

Tharini, V. J., & Shivakumar, B. L. (2023). An efficient pruned matrix aided utility tree for high utility itemset mining from transactional database. *International Journal of Intelligent Systems and Applications in Engineering*, *11*(4s), 46–55.

Tharini, V. J., & Vijayarani, S. (2020). IoT in healthcare: Ecosystem, pillars, design challenges, applications, vulnerabilities, privacy, and security concerns. In *Incorporating the Internet of Things in healthcare applications and wearable devices* (pp. 1–22). IGI Global.

THE 17 GOALS | Sustainable Development. Retrieved, 2025, from https://sdgs.un.org/goals

Ting, D. S. W., Cheung, C. Y. Y., & Lim, G.. (2017). Development and validation of a deep learning system for diabetic retinopathy and related eye diseases using retinal images from multiethnic populations with diabetes. *Journal of the American Medical Association*, *318*(22), 2211–2223. DOI: 10.1001/jama.2017.18152 PMID: 29234807

Ting, D. S., Liu, Y., Burlina, P., Xu, X., Bressler, N. M., & Wong, T. Y. (2018). AI for medical imaging goes deep. *Nature Medicine*, *24*, 539–540. DOI: 10.1038/s41591-018-0029-3 PMID: 29736024

Tita, A. T., Szychowski, J. M., Boggess, K., Dugoff, L., Sibai, B., Lawrence, K., & Andrews, W. W. (2022). Treatment for mild chronic hypertension during pregnancy. *The New England Journal of Medicine*, *386*(19), 1781–1792. PMID: 35363951

Tiwari, P., Warren, J., Day, K. J., & MacDonald, B. (2010). *Some non-technology implications for wider application of robots to assist older people*. Health Care and Informatics Review Online.

Tolosa, E., Garrido, A., Scholz, S. W., & Poewe, W. (2021). Challenges in the diagnosis of Parkinson's disease. *Lancet Neurology*, *20*(5), 385–397. PMID: 33894193

Topol, E. J. (2019). High-performance medicine: The convergence of human and artificial intelligence. *Nature Medicine*, *25*(1), 44–56. DOI: 10.1038/s41591-018-0300-7 PMID: 30617339

Tripathy, S., Singh, R., & Ray, M. (2023). Automation of brain tumor identification using EfficientNet on magnetic resonance images. *Procedia Computer Science*, *218*, 1551–1560. DOI: 10.1016/j.procs.2023.01.136

Truong, Y., & Papagiannidis, S. (2022). Artificial Intelligence as an Enabler for Innovation: A Review and Future Research Agenda. *Technological Forecasting and Social Change*, *183*, 121852.

Tschopp, M. & Ruef, M. (2017). Development of an Artificial Intelligence Quotient. Available at: https://www.iaiqs.org/

Van Alstyne, M., Brynjolfsson, E., & Madnick, S. (1995). Why not one big database? Principles for data ownership. *Decision Support Systems*, *15*(4), 267–284.

van Weel, C.. (2018). Why strengthening primary health care is essential to achieving universal health coverage. *Canadian Medical Association Journal*, *190*(15), E463–E466. PMID: 29661815

Van Woudenberg, J., & O'Flynn, C. (2021). *The hardware hacking handbook: breaking embedded security with hardware attacks*. No Starch Press.

Varhol, R. J., Robinson, S., Lee, C. M. Y., Randall, S., & Boyd, J. H. (2025). Attitudes towards data access and sharing health data for research: A case study of Australian data custodian perspectives. *The HIM Journal*, •••, 18333583251329533. PMID: 40317196

Vayadande, K., Ingale, V., Verma, V., Yeole, A., Zawar, S., & Jamadar, Z. (2022). Ocular disease recognition using deep learning. In *Proceedings of the International Conference on Signal and Information Processing (IConSIP)* (pp. 1–7). IEEE. https://doi.org/DOI: 10.1109/ICoNSIP49665.2022.10007470

Verdejo Espinosa, A., Lopez, J. L., Mata Mata, F., & Estevez, M. E. (2021). Application of IoT in healthcare: Keys to implementation of the sustainable development goals. *Sensors (Basel)*, *21*(7), 2330. PMID: 33810606

Verma, P., Tiwari, R., Hong, W. C., Upadhyay, S., & Yeh, Y. H. (2022). FETCH: A deep learning-based fog computing and IoT integrated environment for healthcare monitoring and diagnosis. *IEEE Access : Practical Innovations, Open Solutions*, *10*, 12548–12563.

Vizitiu, A., Nita, C. I., Puiu, A., Suciu, C., & Itu, L. (2020). Applying deep neural networks over homomorphic encrypted medical data. *Computational and Mathematical Methods in Medicine*, *4*, 1–26. PMID: 32351612

Vorisek, C. N., Lehne, M., Klopfenstein, S. A. I., Mayer, P. J., Bartschke, A., Haese, T., & Thun, S. (2022). Fast healthcare interoperability resources (FHIR) for interoperability in health research: Systematic review. *JMIR Medical Informatics*, *10*(7), e35724. PMID: 35852842

Wang, H., Qi, Q., Sun, W., Li, X., Dong, B., & Yao, C. (2023). Classification of skin lesions with generative adversarial networks and improved MobileNetV2. *International Journal of Imaging Systems and Technology*. Advance online publication. DOI: 10.1002/ima.22807

Wang, J., Yang, L., Huo, Z., He, W., & Luo, J. (2020). Multi-label classification of fundus images with EfficientNet. *IEEE Access : Practical Innovations, Open Solutions*, *8*, 212499–212508. DOI: 10.1109/ACCESS.2020.3040275

Wanriko, S., Hnoohom, N., Wongpatikaseree, K., Jitpattanakul, A., & Musigavong, O. (2021). Risk assessment of pregnancy-induced hypertension using a machine learning approach. In *2021 Joint International Conference on Digital Arts, Media and Technology with ECTI Northern Section Conference on Electrical, Electronics, Computer and Telecommunication Engineering* (pp. 233–237). IEEE.

Wisner, K. (2019). Gestational hypertension and preeclampsia. *MCN. The American Journal of Maternal Child Nursing*, *44*(3), 170. PMID: 31033586

Woebot Health. (2020). *AI in mental health: How Woebot delivers cognitive-behavioral therapy through AI-powered chat*. Woebot Health. https://woebothealth.com

World Health Organization. International Telecommunication Union, & World Intellectual Property Organization. (n.d.). *Global Initiative on AI for Health: Improving health outcomes through AI*. WHO, ITU, & WIPO. Retrieved March 25, 2025, from https://www.who.int/news-room/fact-sheets/detail/ai-for-health

Wubineh, B. Z., Deriba, F. G., & Woldeyohannis, M. M. (2024). Exploring the opportunities and challenges of implementing artificial intelligence in healthcare: A systematic literature review. *Urologic Oncology: Seminars and Original Investigations*, *42*(3), 48–56. DOI: 10.1016/j.urolonc.2023.11.019 PMID: 38101991

Wu, Y. H., Fassert, C., & Rigaud, A. S. (2012). Designing robots for the elderly: Appearance issue and beyond. *Archives of Gerontology and Geriatrics*, *54*(1), 121–126. PMID: 21349593

Xu, P., Song, A., & Wang, K. (2023). Intelligent head-mounted obstacle avoidance wearable for the blind and visually impaired. *Sensors (Basel), 23*(23), 9598. DOI: 10.3390/s23239598 PMID: 38067971

Xu, Y.. (2021). Artificial intelligence is a powerful paradigm for scientific research. *The Innovation, 2*(4), 100179. DOI: 10.1016/j.xinn.2021.100179 PMID: 34877560

Xu, Y.. (2024). *2021; Zhang andTao, 2020; Truong and Papagiannidi; 2022*. Sample.

Yang, G. Z., Cambias, J., & Cleary, K.. (2022). Medical robotics—Regulatory, ethical, and legal considerations for increasing levels of autonomy. *Science Robotics, 7*(66), eabl9514. Advance online publication. DOI: 10.1126/scirobotics.abl9514 PMID: 33157870

Yang, G., Xie, L., Mäntysalo, M., Zhou, X., Pang, Z., Da Xu, L., Kao-Walter, S., Chen, Q., & Zheng, L. R. (2014). A health-IoT platform based on the integration of intelligent packaging, unobtrusive bio-sensor, and intelligent medicine box. *IEEE Transactions on Industrial Informatics, 10*(4), 2180–2191.

Yang, W.-F. (2019). The feasibility of applying artificial intelligence detection technology in predicting the risk of hypertension. *Advances in Artificial Intelligence and Machine Learning, 3*(3), 79–1168.

Yang, Z., Liang, B., & Ji, W. (2021). An intelligent end–edge–cloud architecture for visual IoT-assisted healthcare systems. *IEEE Internet of Things Journal, 8*(23), 16779–16786.

Yan, Y., Zhang, J., Zang, G., & Pu, J. (2019). The primary use of artificial intelligence in cardiovascular diseases: What kind of potential role does artificial intelligence play in future medicine? *Journal of Geriatric Cardiology : JGC, 16*(8), 585–591. PMID: 31555325

Yao, J., Zhang, S., Yao, Y., Wang, F., Ma, J., Zhang, J., & Chu, Y.. (2022). Edge-cloud polarization and collaboration: A comprehensive survey for AI. *IEEE Transactions on Knowledge and Data Engineering, 35*(7), 6866–6886. DOI: 10.1109/TKDE.2022.3156515

Yew, H. T., Ng, M. F., Ping, S. Z., Chung, S. K., Chekima, A., & Dargham, J. A. (2020). February. Iot based real-time remote patient monitoring system. In *2020 16th IEEE international colloquium on signal processing & its applications (CSPA)* (pp. 176-179). IEEE.

Yin, Y.. (2016). The Internet of Things in healthcare: An overview. *Journal of Industrial Information Integration, 1*, 3–13.

Yohannan, A., & Shyam, S. (2020). *Smart cane for blind and visually impaired persons*. https://doi.org/DOI: 10.13140/RG.2.2.10908.51840

Yuehong, Y. I. N., Zeng, Y., Chen, X., & Fan, Y. (2016). The internet of things in healthcare: An overview. *Journal of Industrial Information Integration*, *1*, 3–13.

Yusof, Z. B. (2025). The Role of High-Quality Data in Risk Assessment: Strategies for Ensuring Accuracy, Completeness, and Timeliness in Financial Predictive Analytics. *International Journal of Advanced Computational Methodologies and Emerging Technologies*, *15*(2), 8–16.

Yuste, R.. (2017). Four ethical priorities for neurotechnologies and AI. *Nature*, *551*, 159. DOI: 10.1038/551159a PMID: 29120438

Yu, X., Wang, J., Hong, Q.-Q., Teku, R., Wang, S.-H., & Zhang, Y.-D. (2022). Transfer learning for medical images analyses: A survey. *Neurocomputing*, *489*, 230–254. DOI: 10.1016/j.neucom.2022.05.094

Zhang, J., & Tao, D. J. (2020). Empowering things with intelligence: A survey of the progress, challenges, and opportunities in the artificial intelligence of things. *IEEE Internet of Things Journal*, *8*, 7789–7817.

Zhavoronkov, A., Ivanenkov, Y. A., & Aliper, A.. (2019). Deep learning enables rapid identification of potent DDR1 kinase inhibitors. *Nature Biotechnology*, *37*(9), 1038–1040. DOI: 10.1038/s41587-019-0224-x PMID: 31477924

Zhong, D., Yian, Z., Lanqing, W., Junhua, D., & Jiaxuan, H. (2020). Continuous blood pressure measurement platform: A wearable system based on multidimensional perception data. *IEEE Access : Practical Innovations, Open Solutions*, *8*, 10147–10158.

Zwijsen, S. A., Niemeijer, A. R., & Hertogh, C. M. (2011). Ethics of using assistive technology in the care for community-dwelling elderly people: An overview of the literature. *Aging & Mental Health*, *15*(4), 419–427. PMID: 21500008

About the Contributors

Altaf O. Mulani is a Professor and Head of Electronics and Telecommunication Engineering at SKN Sinhgad College of Engineering, Pandharpur, India. With over 22 years of experience, he has significantly contributed to teaching, curriculum development, academic administration, and research leadership. He has served in key institutional roles including IQAC Coordinator, PG Coordinator, and Examination Coordinator. He is actively associated with reputed international publishers as Guest Editor, Editor and Reviewer for SCI/SCIE and Scopus-indexed journals. His research interests span VLSI, embedded systems, image processing etc. He has published more than 100 research articles, holds 5 UK patents and 2 Indian patent and has successfully organized international conferences with Scopus-indexed proceedings. He received funded research grants from national agencies and continues to mentor research scholars and UG/PG projects, contributing to innovation-driven engineering education.

Korhan Cengiz was born in Edirne, Turkey, in 1986. He received the BSc degrees in Electronics and Communication Engineering from Kocaeli University and Business Administration from Anadolu University, Turkey in 2008 and 2009 respectively. He took his MSc degree in Electronics and Communication Engineering from Namik Kemal University, Turkey in 2011, and the PhD degree in Electronics Engineering from Kadir Has University, Turkey in 2016. Since March 2023, He has been a Senior Researcher in the department of Information Technologies, University of Hradec Kralove, Kralove, Czech Republic. Since September 2022, He has been an Associate Professor in the department of Computer Engineering, Istinye University, Istanbul, Turkey. Since April 2022, he has been the chair of the research committee of University of Fujairah, United Arab Emirates. Since August 2021, he has been an Assistant Professor at the College of Information Technology in University of Fujairah, UAE. Dr. Cengiz is the author of more than 40 SCI / SCI-E articles including IEEE Internet of Things Journal, IEEE Access, Expert Systems with Applications, Knowledge Based Systems and ACM Transactions on Sensor Networks, 5 international patents, more than 10 book chapters, and 1 book in Turkish. He is editor of more than 20 books. His research interests include wireless sensor networks, wireless communications, statistical signal processing, indoor positioning systems, internet of things, power electronics and 5G. He is the Associate Editor of IEEE Transactions on Intelligent Transportation Systems, IEEE Potentials Magazine, Handling Editor of Microprocessors and Microsystems, Elsevier, Associate Editor of IET Electronics Letters, and IET Networks. He serves several reviewer positions for IEEE Internet of Things Journal, IEEE Sensors Journal and IEEE Access. He serves several book editor positions in IEEE, Springer, Elsevier, Wiley and CRC. He presented 40+ keynote talks in reputed IEEE and Springer Conferences about WSNs, IoT and 5G. He is Senior Member, IEEE and Professional Member of ACM. Dr. Cengiz' s awards and honors include the Tubitak Priority Areas PhD Scholarship, the Kadir Has University PhD Student Scholarship, best presentation award in ICAT 2016 Conference and best paper award in ICAT 2018 Conference.

Suman Lata Tripathi is working as Professor in Department of Electronics and Telecommunication Engineering, Symbiosis Institute of Technology, Symbiosis International (Deemed University), Pune with more than 23 years of experience in academics and research. She has completed her Ph.D. in the area of microelectronics and VLSI Design from MNNIT, Allahabad. She did her MTech in Electronics Engineering from UP Technical University, Lucknow and BTech in Electrical Engineering from Purvanchal University, Jaunpur. She is also a remote post-doc researcher at Nottingham Trent University, London, UK in the year 2022. She has published more than 225 research papers in refereed Springer, Elsevier, IEEE, Wiley and IOP science journals, conference proceeding and e-books. She has also published 13 Indian patents and 4 copyright. She has guided 8 PhD scholar and 4 are under submission stage. She has organized several workshops, summer internships, and expert lectures for students. She has worked as a session chair, conference steering committee member, editorial board member, and peer reviewer in international/ national IEEE, Springer, Wiley etc Journal and conferences. She has received the "Research Excellence Award" in 2019 and "Research Appreciation Award" in 2020, 2021, 2023 at Lovely Professional University, India. She is recipient of IGEN Women's for Green Technology "Women's Achievers Award" on International Women's Day, 8th March-2023. She had received the best paper at IEEE ICICS-2018. She has also received funded project from SERB DST under the scheme TARE in the area of Microelectronics devices. She has edited and authored more than 35 books in different areas of Electronics and electrical engineering. She is associated for editing work with top publishers like Elsevier, CRC Taylor and Francis, Wiley-IEEE, SP Wiley, Nova Science and Apple academic press etc. She is also working as book series editor for title, “Smart Engineering Systems” CRC Press, “Engineering system design for sustainable developments” & “Decentralized Systems & Next Generation Internet” Wiley-Scrivener, and conference series editor for “Conference Proceedings Series on Intelligent systems for Engineering designs” CRC Press Taylor & Francis. She is serving as academic editor of the journals “Journal of Electrical and Computer Engineering”, “International Journal of Reconfigurable Computing”, and “Active and Passive Electronic Component”, Wiley, USA. She is associated as senior member IEEE, Fellow IETE and Life member ISC and is continuously involved in different professional activities along with academic work. Her area of expertise includes microelectronics device modelling and characterization, low power VLSI circuit design, VLSI design of testing, and advanced FET design for IoT, Embedded System Design, reconfigurable architecture with FPGAs and biomedical applications etc.

***

A Aruna having 7+ years of experience as Assistant professor in the department of computer science and engineering. She is currently pursuing her Ph.D in the area of EHR security. She has authored and co authored various research publications and patents.

A. Ramathilagam is working as a Professor in the Department of Computer Science and Engineering at P.S.R. Engineering College, Sivakasi. She has 21 years of teaching experience. She completed her Ph.D. in Information and Communication Engineering from Anna University in the year 2018. She obtained her M.E Computer Science, Engineering in the year 2004, B.E Computer Science, and Engineering in the year 1999 from Arulmigu Kalasalingam College of Engineering, Krishnankovil. She has authored many book chapters in the reputed publishers like springer, CRC Press etc. She has published 15 papers in reputed international/national journals and presented 20 papers in National and International conferences. Her research interests are Computer Network, Security, Cloud Computing, Big Data Analytics, Machine Learning and Data Science. She is the reviewer of Journal of Communication systems (Wiley publishers), Journal of Super Computing (Springer), and Journal of Intelligent System (Wiley publishers). She has published seven patents. She has received Rs.3 Lakhs from AICTE for organizing STTP. She also holds professional membership in ACM and Life Member in ISTE.

A.Sathya, Associate Professor, Department of Artificial Intelligence and Data Analytics, Sri Ramachandra Faculty of Engineering and Technology,SRIHER has 17 Years of teaching experience. She has undertaken and guided many social relevant project works. A patent has been filed in her name and authored book chapters in reputed publications like springer and Wiley. She published more than 25 papers in conferences and journals. Her area of interest includes Cloud security, Data Analytics. She also worked in a consultancy project in the area of machine vision, image processing, web application, mobile application and cloud computing.

Kashvi Chaturvedi, is studying B.Tech, specialisation in Artificial Intelligence and Data Science at Ajeenkya DY Patil University. She started solidifying her programming skills by completing various certification courses like Data Structures in C, Tableau functions and Operating Systems along with doing few projects using languages like Python, C, C++ and creating Web Page using HTML, CSS and Java Script. She had also attended an Arduino-Based Automation course at Dolphin Labs to enhance her software knowledge. There, she learned how to work with sensors, microcontrollers, and circuit design. She has also written multiple review papers on topics such as Geographic Information Systems, Comparative Analysis of BJT Configurations, Swiss Bank vs. European Central Bank: Data Analysis. She is also researching on and learning many topics such as Small Modular Reactors, Bibliometric Analysis, UNSDGs etc. Because of her interest in latest technologies, she also participated in Global Hyperloop Competition hosted by IIT Madras representing her college as team Vac-Vectoor where she learnt more about various subtopics from the mentors.

D. Dhinakaran (M'84) was born in Chennai, Tamilnadu, India, in 1984. He is a distinguished scholar and educator with a passion for advancing the fields of Computer Science and Engineering. Dr. Dhinakaran earned his B.E degree in Computer Science and Engineering from Anna University, Chennai, in 2006, showcasing early dedication to his academic pursuits. Building upon his foundation, he pursued and obtained the M.E degree in the field of Computer Science and Engineering from Anna University, Trichy, in 2009. Demonstrating a commitment to academic excellence, Dr. Dhinakaran completed his Ph.D. in Computer Science and Engineering from Anna University, Chennai, further solidifying his expertise in the field. Currently serving as an Associate Professor in the Department of Computer Science and Engineering at Vel Tech Rangarajan Dr. Sagunthala R&D Institute of Science and Technology, Chennai, Dr. Dhinakaran continues to inspire students and colleagues alike. His areas of specialization encompass Privacy-Preserving Data Mining, Artificial Intelligence, Internet of Things (IoT), Mobile Ad Hoc Networks (MANET), Cloud Computing, and Image Processing, reflecting his diverse and extensive contributions to cutting-edge technologies. Dr. Dhinakaran is a prolific researcher, having presented more than 30 papers at various National and International Conferences. His commitment to advancing knowledge is evident through his membership in esteemed professional societies such as IAENG (International Association of Engineers), IFERP (International Foundation for Engineering Research and Publications), and CSTA (Computer Science Teachers Association). Notably, Dr. Dhinakaran has made significant contributions to academic literature, with publications in 50 different international journals and the successful filing of two patents. His work demonstrates a keen interest in addressing contemporary challenges and pushing the boundaries of technological innovation. As an accomplished academic, researcher, and member of professional societies, Dr. Dhinakaran continues to play a pivotal role in shaping the future of Computer Science and Engineering, leaving an indelible mark on both academia and the broader technological landscape.

Susanta Das is a seasoned educator with a proven record of teaching and mentoring diverse students, working at multiple institutions, and providing service to the various initiatives of organizations. He received his Ph.D. and M.A. degrees from Western Michigan University (WMU), USA, and M.Sc. degree from Banaras Hindu University (BHU), India all in Physics. He continued his post-doctoral research as a Marie-Curie post-doctoral fellow at Stockholm University Stockholm, Sweden on beam diagnostics for the DESIREE (Double ElectroStatic Ion Ring ExpEriment) in the project DITANET (Diagnostic Techniques for particle Accelerators – a Marie-Curie initial training NETwork), at the Indian Institute of Science Education and Research-Kolkata, India on high-pressure physics as a Project Scientist-B, and at the University of Electro-Communications, Tokyo, Japan on ion-surface interactions as a Post-doctoral fellow. Throughout his career, Dr. Das worked and collaborated with many researchers, Ph.D., master, and visiting students from different countries. He further visited many countries to discuss research and an international conference participant (UK, Italy, Germany, Greece, Belgium, Bulgaria, Romania, Brazil etc.). He co-authored several research articles in WoS/Scopus indexed international journals, conference proceedings, and scholarly book chapters published by renowned international publishing houses. Beyond his research endeavors, Dr. Das has a storied history of service to academic and administrative committees, exhibiting his commitment to the growth and development of educational institutions. His experience includes tenure at Central University South Bihar, Sri Sri University, and P.K. University before assuming his current role at Ajeenkya DY Patil University. He received the Marie-Curie post-doctoral fellowship in Sweden, Science Academies' Summer Research Fellowship in India, Gwen Frostic Doctoral Fellowship, Department Graduate Research and Creative Scholar Award by WMU, and Leo R. Parpart Doctoral Fellowship by Dept. of Physics, WMU, among many others, throughout his academic journey. At present, Dr. Das continues to delve into cutting-edge fields, with a keen interest in nanotechnology, quantum computing, and data science. His multifaceted contributions, spanning teaching, research, and administrative leadership, showcase a dedicated professional who is instrumental in advancing the vision and mission of the institutions he serves.

Himadri Sekhar Das is presently working as Assistant professor in Haldia Institute of Technology. He did his post doc from Haldia Institute of Technology. He got his Ph. D degree from Indian Institute of Engineering Science and Technology (IIEST), Shibpur in 2021, M. Tech from Maulana Abul Kalam Azad University of Technology, West Bengal in 2010. M.Sc and B.Sc from Vidyasagar University in 2006 and 2008 respectively. His research area was Doped ZnO based thin Film for different optoelectronics applications. Synthesis and characterization of organic-inorganic Perovskite material for Solar cell. ZnO based transparent conducting oxide thin film for mesoporous TiO2 based dye sensitized solar cell. Solid state electrolyte based dye sensitized solar cell: stability and device performance. Solvo thermal synthesis of ZnO nanoparticle. Polymer based Organic Solar Cell, Photonic Materials and devices (LED & Thin Film Display). He has published more than 40 research articles and 2 book and 10 book chapter. He is also DST Fellow and life member and Fellow of Indian Chemical Society (FICS) and Indian Photobiology society (IPS) also the Member of Royal Society of Chemistry-UK.

Pooja Dehankar is working as an Assistant Professor at Ajeenkya DY Patil School of Engineering, Savitribai Phule Pune University, Pune. She has completed BE in Computer Engineering from Priyadarshini College of Engineering, Nagpur, and ME in Information Technology from Sinhgad College of Engineering, Pune. She has done Post Graduate Diploma in Advance Computing. She has 15 years of experience in academics. Her areas of interest are Artificial Intelligence, Cyber Security, and Data Mining. She has published papers in Scopus Journals. She actively participates in workshops, faculty development programs, short-term training programs, conferences, and webinars. She is pursuing Ph.D. from Symbiosis Center for Research and Innovation, Symbiosis International (Deemed University).

Harsh Deshmukh is pursuing BTech in Computer Scienec and Engineering at Rajarambapu Institute of Technology, Islampur, India

Nagaraj V. Dharwadkar obtained B.E. in Computer Science and Engineering in 2000, from Karnataka University Dharwad, M.Tech. in Computer Science and Engineering in the year 2006 from VTU, Belgum and Ph.D. in Computer Science and Engineering in 2014 from National Institute of Technology, Warangal . He is Associate Professor in the department of Computer Science at Central University of Karnataka, Kadaganchi. He had 23 years of Teaching Experience at Professional Institutes across India and published 100 papers in various International Journals and

Conferences. His area of research interest is Multimedia Security, Image Processing, Big Data Analytics and Machine Learning.

Raghavendrasingh Dharwadkar is Assistant Professor in the department of Neurology Physiotherapy, KAHER Institute of Physiotherapy Belagavi. His domain of expertise is neurology and expert in Physiotherapy.

Jeno Jasmine, Associate Professor, Department of Computer Science and Engineering in Vel Tech High Tech Dr. Rangarajan Dr. Sakunthala Engineering College. She has completed her Ph.D. in Information and Communication Engineering from Anna University-Chennai in the year 2020. She obtained her M.E. (Network Engineering) in the year 2008 from Arulmigu Kalasalingam College of Engineering, Krishnankovil and her B.E. (Information Technology) in the year 2006 from Karunya Institute of Technology and Science, Coimbatore. She has thirteen plus years of teaching experience. Her area of interests is on Computer Networks. She has published more than 6 research articles in journals, conferences and a patent.

Vishnulakshmi K is working as assistant professor in Dr.N.G.P Institute of Technology, from 11-12-2023 onwards. She has completed masters in Medical Electronics and completed Undergraduate in Electronics and communication Engineering. She has 3.5 years of Teaching experience and published journal paper Genetic Algorithm Based Brain Tumor Detection and Segmentation.

Vijay H. Kalmani holds an M.Tech in Computer Science and Engineering from Gogte Institute of Technology, Belagavi, affiliated with Visvesvaraya Technological University, and a Ph.D. in Computer Science and Engineering from Suresh Gyan Vihar University, Jaipur, India, obtained in 2016. Currently, he serves as a Professor in the Department of Computer Science and Information Technology at Rajarambapu Institute of Technology, Islampur, Sangli, India. His expertise lies in Cloud Security, Artificial Intelligence, and Machine Learning.email:vijay.kalmani@ritindia.edu

Tawanda Mushiri has research areas in Artificial Intelligence, Medical Robotics and Biomedical Engineering. His main research focus is on the Robotic First Aid (RFA) systems to reduce Road Traffic Accidents (RTA) and Disease Prediction Modelling using Artificial Intelligence. He is in the process of finalizing his patent for Robotic First Aid in passenger vehicle, which will reduce deaths in the global society at scenes where accidents occur. He is the point person for Artificial Intelligence at University of Zimbabwe. He has managed to do projects and grants up to USD$3,5m. He is Currently the Coordinator and an Associate Professor in the Department of Biomedical Informatics and Biomedical Engineering (BIBE) in the Faculty of Medicine and Health Sciences (FMHS) at UZ. Tawanda has worked under University of Zimbabwe in developing a number of currently working plants which are Number Plate, Edible Oil, Feed, Bakery and Sanitiser design, procurement of raw materials upto implementation. Tawanda is a Corporate Member of the Zimbabwe Institute of Engineers (ZIE) and the Engineering Council of Zimbabwe. He has supervised more than 380 students' undergraduate projects, 116 master's Students to completion, 1 MPhil and 5 PhD students in progress, 1 MPhil and 2 PhD students completed. He has also published 5 books, 14 chapters in a book, 25 journals in highly accredited publishers, 87 conferences in peer reviewed publishers and 1 patent. In the Global world, Tawanda supervises FIRST GLOBAL students for Robotics club, was a Senior Research Associate in the Department of Quality and Operations Management from 1 November 2017 – 31 October 2020 at UJ, has been a reviewer of journals and conferences in the academic world and an external reviewer of MPhils and DPhils in different universities. He is currently an External Examiner for National University of Science and Technology (NUST) ZW and Harare Institute of Technology (HIT). Tawanda Mushiri is a Senior Research Associate Research Fellow (SRARF) in the Faculty of Health Sciences, Biomedical Engineering and Healthcare Technology (BEAHT) Research Centre at UJ. He is a consultant Biomedical Engineer with Global Health since April 2020 to date working with medical equipment for Nyadire, Mutambara and Old Mutare Hospital in maintenance issues and procuring new equipment.

Thiyagarajan N, is working as Assistant Professor in the Department of ECE, KGiSL Institute of Technology, Coimbatore, Tamil Nadu, India. His research interests include wireless sensor networks, meta heuristic optimization algorithms and machine learning. This author has 12 years of experience in teaching and 3 years in research

Veena Raj received the bachelor's degree in electronics and communication Engineering and master's degree in applied electronics from Anna University in Chennai, India. She received the Ph.D. degree in systems engineering from the Faculty of Integrated Technologies, Universiti Brunei Darussalam. She is currently working as a lecturer in Info Communication System at the Faculty of Integrated Technologies, Universiti Brunei Darussalam. Her research primarily focuses on applying Artificial Intelligence to design and manage renewable energy systems. She is also keen on using various machine learning techniques to solve complex real-life problems. She has published over 40 technical papers.

B. Narendra Kumar Rao is currently working as Professor and Program Head, Department of AI&;ML in the School of Computing, Mohan Babu University, Tirupati. He is a Member of Research Advisory Committee and also Doctoral

Supervisor Cluster Head in School of Computing, Mohan Babu University. His Research interests include Software Testing, Embedded Systems and Machine Learning. He has been part of several International Conferences as Convener and Conference Chair for THREE International Conferences. Has published articles in reputed Journals and Conferences. He was the convener for International Conference on Data Analytics, Intelligent Computing and Cyber Security-2021, He is editor for two Proceedings by Springer published in the year 2018 and 2022. He has been associated with IEEE, ACM, CSTA and IAENG. He has won Best Faculty Recognition, Nava Bharat Nirman Award by Information Technology Association of AP; India Servers, October, 2019 and Best Researcher Award by Integrated Research Group(IRG), Chennai for research work carried out, January, 2018. He received his Ph.D in CSE from Jawarharlal Nehru Technological University, Hyderabad.

S. David Samuel Azariya is working as an Assistant Professor in the Department of Information Technology at Sona College of Technology. He is currently pursuing a Doctorate in Anna University, Chennai, Tamil Nadu, India. He has completed Diploma in Electronics and Communications and Bachelor of Engineering degree in Information Technology and Master of Engineering in Computer and Communication Engineering. He is actively engaged in the research area of data visualization, computer vision, deep learning and IoT. He has published various research papers in Springer and IEEE conferences related to research domain. He is the member of IEI and ISTE professional society.

S. Edwin Raja, Associate Professor, Department of Computer Science and Engineering in Vel Tech Rangarajan Dr.Sagunthala R&D Institute of Science and Technology, Chennai. He has completed his Ph.D. in Information and Communication Engineering from Anna University-chennai in the year 2021. He obtained his M.Tech. (Network Engineering) in the year 2010 from Kalasalingam University, Krishnan kovil and B.E. (Computer Science and Engineering) in the year 2006 from C.S.I Institute of Technology, Thovalai. He has more than thirteen plus years of teaching experience and his area of interests are Cyber Security, Big Data Analytics, Machine Learning & Computer Networks. He has published more than 4 research articles in various journals and conferences. Also, he has published 3 patents, acted as reviewer in reputed journals.

Venkatasubramanian S has 24 years of teaching experience. He is currently pursuing doctoral research in mobile Ad hoc networks. His areas of interest include mobile networks, Network Security and software Engineering. He has published several papers in the international journals, international conferences, filed six patents and authored 7 textbooks. At present he is working as an Associate Professor in

Department of Computer Science and Business Systems at Saranathan college of Engineering, Trichy, India. He has also received Dr.Sarvepalli Radhakrishnan Lifetime achievement National award, Academic Excellence Award 2022 and Global teachers awards.

Swagat Samantaray is an Assistant professor Senior at School of Computing Sciences and Engineering, VIT Bhopal University, India.

Rizwan Shaikh is a distinguished academician, researcher, and software consultant with over 30 years of rich experience. He holds a Ph.D. in Computer Applications from Pune University, India. His doctoral work focused on the evaluation and analysis of e-Governance systems. Dr. Rizwan currently serves as Professor (Computer Applications) in prestigious D Y Patil Group of Institutes, Pune. He was Director (R&D, Science and Technology) at Anam Green Revolution (AGR) IT Solutions LLP. As a Board of Studies (BoS) member and syllabus designer, he contributed to curriculum reforms at RTM University and SPPU. He has authored and co-authored over 25 research papers on e-Governance, CRM, semantic web, and cloud computing. He has received research grants from BCUD, University of Pune, and holds a patent on electronic assessment systems. He has presented research at international conferences organized by IIM Bangalore, CSIR-IPR, and London Business School. Dr. Rizwan is an active member of professional bodies including INETA, CSI, ISTE, and the National Entrepreneurship Network (NEN). He played a pioneering role in establishing EDP cells in collaboration with IIM Bangalore and IIT Mumbai. He has served as coordinator for MBA online exams across 153 institutions affiliated with SPPU since 2013. As an educator, he has taught Computer Science, Management, Physics, and Engineering subjects. His contributions span academic leadership, accreditation processes (NAAC, NBA), and institutional development. He is a passionate advocate for value-based education and digital transformation in governance. With his cross-disciplinary expertise, he mentors students, faculty, and professionals in research and innovation. His vision is to create impactful digital ecosystems through governance, education, and technology.

Jeevika Tharini received the B.C.A degree from Mother Teresa Women's University, Tamilnadu, India, in 2016, and the M.Sc. Computer Science and M.Phil Computer Science from Bharathiar University, Coimbatore, Tamilnadu, India. She is a Ph.D. Research Scholar with the Department of Computer Science from Sri Ramakrishna College of Arts and Science (Formerly SNR), Coimbatore, Tamilnadu, India. She has 4 years of teaching and 5 years of research experience. Her current research interests include utility mining, privacy-preserving, business intelligence, machine learning, IoT, and optimization techniques. She has published papers in international journals and conferences.

Devaki V has 5+ years of teaching and research experinces. Her academic journey is deeply rooted in English Language Teaching and Applied Linguistics, having cleared the National Eligibility Test (UGC-NET). She has also cleared the National Eligibility Test (UGC-NET). she has an experienced researcher in the field of English Language Teaching and Applied Linguistics, having worked for 3 years at the National Institute of Technology Tiruchirappalli, India. Ms. Devaki holds a Master of Philosophy in English Language Teaching from Anna University, Chennai, and a Master in Comparative Literature from Pondicherry Central University. She has worked as an Assistant Professor of English at Vels Institute of Science and Technology (VISTAS) deemed University, Chennai from 2017 to 2019, and at Rajalakshmi Institute of Technology, Chennai from 2021 to 2023. She has worked at Vignan University from 2023 to 2024. Her outstanding performance was recognized with an Appreciation Award for the Best Utilization of Library Facilities at Vels University in 2018. Her academic interests lie in English for Specific Purposes, Applied Linguistics, LGBT studies, Postcolonial Literature, Modernism, and Narratives. She has published more than 20 high-quality research articles in internationally and nationally recognized peer-reviewed and refereed including Scopus and Web of Science-indexed journals. Additionally, she has authored several book chapters with ISBNs and presented research papers at both international and national conferences. She has also served as a reviewer in over four international journals in English Literature and Language Teaching and as an editorial board member in the Journal of English Language, Literature & Culture. Furthermore, she has completed a one-month residential induction training program at IIT Bombay, organized by Pandit Mandan Malvaliya National Mission on Teachers and Teaching (PMMNMTT), MHRD, Government of India, from November to December 2017. She has also received certificates for online courses through Coursera from various international universities worldwide, such as the University of Houston, Colorado, Wesleyan, and Arizona State University.

Loganathan V has research interests that lie at the intersection of biomedical Instrumentation and rehabilitation sciences. He is particularly interested in integration of artificial intelligence and machine learning in personalized rehabilitation therapies, Development of wearable sensors for monitoring and enhancing physical therapy outcomes, Design and optimization of assistive devices for individuals with mobility impairments, and Implementation of non-invasive techniques for neurological rehabilitation. His goal is to push the boundaries of biomedical engineering to positively impact global healthcare delivery.

Index

A

B

C

D

E

F

G

H

I

M

O

P

R

S

T

www.ingramcontent.com/pod-product-compliance
Lightning Source LLC
LaVergne TN
LVHW080908300926
849162LV00003B/595